Medical Management of Acute and Chronic Low Back Pain.
An Evidence-Based Approach

Pain Research and Clinical Management

Pain Research and Clinical Management

Volume 13

Medical Management of Acute and Chronic Low Back Pain.
An Evidence-Based Approach

By

Nikolai Bogduk
University of Newcastle, Royal Newcastle Hospital,
Newcastle, NSW 2300, Australia

Brian McGuirk
Hunter Area Health Service, Royal Newcastle Hospital,
Newcastle, NSW 2300, Australia

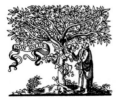

2002

ELSEVIER

AMSTERDAM • BOSTON • LONDON • NEW YORK • OXFORD • PARIS • SAN DIEGO •
SAN FRANCISCO • SINGAPORE • SYDNEY • TOKYO

ELSEVIER SCIENCE B.V.
Sara Burgerhartstraat 25
P.O. Box 211, 1000 AE Amsterdam, The Netherlands

First edition 2002

Library of Congress Cataloging in Publications Data
A catalog record from the Library of Congress has been applied for.

ISBN: 0-444-50845-7 (hardbound)
ISBN: 0921-3287 (series)

⊗ The paper used in this publication meets the requirements of ANSI/NISO Z39.48-1992 (Permanence of Paper).
Printed in The Netherlands.

Foreword

I feel privileged being asked to write the foreword to this book, which will influence and possibly dictate future management of low back pain. Costs of low back pain (in dollars, diminishing quality of life and loss of skilled workforce) continue to escalate and become an increasing burden to governments, the private sector and society in general.

As we enter the 21st Century, the book comes at an opportune time as it challenges traditional dogma, orthodox and alternative medicine, institutionalised practices and political correctness. The text is challenging and at times provocative and controversial with its thought-stimulating approach. The style reflects the authors' personae, is user friendly, and promotes communication.

The introduction sets the scene not dissimilar to a novel with a medical setting that incites the reader to continue. It is an excellent review for graduates and a clinical relevant text for students.

The book is a must for undergraduates and an indispensable reference to all who practice musculoskeletal medicine. It is a tool of trade in the treatment of acute and chronic low back pain.

Tommasino Mastroianni FAFOM(RACP)
Recovre–Allianz Insurance
Level 11, 2 Market Street
Sydney, NSW 2000
Australia
E-mail: lanej@allianz.com.au

Contents

Medical Management of Acute and Chronic Low Back Pain. An Evidence-Based Approach
Pain Research and Clinical Management, Vol. 13
Nikolai Bogduk and Brian McGuirk
© 2002 Elsevier Science B.V. All rights reserved

CHAPTER 1

Introduction

This text is designed to serve two cardinal purposes. It is at the same time a compendium of the contemporary evidence on the medical management of low back pain, and a reference manual for the management of this condition. For scholars and teachers it should serve in both respects. For primary care practitioners its role as a reference manual is paramount.

1. Compendium

As a compendium of the literature, this text is not a systematic review. It does not include the formalities of listing, grading, and discussing individual publications, nor does it dwell on the methodology of systematic reviews. That has been done elsewhere [1]. Instead, the present text capitalises on the results of systematic reviews, where available, supplemented by additional and more recent publications. As a compendium the present text offers readers a digest of the literature. Through its reference lists, it directs interested readers to the source literature, but spares them the labour of having to pursue that literature.

In drawing conclusions and making recommendations, the text unashamedly has adopted a sceptical and conservative position. It offers, and is bound by, no allegiance to any particular craft group or traditional method of management. It relies on the evidence, as interpreted by the authors.

In defining evidence-based medicine, the text is less conciliatory than some other definitions [2]. It follows the definition that:

Evidence-based medicine is medical practice that uses techniques with proven reliability, validity, and efficacy, while shunning those that patently lack reliability, validity, or efficacy.

In the body of the text, it is assumed that readers are familiar with the concepts of reliability, validity, and efficacy, and their parameters, such as kappa scores, likelihood ratios, effect sizes and number needed to treat. For those not familiar with these concepts, a précis is provided in Appendix 1.

When assessing evidence, the text pursues a high standard of expectation. It does not accept a P-value of less than 0.05 as the singular hallmark of significance. It looks also for clinical significance, and what the results mean for consumers. In this context, consumer means both the patient and the practitioner, the latter being someone who is a consumer of information in the interest of securing the best management for the patients.

In adopting a high standard before accepting a practice, the present text may offend some practitioners when they find that their favourite practice is not endorsed. That is not to say that such practices are not reliable, valid, or effective; it is just that evidence to that effect is lacking. The text avoids endorsing practices for which evidence is lacking, regardless of how enthusiastically others might support them.

Yet the text is not nihilistic. Where it might decline certain traditional or accepted practices, it does not leave a void. It offers a replacement from amongst those practices for which there is evidence of reliability, validity, or efficacy.

2. Manual

The text is laid out in a conceptual and chronological manner. It is designed to correspond, in the order in which they would occur, to the thoughts and actions that a practitioner might have or undertake when faced with a patient with low back pain.

Thus, the opening chapters deal with theoretical issues: the background knowledge that should be prompted when the practitioner first learns that they are about to see a patient with back pain. Subsequent chapters deal with the assessment and treatment of the patient with acute low back pain. The final chapters address chronic low back pain, in a fashion previously not seen in a textbook on back pain. It may well be perceived as both contentious and stimulating. If that proves to be the case, then the text will have achieved its (primary) aim.

Specifically, each chapter has been designed to answer theoretical and practical questions that, overtly or subconsciously, should arise in the practitioner's mind, as they progress through their interaction with the patient, or as the patient's problem progresses from acute to chronic.

Theoretical issues

Is it low back pain? Readers confident of the answer to this question can move on to other chapters. Those interested in checking their answer should read Chapter 2.

What could be causing it? Chapter 3 reviews the theoretical background of the possible causes of acute low back pain that the practitioner can expect to encounter.

What is the nature of back pain? Chapter 4 explores the natural history of acute low back pain, and provides a background of what the practitioner can expect to happen to the patient over time, perhaps even regardless of what the practitioner does.

Will it be a case that will not get better? Chapter 5 summarises the prognostic risk factors that determine chronicity. It introduces the concept of psychosocial factors, and heralds the clinical features that should be addressed both in assessment and in management.

Acute low back pain

What to look for in a history? Chapter 6 outlines a protocol for taking a meticulous history in a disciplined manner. It emphasises the importance of history in formulating a provisional diagnosis. It elaborates the concept of 'red flags', and provides a survival device by which practitioners can protect themselves from missing a serious cause of acute low back pain, without resorting to unnecessary investigations.

What should I examine? Many practitioners might believe that there are special tests and techniques of examination that will allow them to diagnose acute low back pain. Chapter 7 describes the lack of reliability and validity of common and not so common techniques. While not denying the propriety of physical examination, this chapter argues against drawing diagnostic conclusions from the results.

Should I take an X-ray? Chapter 8 argues against medical imaging for acute low back pain. X-rays are rarely diagnostic. When taken 'just in case', they create a false sense of security. Because X-rays constitute a health hazard, patients can be dissuaded from wanting an X-ray.

What about EMG? Chapter 9 explains why EMG is not indicated in the assessment of low back pain.

So, what do I diagnose? Psychosocial assessment is critical in the assessment of patients with acute low back pain. It serves to identify factors and features that potentially interfere with recovery. Chapter 10 outlines the theory and practice of psychosocial assessment.

How should I treat? Chapter 11 outlines in detail an algorithm for the treatment of acute low back pain, based on the best available evidence.

What about other treatments? The evidence supporting the algorithm for treatment, and the evidence against other interventions is collated in Chapter 12.

Chronic low back pain

What do I do if the patient develops chronic low back pain or presents with chronic pain? Chapter 13 provides an introductory outline to the problem of chronic low back pain.

What is the cause? Chapter 14 establishes that many of the purported causes of chronic low back pain are not valid, but newly recognised entities account for most cases.

What should I look for? Although the assessment of chronic low back pain is similar in principle to the assessment of acute low back pain, certain differences apply. These are explained in Chapter 15.

How should I treat it? Chapter 16 sets the scene for the various options for treating chronic low back pain.

Various individual treatments are assessed in Chapter 17, and multidisciplinary treatment is considered in Chapter 18.

Special techniques of investigation, designed for making a precision diagnosis are described in Chapter 19, followed by an algorithm for their application in Chapter 20.

Chapter 21 outlines the treatment options available for patients in whom a precision diagnosis is made.

How do I handle all this conflicting information? Chapter 22 offers an algorithm for the management of chronic low back pain. It distils the best options, and deals with the differences between definitive treatment and palliative treatment.

Two appendices are provided at the end of the text. The first deals with elementary biostatistics and the definitions of evidence, and is designed to acquaint readers with the principles and devices used in the body of the text to evaluate the published evidence. The second revisits the issue of taxonomy, and suggests how to label acute low back pain.

References

1   Nachemson AL, Jonsson E (eds). Neck and Back Pain. The Scientific Evidence of Causes, Diagnosis and Treatment. Lippincott Williams and Wilkins, Philadelphia, PA, 2000.
2   Sackett DL, Rosenberg WMC, Gray JAM, Haynes RB, Richardson WS. Evidence based medicine: what it is and what it isn't. Br Med J 1996; 312: 71–72.

Medical Management of Acute and Chronic Low Back Pain. An Evidence-Based Approach
Pain Research and Clinical Management, Vol. 13
Nikolai Bogduk and Brian McGuirk
© *2002 Elsevier Science B.V. All rights reserved*

CHAPTER 2

Definition

1. Introduction

Experienced practitioners may feel confident that they know how to recognize back pain. Ostensibly everyone can tell when a patient is indicating pain in their back. However, not everyone agrees. Formal research has shown that two observers have difficulty agreeing on whether or not a patient is actually complaining of back pain. The issue at hand is not whether or not the patient's complaint is genuine, but simply: where do they complain of pain?

In a study of 83 patients, McCombe et al. [1] found that neither two orthopaedic surgeons nor an orthopaedic surgeon and a physiotherapist could agree on whether the patients were complaining of back pain or another site of pain. On this question they had kappa scores of only 0.16 and 0.18, respectively.

Recognising whether a patient has back pain or some other complaint is fundamental to the further assessment of the patient. Actions pertinent to the assessment of back pain may be inappropriate for other complaints. Other complaints may require actions that are totally inappropriate for a patient with back pain.

For these reasons, the International Association for the Study of Pain (IASP) was very particular in defining back pain, in its taxonomy of pain [2]. It adopted a topographic basis for definition. It asked that practitioners pay attention to where patients indicated that they perceived their pain. The ensuing definitions related exclusively to the location of the pain, without regard to any inferences or deductions as to its cause. Even if subsequent investigations proved that the cause of pain was elsewhere, the presenting complaint was to be defined according to where the patient perceived their pain.

2. Low back pain

The taxonomy [2] does not recognise the colloquial term back pain, but instead refers to different forms of spinal pain.

Lumbar spinal pain is pain perceived as arising anywhere within a region bounded superiorly by an imaginary transverse line through the tip of the last thoracic spinous process, inferiorly by an imaginary transverse line through the tip of the first sacral spinous process, and laterally by vertical lines tangential to the lateral borders of the lumbar erectores spinae (Fig. 1C).

Sacral spinal pain is pain perceived as arising anywhere within a region bounded superiorly by an imaginary transverse line through the tip of the first sacral spinous process, inferiorly by an imaginary transverse line through the posterior sacrococcygeal joints, and laterally by imaginary lines passing through the posterior superior and posterior inferior iliac spines (Fig. 1C).

The two definitions were provided because when a patient indicates sacral spinal pain but not lumbar spinal pain, practitioners should not presume or assume that this pain is referred from the lumbar spine, unless and until corroborating evidence is to hand.

Without such evidence, sacral spinal pain should be identified as sacral spinal pain.

For pain overlapping between the lumbar and sacral regions, the IASP have provided another definition:

Lumbosacral pain is pain perceived as arising from a region encompassing or centred over the lower third of the lumbar region, as described above, and the upper third of the sacral region, as described above.

Lumbar spinal pain, sacral spinal pain, or lumbosacral pain, or any combination thereof, legitimately constitute what colloquially might be referred to as 'low back pain'. These definitions explicitly locate the pain as perceived in the lumbar and/or sacral regions of the spine. Pain in other, but adjacent, regions does not constitute low back pain.

3. Not low back pain

Pain perceived in regions adjacent to either the lumbar spinal region or the sacral spinal region does not constitute back pain. Pain above the T12 spinous process is located in the thoracic region. If it is located over the vertebral column and back muscles it is properly known as *thoracic spinal pain*[2] (Fig. 1B) If it lies substantially over the ribs, it should be referred to as posterior thoracic wall pain. Pain in a sector centred on the greater trochanter and spanning from the posterior inferior iliac spine to the anterior superior iliac spine is *gluteal pain*[2] (Fig. 1B). Pain perceived over the posterior region of the trunk but lateral to the erector spinae is *loin pain*[2] (Fig. 1D).

Loin pain should be distinguished from low back pain not only because loin pain requires consideration of visceral disorders, notably of the urinary tract, but also because it does not require, in the first instance, investigation of the lumbar spine. Mistaking loin pain for back pain may result in delays in recognising a serious visceral disorder.

Gluteal pain is probably the complaint that is most easily and most commonly mistaken for back pain. It is true that pain from the lumbar spine may be referred to the gluteal region (see Chapter 6), but

in the absence of lumbar spinal pain as a cue, gluteal pain should not be assumed to be lumbar in origin. Local causes of gluteal pain should be considered first. Patients who present with a complaint of so-called 'back pain' after exertion or a bout of lifting may actually have pain from the gluteal muscles, for these muscles will have been exerted as much as, or even more than, the back muscles. The distinction of gluteal pain is that it is centred distal to the concavity of the iliac crest, in the absence of pain in the lumbar or sacral spinal regions.

Most critically, low back pain should not be confused with, or regarded as synonymous with 'sciatica', more correctly known as radicular pain. Although the latter may be caused by disorders in the lumbar spine, it is a pain felt in the lower limb; and although radicular pain often occurs in conjunction with back pain, their causes are not necessarily the same, nor are their mechanisms. The investigations and management of radicular pain are different from those for back pain, as is the evidence-base for each of the two conditions. In that regard, the present text pertains strictly to the complaint of low back pain. Sciatica and radicular pain are addressed elsewhere[3].

4. Acute, subacute, and chronic

There are many ways in which the terms acute, subacute, and chronic are used and defined. Some definitions gravitate to chronic pain being characterised by its persistent and intractable nature[4]. However, the traditional and most common definitions are based on time. That system of definition is used for present purposes.

The IASP[2] recognises chronic pain, in general, as any pain that has persisted for longer than 3 months, although for research purposes it prefers 6 months as the defining period. By implication, acute pain is pain that has lasted for less than 3 months.

Some authorities use an additional term, subacute pain, to refer to pain that has persisted for longer than a brief period but not yet 3 months. Different authorities have recommended different critical periods, but the one that has dominated the literature on

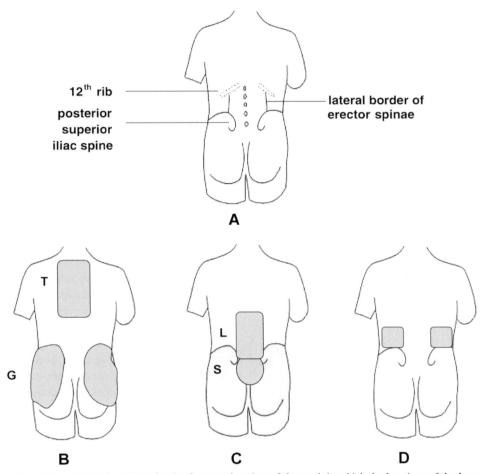

Fig. 1. The definition of low back pain. (A) A sketch of a posterior view of the trunk in which the locations of the lower ribs and iliac crest are indicated. (B) Thoracic spinal pain (T) and gluteal pain (G). (C) Lumbar spinal pain (L) and sacral spinal pain (S). (D) Loin pain.

back pain is 5 to 7 weeks[5]. Furthermore, most of the literature on the efficacy of treatment has been segregated on the same basis. Accordingly, the definitions used in the present text are:

Acute low back pain. Low back pain that has been present for less than 3 months.

Subacute low back pain. Low back pain that has been present for longer than 5 to 7 weeks but not longer than 12 weeks.

Chronic low back pain. Low back pain that has been present for at least 3 months.

Distinguishing between acute, subacute, and chronic low back pain is important because the biological basis, natural history, and response to therapy are different for each category. Interventions applicable to, and recommended for, acute or subacute low back pain are not necessarily appropriate for chronic low back pain. Nor are interventions for chronic back pain, as a rule, applicable for acute low back pain.

More difficult to define are the entities of 're-current' low back pain, and 'acute on chronic' back pain. In these presentations, the patient does not suffer persistent or continuous pain, but has periods relatively free of pain punctuated by episodes that, in a different context, would constitute acute back pain.

When a patient suffers recurrent episodes of pain, but each is separated by a pain-free period of at least 3 months, each episode satisfies the definition of acute low back pain.

When a patient suffers a continuous, or essentially continuous, but low level of back pain punctuated by exacerbations of pain (each of which might be referred to as 'acute' but in the sense of being severe), the patient is most comfortably defined as having chronic back pain, on the grounds that the adjectives acute or chronic refer to the duration of pain, not its severity.

Episodes of pain that recur within periods less than 3 months in duration do not lend themselves to classification as acute or chronic. These are perhaps best defined as recurrent back pain, with the descriptors acute or chronic, being promoted to define the length of period over which the recurrences have occurred. Unfortunately no studies have been published that constitute an evidence-base for the interpretation or management explicitly of recurrent back pain. So, for practical purposes, there is little point in recognising this category beyond simply describing the patient's pattern of pain.

5. Referred pain

In its broadest sense, referred pain is pain perceived in a region displaced or remote from the actual source of pain. More strictly and accurately, referred pain is defined as pain perceived in a region innervated by nerves other than the ones that innervate the actual source of pain[2].

Referred pain can occur by either of two mechanisms, depending on the nature of the stimulus that produces the pain. Understanding the difference can be critical in predicating which investigations to undertake, or perhaps more significantly, which investigations not to undertake.

Visceral referred pain is referred pain whose source lies in one of the organs or blood vessels of the body. *Somatic referred pain* is referred pain whose source lies in one of the tissues or structures of the body wall (soma) or limbs. Both in visceral and in somatic pain the primary pain is evoked by the stimulation of the peripheral endings of nociceptive afferent fibres. The referred pain is evoked when these afferents converge on second-order or third-order neurons in the central nervous system that happen also to receive afferents from the region to which the pain is referred.

In contrast, *neurogenic pain* is pain evoked by the stimulation of peripheral axons or their cell bodies (rather than their peripheral endings). *Radicular pain* is a subset of neurogenic pain, in which pain is evoked by stimulation of the nerve roots or dorsal root ganglion of a spinal nerve[2]. In neurogenic pain, the pain is perceived in the peripheral territory of the affected nerve. In as much as the pain is perceived in a region remote from the actual source of pain, neurogenic pain is, by definition, a form of referred pain. It differs, however, from somatic and visceral referred pain in that it does not involve the stimulation of nerve endings, and does not involve convergence. Rather, it is perceived as arising from the periphery because the nerves from that region are artificially stimulated proximal to their peripheral distribution.

5.1. Visceral referred pain

In the context of low back pain, visceral pain may be referred to the lumbar spinal region or sacral spinal region from pelvic viscera, notably the uterus, and from abdominal structures, notably the abdominal aorta. Certain conditions, such as pancreatitis and infections of abdominal viscera, may sometimes be associated with low back pain, but it is not certain if the back pain is actually referred from the affected organ. It may be that the back pain is produced by irritation of the posterior abdominal wall by pus, blood, or leaking enzymes, in which case the back pain is not referred but is arising directly from the anterior aspect of the back.

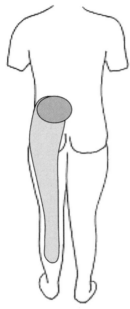

Fig. 2. The distribution of somatic referred pain from the lower lumbar zygapophysial joints.

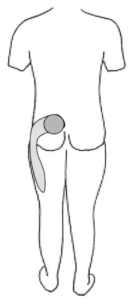

Fig. 3. The distribution of somatic referred pain from the sacroiliac joint.

5.2. Somatic referred pain

It has been established, in experiments in normal volunteers and in clinical studies, that somatic referred pain can arise from a number of structures in the lumbar spine and sacrum. Noxious stimulation of the lower lumbar zygapophysial joints produces pain in the gluteal region, thigh, and even into the leg and foot [6-8] (Fig. 2). Noxious stimulation of the lumbar intervertebral discs produces pain in the gluteal region, thigh, and leg [9]. Discogenic pain may even be perceived in the leg without involvement of the buttock or thigh [9]. Stimulating the sacroiliac joint with a noxious stimulus produces pain in the gluteal region [10] (Fig. 3). In so far as it has not been recorded in experiments in normal volunteers, or reported in clinical studies, it is not known if referred pain from the sacroiliac joint can be referred beyond the gluteal region.

In all these instances, the referred pain is produced by noxious stimulation of the nerve endings in a lumbar or sacral structure. Therefore, each constitutes an example of somatic referred pain. However, each also superficially resembles what has tradition-

ally been described as 'sciatica', in as much as the pain appears to extend into the lower limb, along the course of the sciatic nerve.

Failure to distinguish somatic referred pain from radicular pain is perhaps one of the oldest and still persisting pitfalls in the assessment of low back pain. It leads to inappropriate investigations, such as CT scanning and EMG, and it can result in inappropriate treatment, such as laminectomy and excision of bulging (but asymptomatic) intervertebral discs. For this reason, the distinction between somatic referred pain and radicular pain is emphasized in Chapter 6, in the context of taking a history. However, the matter is of such importance that the underlying principles bear preliminary emphasis here.

Pain radiating from the lumbar spine into the lower limb is not necessarily radicular pain (i.e. 'sciatica'). It may be somatic referred pain. Indeed, radicular pain is uncommon compared to the prevalence of low back pain and somatic referred pain [3]. Consequently, just on epidemiological grounds, pain in the lower limb is, in the first instance, more likely to be somatic referred pain.

The clinical distinction between radicular pain and somatic referred pain lies in its distribution and behaviour.

- It is not true that pain distal to the knee must be radicular pain. Somatic pain from the lumbar zygapophysial joints[6–8] or from the lumbar intervertebral discs[9] can be referred distal to the knee.
- Radicular pain tends to be shooting, lancinating, or electric in quality[11], whereas somatic referred pain is typically a dull, deep ache or pressure-like in quality[12,13].
- Radicular pain is distributed along a narrow band, no more than 2 inches wide[11]. In contrast, somatic referred pain is distributed in wide areas, the boundaries of which may be difficult for the patient to perceive exactly, but the centres of which can be quite confidently indicated[6,7,12,13].
- Radicular pain travels into the lower limb[11], whereas somatic referred pain tends to be fixed in location. Although initially it may feel like an expanding pressure extending into the lower limb, once established it remains in the same location and does not travel; it may wax and wane in intensity but does so in the same location.

It is possible for somatic pain to be referred without any clinical evidence of its spinal origin, i.e. the patient does not feel any back pain; but such cases are uncommon if not rare. Pain in the lower limb in the absence of back pain, therefore, invites a consideration of local causes in the lower limb, such as peripheral vascular disease, neurological disorders, disorders of the hip or knee, and disorders of the muscles of the lower limb. As emphasised previously, gluteal pain in the absence of back pain invites a consideration of disorders of the gluteal muscles and hip joint, before mistaking gluteal pain for low back pain or assuming a spinal or sacroiliac origin.

Key points

- Low back pain is pain perceived in the lumbar spinal region or sacral spinal region.
- Low back pain should be distinguished from thoracic spinal pain, loin pain, and gluteal pain.
- Acute pain is pain that has been present for less than 12 weeks.
- Subacute pain is pain that has been present for less than 12 weeks but longer than 5 to 7 weeks.
- Chronic pain is pain that has been present for longer than 12 weeks.
- Low back pain may be referred into the lower limb, but
- somatic referred pain should be distinguished from radicular pain.

References

1. McCombe PF, Fairbank JCT, Cockersole BC, Punsent PB. Reproducibility of physical signs in low-back pain. Spine 1989; 14: 908–918.
2. Merskey H, Bogduk N (eds). Classification of Chronic Pain. Descriptions of Chronic Pain Syndromes and Definitions of Pain Terms, 2nd edn. IASP Press, Seattle, WA, 1994.
3. Bogduk N, Govind J. Medical Management of Acute Lumbar Radicular Pain: An Evidence-Based Approach. Newcastle Bone and Joint Institute, Newcastle, 1999.
4. Waddell G. The Back Pain Revolution. Churchill Livingstone, Edinburgh, 1998: 33.
5. Van Tulder MW, Koes BW, Bouter LM. Conservative treatment of acute and chronic nonspecific low back pain: a systematic review of randomized controlled trials of the most common interventions. Spine 1997; 22: 2128–2156.
6. Mooney V, Robertson J. The facet syndrome. Clin Orthop 1976; 115: 149–156.
7. Fairbank JCT, Park WM, McCall IW, O'Brien JP. Apophyseal injections of local anaesthetic as a diagnostic aid in primary low-back pain syndromes. Spine 1981; 6: 598–605.
8. Fukui S, Ohseto K, Shiotani M, Ohno K, Karasawa H, Naganuma Y. Distribution of referred pain from the lumbar zygapophyseal joints and dorsal rami. Clin J Pain 1997; 13: 303–307.
9. O'Neill C et al. Spine (in press).
10. Fortin JD, Dwyer AD, West S, Pier J. Sacroiliac joint: pain

referral maps upon applying a new injection/arthrography technique, Part I. Asymptomatic volunteers. Spine 1994; 19: 1475–1482.

11 Smyth MJ, Wright V. Sciatica and the intervertebral disc. An experimental study. J Bone Joint Surg 1959; 40A: 1401–1418.

12 Kellgren JH. On the distribution of pain arising from deep somatic structures with charts of segmental pain areas. Clin Sci 1939; 4: 35–46.

13 Feinstein B, Langton JNK, Jameson RM, Schiller F. Experiments on pain referred from deep somatic tissues. J Bone Joint Surg 1954; 35A: 981–987.

Medical Management of Acute and Chronic Low Back Pain. An Evidence-Based Approach
Pain Research and Clinical Management, Vol. 13
Nikolai Bogduk and Brian McGuirk
© *2002 Elsevier Science B.V. All rights reserved*

CHAPTER 3

Differential diagnosis

For many, if not most, conditions in medical practice, practitioners will rely, overtly or subconsciously, on pre-test probability when making a diagnosis. Pre-test probability is a biostatistics term that pertains to the prevalence of a condition, and relates to the aphorism 'common things occur commonly'. Whether based on formal epidemiological data, or acquired by experience, practitioners will harbour an intuition or knowledge about what the most likely cause is of a presenting complaint. This knowledge predicates and often determines how they will investigate and manage that complaint. It is more efficient to pursue common causes of a complaint, in the first instance, than routinely to pursue a rare or exotic cause, which is unlikely to be present.

There would seem to be utility, therefore, in knowing what the common and most likely causes are of low back pain. However, although the literature abounds with suggestions and proclamations about what the causes may be, compelling data are scarce.

Systematically, the possible causes of low back pain can be summarised in an anatomical–pathological matrix (Table I). However, it is not the intention of this chapter to debate if and how particular entities cause back pain, nor is it to evaluate the strength of the literature concerning each putative or alleged cause. That has been done elsewhere [1].

TABLE I

A summary of the possible causes of low back pain in terms of anatomy and pathology

Pathology	Anatomical site					
	Muscle	Fascia	Ligament	Bone	Joint	Disc
Trauma	sprain	tear	sprain	fracture	sprain	sprain
Fatigue failure				fracture		internal disc disruption
Infection	abscess			osteomyelitis	arthritis	discitis
Inflammation	myositis		enthesopathy		arthritis	
Tumour	sarcoma			primary metastatic	primary	
Mechanical/ physiological	spasm trigger points	compartment syndrome			dysfunction	

'Muscle' refers to any of the muscles of the lumbar spine. 'Fascia' refers to the thoracolumbar fascia. 'Ligament' refers to the interspinous and iliolumbar ligaments. 'Bone' refers to any part of the lumbar vertebrae or sacrum. 'Joint' refers to the lumbar zygapophysial joints or the sacroiliac joint. 'Disc' refers to the intervertebral discs.
Not included in the table are metabolic disorders of bone, such as osteoporosis, which are not known to cause pain in their own right.

The facts are that the evidence for these various causes of back pain is absent, poor, or contentious [1]. Moreover, essentially and effectively, no patho-anatomic diagnosis of low back pain can be made clinically, i.e. on the basis of history and examination alone, without special investigations (see Chapters 6, 7, and 8). Those investigations that can pinpoint a diagnosis are invasive, and although appropriate for the investigation of chronic low back pain (see Chapter 19), they are not appropriate for acute low back pain, on the grounds that acute low back pain has a favourable prognosis (see Chapter 4), and can be managed quite adequately without establishing a patho-anatomic diagnosis (q.v.).

Consequently, there is no evidence base for the differential diagnosis of acute low back pain, but there is no need for one. The management of acute low back pain can be undertaken without a knowledge of the pre-test probability of its exact cause. Those considerations pertain only if and once the complaint becomes chronic or threatens to become so.

Accordingly, practitioners should not feel disadvantaged if they do not know what the possible causes of acute low back pain are; they would not be able to make the diagnosis even if they were. Nor should practitioners feel deficient or delinquent if they do not understand and cannot make a diagnosis of 'myofascial pain', 'segmental dysfunction', or other such entities. These entities have no proven validity, and their diagnosis lacks reliability (see Chapter 7).

In the context of acute low back pain, the leading responsibility of a practitioner is to distinguish serious from non-serious, possible causes of back pain. Table I lists certain serious causes of back pain, such as tumours and infections, that are important because they pose an immediate threat to the patient's health, and fractures, which may pose a threat to the integrity of the patient's spine and central nervous system. These conditions are typically associated with features, other than just pain, that should draw attention to the possibility of a serious condition. Collectively these features have become known as 'red flags' on the grounds that any hint of their presence in a patient should sound an alarm to the treating practitioner, as if an imaginary red flag were to wave in their mind. By the same token, serious causes of low back pain can be collectively referred to as 'red flag conditions', for it is important that they be detected early. A dependable method by which to acquit this responsibility is elaborated in Chapter 6.

Otherwise, Table I lists conditions attributed to minor trauma or fatigue failure, or to idiopathic mechanical or physiological disturbances. In contrast to red flag conditions, these conditions do not constitute a major threat to the patient. For practical purposes, they do not need to be recognised explicitly or specifically.

The one problem that remains is that, if and once a practitioner is satisfied that the patient does not have a red flag condition, and if is both pointless and impossible to establish a specific patho-anatomic diagnosis, what label should be applied to the patient. For the moment, let the diagnostic label be simply low back pain. What else it might or should be called is a contentious and vexatious issue. That is explored in Appendix 2.

Key points

- Practitioners do not need to be armed with the pre-test probabilities of the differential diagnosis of acute low back pain.
- The leading requirement is to identify red flag indicators.

References

1   Bogduk N. Clinical Anatomy of the Lumbar Spine and Sacrum, 3rd edn. Churchill Livingstone, Edinburgh, 1997: 187–213.

Medical Management of Acute and Chronic Low Back Pain. An Evidence-Based Approach
Pain Research and Clinical Management, Vol. 13
Nikolai Bogduk and Brian McGuirk
© *2002 Elsevier Science B.V. All rights reserved*

CHAPTER 4

Natural history

1. Introduction

Some practitioners might consider epidemiology to be a subject that is irrelevant to their practice needs. They might view the subject as an exercise simply in counting patients and describing diseases as opposed to the real problems of diagnosing and treating those conditions. However, some elements of epidemiology are intellectually pertinent to everyday practice.

The natural history of a disorder is a major determinant of its prognosis. If the natural history is known to be favourable, a practitioner does not need to be artificially reassuring. The practitioner can legitimately reassure patients that they are likely to recover. Doing so would constitute evidence-based practice, if the evidence is available to indicate a favourable prognosis. On the other hand, if the evidence is less favourable, the practitioner might need to be more guarded about simply reassuring patients, and might need to implement additional measures so as to optimise outcome.

The natural history is also a determinant of outcome. If it is the nature of a disorder to resolve with time, this will contribute to the outcome of any treatment that may be applied. In some disorders, natural history may be the major, or even sole, determinant of outcome. Practitioners should know that this is the case lest they wrongly infer that good outcomes were due to treatment as opposed to the natural history.

Both of these considerations apply to acute low back pain. Practitioners should be aware of its natural history so that they can responsibly plan their management, and so that they do not suffer any illusions about the effectiveness of available treatments.

2. Epidemiological data

It has been traditional wisdom that most patients with low back pain will recover. Rules such as '90% of patients recover within two months' have been endorsed by various authorities (see Von Korff[1,2] for review). The data on which these rules have been based, however, are confounded by insufficient follow-up.

Although one study in a primary care setting did find that 90% of patients with acute low back pain recovered within 2 weeks[3], it enrolled patients within 2 weeks of onset but followed them for only 4 weeks. Others found lesser rates of recovery within this time of 62%[4], 28%[5] or 33%[6]. Furthermore, most studies that have attempted to describe the natural history of acute low back pain have followed their patients for only 1[3,6], 3[5,7], or 6[8] months. One study[9] that did follow patients for 12 months reported that the status of patients at 2 months was an indicator of their status at 12 months, but that only 7.3% of their inception cohort became chronic. However, this may be an underestimate because these investigators followed through 2 months and 12 months only 123 of their original 300 patients.

In contrast to this literature that suggests a favourable prognosis, Von Korff et al.[10] referred to earlier studies that indicated that some 40% of patients remain in pain at 6 months, or that 62% of patients suffer a relapse within 1 year. Their own study[10] provided detailed data. During the 12 months following the onset of back pain, the patients whom they followed achieved various endpoints, with respect to intensity of pain and degree of dis-

TABLE I

Outcome of low back pain, 12 months after first consultation, based on Von Korff et al. [10]

Onset of back pain	Proportion of patients by pain status at 12 months				
	No pain	Low disability, low intensity	Low disability, high intensity	High disability, moderately limiting	High disability, severely limiting
Recent	0.21	0.55	0.10	0.06	0.08
Non-recent	0.12	0.52	0.16	0.11	0.09

Recent onset was defined as pain commencing within 6 months of first interview.

ability (Table I). The figures that emerged indicated that only a minority of patients actually recover fully; most retain some pain and some disability. These figures, however, may be unduly pessimistic because the inception cohort consisted of patients who had been in pain for up to 6 months. However, other studies bear out the same pattern.

A British study [11] underscored the illusion that arises when practitioners believe that if a patient has not returned to see their doctor they must have recovered. Of 463 patients presenting with a new episode of low back pain, 59% had only a single consultation, and 32% had a repeat consultation confined to the 3 months after the initial consultation. However, independent review at 3 months and at 12 months revealed that only 21% and 25%, respectively, had completely recovered. These proportions echo the figures of Von Korff et al. [10] in the United States.

More optimistic figures arise from a Dutch study [12] of 443 patients, 342 of whom had an onset of pain within the preceding 7 weeks. The median time to recovery was 7 weeks (interquartile range: 3–16 weeks), with 70% still having pain at 4 weeks, 48% at 8 weeks, and 35% after 12 weeks. At 12 months, 10% of the patients still had back pain. Strikingly, however, the recurrence rate was high. Some 76% of patients endured a relapse. The median number of relapses was two (interquartile range: 1–3), with a median time to relapse of 7 weeks (interquartile range: 5–12), and a median duration of 3 weeks for the first relapse, 2 weeks for the second and third, and 1 week for the fourth.

These international figures stand in contrast to recent Australian data [13]. The outcomes were monitored of 547 patients with acute low back pain managed in special evidence-based clinics, and 101 patients with acute low back pain managed under usual care by their general practitioner. At 3 months, 67% of clinic patients and 49% of usual care patients had fully recovered. At 12 months the respective figures were 71% and 56%. Recurrence rates were only 16% and 6%, respectively, at 6 months and 7% and 27%, respectively, at 12 months. The differences in recovery rates and recurrence rates between the international data and the Australian data may be due partly or largely to the fact that the Australian study excluded patients with workers compensation claims. As such they may reflect, better than the international data, what the natural history is of low back pain uncomplicated by compensation issues.

3. Implications

The preceding figures allow the practitioner to be optimistic, although guarded, about prognosis. They can advise patients that they are likely to recover from the presenting episode; but practitioners should also plan for recurrences, for these are possible, if not likely. The window of therapeutic opportunity seems to be about 2 months. Patients who have not recovered, or are not recovering by this time, will require more concerted effort in management.

Key points

- The data on the natural history of acute low back pain are conflicting.

According to studies in Britain, The Netherlands, and the USA,

- patients are likely to recover from their presenting episode of back pain,
- the median time to recovery is about 7 weeks, but
- relapses are common.
- The status of the patients at 2 months is an indicator of their status at 12 months, and
- up to 80% of patients may remain disabled to some degree at 12 months, although
- perhaps only 10%–15% will be highly disabled.
- When patients do not return for treatment or for follow-up, they have not necessarily recovered. In fact, it is likely that they have not recovered, and simply do not return.

A study in Australia, of patients without a compensation claim found that

- up to 70% of patients can expect to recover and remain so at 12 months,
- with a low risk of recurrence.

References

1 Von Korff M. Studying the natural history of back pain. Spine 1994; 19: 2041S–2046S.

2 Von Korff M, Saunders K. The course of back pain in primary care. Spine 1996; 24: 2833–2839.

3 Coste J, Delecoeuillerie G, Cohen de Lara A, Le Parc JM, Paolaggi JB. Clinical course and prognostic factors in acute low back pain: an inception cohort study in primary care setting. Br Med J 1994; 308: 577–580.

4 Dillane JB, Fry J, Kalton G. Acute back syndrome — a study from general practice. Br Med J 1966; 2: 82–84.

5 Chavannes AW, Gubbels J, Post D, Rutten G, Thomas S. Acute low back pain: patients' perceptions of pain four weeks after initial diagnosis and treatment in general practice. J R Coll Gen Pract 1986; 36: 271–273.

6 Roland M, Morris R. A study of the natural history of low-back pain. Part II: development of guidelines for trials of treatment in primary care. Spine 1983; 8: 145–150.

7 Lanier DC, Stockton P. Clinical predictors of outcome of acute episodes of low back pain. J Fam Pract 1988; 27: 483–489.

8 Carey TS, Garrett J, Jackman A, McLaughlin C, Fryer J, Smucker DR. The outcomes and costs of care for acute low back pain among patients seen by primary care practitioners, chiropractors, and orthopaedic surgeons. N Engl J Med 1995; 333: 913–917.

9 Klenerman L, Slade PD, Stanley IM, Pennie B, Reilly JP, Atchison LE, Troup JDG, Rose MJ. The prediction of chronicity in patients with an acute attack of low back pain in a general practice setting. Spine 1995; 20: 478–484.

10 Von Korff M, Deyo RA, Cherkin D, Berlow W. Back pain in primary care: outcomes at 1 year. Spine 1993; 18: 855–862.

11 Croft PR, Macfarlane GJ, Papageorgiou AC, Thomas E, Silman AJ. Outcome of low back pain in general practice: a prospective study. Br Med J 1998; 316: 1356–1359.

12 Van den Hoogen HJM, Koes BW, van Eijk JThM, Bouter LM, Deville W. On the course of low back pain in general practice: a one year follow up study. Ann Rheum Dis 1998; 57: 13–19.

13 McGuirk B, King W, Govind J, Lowry J, Bogduk N. Safety, efficacy, and cost–effectiveness of evidence-based guidelines for the management of acute low back pain in primary care. Spine 2001; 26: 2615–2622.

Medical Management of Acute and Chronic Low Back Pain. An Evidence-Based Approach
Pain Research and Clinical Management, Vol. 13
Nikolai Bogduk and Brian McGuirk

CHAPTER 5

Prognostic risk factors

1. Introduction

Prognostic risk factors are features exhibited by patients with back pain early in the course of their problems that correlate statistically with whether or not they are likely to develop chronic disability because of back pain. Prognostic risk factors, which predict chronicity, should not be confused with standard risk factors, which predict whether or not an unaffected individual will develop back pain in the first instance.

2. Relevance

The pursuit of prognostic risk factors in back pain has been driven by the prospect that appropriate intervention, early in the course of the problem, directed at the risk factor may reduce chronic disability. Being aware of the prognostic risk factors of back pain is, therefore, potentially of value to the practitioner, for it can direct management into domains that might not otherwise, or conventionally, be considered.

3. The factors

Two broad categories of prognostic risk factors can be described. These are (1) *biological factors* that encompass the patient's demographic and clinical features, and (2) *psychosocial factors* that encompass how the patient thinks, feels and behaves (Fig. 1).

In each category there are immutable and potentially remediable factors. Immutable biological factors might include age, gender and race. Even if these were cardinal predictors of chronicity, they cannot be changed.

Potentially remediable biological factors include:

diagnostic features of specific conditions that can be corrected, such as fractures and infections, but by and large, these occur only in the minority of cases that are categorised as 'red flag' conditions (see Chapter 6).

associated features, such as muscle weakness, immobility or lack of fitness. It is these features that have attracted interventions such as exercise and functional restoration (see Chapter 12).

Immutable psychosocial factors include personality type and past history of psychological distress. One cannot change the patient's personality, and one cannot change the past.

Relatively immutable psychosocial factors might include socio-economic status, intelligence, job dissatisfaction and education. Although these factors might possibly be changeable, it may be too impractical to change them, or beyond the province and power of Medicine to do so.

Potentially remediable psychosocial factors include beliefs, cognitions, and fears. It is these latter features that have attracted attention in the contemporary management of back pain, in parallel with remediable biological factors.

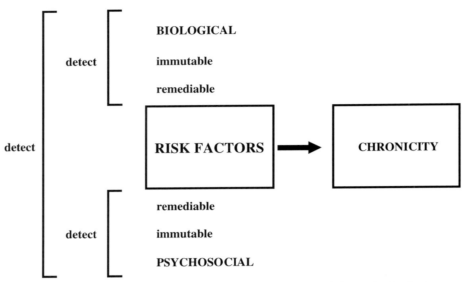

Fig. 1. A model of prognostic risk factors. The objectives of research are to detect the risk factors for the development of chronicity of back pain. The factors may be biological or psychosocial, and immutable or remediable. Research may focus on detecting psychosocial or biological factors or both.

4. The factors

In the search for prognostic risk factors, the frailties of poor clinical epidemiology obtain. Observer bias, deliberate or subconscious, can affect what is detected. The results of epidemiological surveys are constrained by the devices used. Any questionnaire will contain a finite number of possible factors. Any that emerge as statistically significant must, by definition, have been asked about in the questionnaire. If an investigator does not consider and include a particular factor, he or she will not find that factor to be significant. Thus, the results of any survey will be a function of what is asked. In broad terms, if a survey focuses on psychosocial factors it will likely find one or more to be significant but, by definition, will find no biological factors to be significant, for no biological factors were asked about. Conversely, if a survey addresses only biological factors it will never find psychosocial factors to be significant.

Illustrative in this regard are two studies from the same unit. The first study[1] addressed only demographic and clinical features, and found frequency of pain, duration of pain, playing adult sport, in-

ability to perform sit-ups, inappropriate signs, and leg pain to be significant predictors of poor outcomes. However, the second study[2] included psychosocial factors and found depressive symptoms, coping strategies, somatic perception, as well as leg pain and duration of pain, to be significant predictors of poor outcome.

Factors that appear significant when a small list of possibilities is considered may not remain significant if diluted in a larger list of possibilities; and factors that appear significant on univariate analysis may lose their significance on multivariate analysis. Reliable are only the most rigorous studies that consider an initial large number of possible factors and submit them to multiple regression analyses in order to eliminate the spurious factors and identify the dominant factors.

Thereafter, it is the responsibility of the investigators to determine how much of the variation between patients is accounted for by the factor or factors identified as significant. This has rarely been done in the back pain literature. Instead, authors have been satisfied to take factors that are statistically significant and promulgate them as if they were major determinants of chronicity, almost as if they were 'the answer to chronic back pain'; yet the factor may account for only a small proportion of the variance amongst patients. Although it may be worthwhile to identify potentially remediable factors, the eventual impact will be small if the factor accounts for only a small proportion of the problem.

Epidemiological studies that have looked for prognostic risk factors for back pain have varied in methodological rigour, from consensus summaries to exhaustive iterations of regression models[1-20]. No study is perfect. What it may make up for in methodological rigour may be compromised by an inappropriate or unfair selection of putative factors. Indeed, factors found in weaker studies have usually been denied in more rigorous studies that addressed the same putative factors but included others that proved to be more discriminating.

Without venturing to rank individual studies for rigour and reliability, the cardinal prognostic risk factors that have been identified for chronicity of back pain are listed in Table I. Those factors iden-

tified in methodologically more rigorous studies are shown in upper case, while those factors found in less robust studies are shown only in lower case. Factors detected in weaker studies but explicitly denied in stronger studies have been excluded.

What is evident from this table is that the strongest and potentially remediable factors are clustered in the psychosocial category. They paint the picture that those patients at risk of developing chronicity tend to be those who are depressed, focused on their complaints, are unable to cope with their pain and, most significantly, who are fearful of aggravating their pain. It is this constellation of factors that has generated contemporary interest in psychosocial management of back pain (see Chapter 12). However, before endorsing that paradigm, it is salutary to recognise the strength of these risk factors.

Bigos et al.[11] reported that individuals with high scores on scale 3 of the Minnesota Multiphasic Personality Inventory had an 18.6% chance of reporting back pain during a 3-year period, com-

TABLE I

Prognostic risk factors for chronicity of back pain

	Biological	Psychosocial
Immutable	frequency of attacks playing adult sport DURATION OF BACK PAIN PAST HISTORY OF BACK PAIN	marital status family status
Relatively immutable	severity job demands LEG PAIN	compensation employment wage occupation somatisation JOB DISSATISFACTION EDUCATION MMPI
Potentially remediable	smoking BMI inability to sit-up WORK CAPACITY DISABILITY	inappropriate signs lack of understanding SICKNESS IMPACT DEPRESSION COPING DISTRESS RATING OF LOADS FEAR

pared with 5.5% for individuals with low scores. Further analysis [15], however, showed that of patients with scores in the highest quintile, only 12% reported back injury.

Burton et al. [2] found that conventional clinical information correctly predicted outcome in only 10% of patients with acute back pain, but psychosocial factors correctly predicted 59%. Collectively those factors were: depression, coping strategies, and somatic perception.

Troup et al. [19] determined that a battery of psychophysical lifting tests, including rating what constituted an acceptable load, was predictive of whether a patient had no pain, acute back pain, mild back pain or chronic back pain. These factors had an overall accuracy of 35% for men and 37% for women.

Croft et al. [5] reported that psychological distress, as measured by the General Health Questionnaire, predicted 16% of recurrences of back pain in their sample.

Klenerman et al. [17] found that demographic, historical and fear–avoidance factors accounted for 12%, 15% and 14%, respectively, of the variance in predicting outcome from acute pain to pain and disability at 12 months.

Thus, although these factors are statistically significant and substantial predictors of chronicity, none alone is the predominant factor. Each still accounts for only a small proportion of the influences that determine chronicity. This has ramifications for any interventions based on trying to correct these factors. If the factor accounts for only a small proportion of the variance between patients who recover and those who become chronic sufferers, even the most efficacious intervention is destined to have only a minor impact on the overall burden of illness.

It should also be recognised that a single risk factor alone carries little prognostic significance. In this regard, Thomas et al. [21] highlighted the importance of multiple, simultaneous factors. In that study, the cardinal risk factors identified for chronicity were history of low back pain, dissatisfaction with cur-

rent employment or work status, widespread pain, radiating leg pain, restriction in two or more spinal movements, and gender. Of patients with none, one or two risk factors, only 6% became chronic sufferers. The corresponding percentages for those with three or four factors were 27% and 35%, but of patients with five or six factors, 70% became chronic. Consequently, prognostic risk factors become major determinants of chronicity only when several are present simultaneously.

5. The fear–avoidance model

Eminent authorities have taken pains to point out that psychosocial risk factors do not mean that the patient has psychogenic pain [22]. Rather, distress and illness behaviour are secondary to the physical disorder, but physical disorder, distress, and illness behaviour combine to produce disability [23,24].

Whereas disability might, in the first instance, be considered a biological factor in that the patient appears physically to be unable to execute certain activities, there is growing evidence that such intolerance of activity may have a substantial behavioural basis and, therefore, more appropriately constitutes a psychosocial factor.

The relationship between disability in activities of daily living and severity of low back pain is weak. Severity of pain accounts for only some 10–14% of the variance of physical disability [22,25] and only 5% of the variance for work lost [22]. Rather, much of the variance can be explained by a combination of severity of pain, depression and illness behaviour [26]. In turn, cognitive measures, particularly catastrophising, explained 35% of the variance of the depressive symptoms associated with chronic low back pain [26].

Such relationships have led to the generation of a fear–avoidance model that incorporates various psychosocial factors to explain how they bear on the patient's complaint of pain and their behaviour. This model has been developed and promulgated in the context of back pain by a variety of separate groups [17,22,27–30], and its key elements are summarised in Fig. 2.

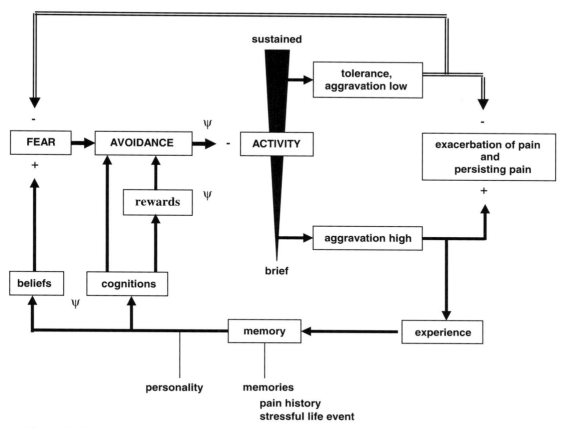

Fig. 2. The fear–avoidance model of back pain. Sites at which behavioural therapy might be applied are marked Ψ.

The model maintains that a patient's disability is a function not only of their pain but also of their response to it. The model does not stipulate that psychological factors generate the pain. Indeed, the evidence is that disability is independent of the severity of the pain [30]. Rather, disability seems to arise because patients seek to avoid exacerbations of their pain. Consequently, avoidance behaviour dominates their activities of daily living. Avoidance patently does not reduce the intensity of persisting, chronic pain — the patient always has that — but it is the aggravation of pain that patients seek to avoid.

The model maintains that avoidance behaviour is based on experience, memory, cognitions and beliefs. It is largely the experience of patients that attempting activities aggravates their pain. How they deal with this experience and its memory depends on a variety of other factors.

Cognitions are reasoned thoughts that the patients may have about their pain; they are logical but may be based on limited knowledge or understanding. Thus, a patient may reason logically that 'if activity aggravates my pain I should avoid it', but they may not be informed that activity is beneficial. The patient may reasonably believe that rest promotes healing and that activity disrupts healing. Cognitions may be reinforced if avoidance of activity is rewarded by attention or excuse from social obligations.

Beliefs are less rational thoughts that may be related to emotions. Fear is one such emotion. Thus, patients may avoid activity for fear of aggravating their pain, as opposed to reasoning logically that activity will lead to aggravation. They may believe that pain is a sign of impending disaster, and therefore reason that avoiding pain will avoid disaster. They may fear that they will not be able to cope.

Beliefs can be influenced by other factors such as past history of pain, and previous stressful life events [29,30], and personality. It is believed that hypochondriasis and hysteria, as measured by the MMPI, serve to reinforce avoidance [27].

As a result of these influences, patients consciously or unconsciously may elect either to confront or to avoid their problem with pain. So-called 'confronters' will view their pain as a temporary nuisance, will be motivated to return to activities, and are prepared to address how to manage their pain [27]. 'Avoiders' avoid the pain experience and avoid painful activities [27].

Several deleterious consequences are believed to arise from avoidance behaviour [30]. First, because it does not reduce pain, it is unproductive. Secondly, avoidance behaviour reduces physical and social activity and may lead to 'invalid' status [28]. Fear–avoidance beliefs correlate strongly with self-reported disability in activities of daily living and with work loss, and account for 23% of variance of disability in activities of daily living, and 26% of the variance of work loss [22].

The irony of fear avoidance is that some evidence indicates that forced exposure to aversive stimuli actually increases tolerance [30], and, therefore, reduces the experience that activity aggravates pain. This is in keeping with beliefs in Musculoskeletal Medicine and Pain Medicine that persisting with movement despite pain facilitates recovery (see Chapters 11 and 12) and with the principles of therapy for phobias [30].

The predictions of the fear–avoidance model [30] are that:

preventing withdrawal and avoidance, and encouraging repeated graded exposures to stimuli previously avoided will lead to the greatest reduction in avoidance behaviour, and to the largest shifts in self-efficacy, judgements, and expectations; and

behavioural therapy should be efficacious by encouraging increased activity, and by providing cognitive skills.

For these reasons behavioural and cognitive therapy approaches have been developed by physicians and by psychologists for the management of back pain (see Chapter 12).

Questionnaires have been developed to screen for fear–avoidance behaviours [22,28,29], and constitute suitable checklists for physicians wishing to identify systematically indicators of fear–avoidance behaviour in their patients (see Chapter 10).

Key points

- Prognostic risk factors are features that correlate statistically with the risk of acute low back pain becoming chronic.
- The principal risk factors for chronicity of back pain are psychosocial in nature.
- Psychosocial factors, however, are not major determinants of chronicity, unless several are present simultaneously.
- Avoidance of activity, for fear of aggravating pain or fear of worsening the pathology, is a significant cause of disability.
- Reducing fear and reducing avoidance of activity offers the prospect of reducing disability.

References

1   Burton AK, Tillotson KM. Prediction of the clinical course of low-back trouble using multivariate models. Spine 1991; 16: 7–14.

2   Burton AK, Tillotson M, Main CJ, Hollis S. Psychosocial predictors of outcome in acute and subchronic low back trouble. Spine 1995; 20: 722–728.

3   Frymoyer JW, Cats-Baril W. Predictors of low back pain disability. Clin Orthop 1987; 221: 89–98.

4   Cherkin DC, Deyo RA, Street JH, Barlow W. Predicting poor outcomes for back pain seen in primary care using patients' own criteria. Spine 1996; 21: 2900–2907.

5   Croft PR, Papageorgiou AC, Ferry S, Thomas E, Jayson MIV, Silman AJ. Psychologic distress and low back pain: evidence from a prospective study in the general population. Spine 1996; 20: 2731–2737.

6   Goertz MN. Prognostic indicators for acute low-back pain. Spine 1990; 15: 1307–1310.

7   Lacroix JM, Powell J, Lloyd GJ, Doxey NCS, Mitson GL, Aldam CF. Low-back pain: factors of value in predicting outcome. Spine 1990; 15: 495–499.

8   O'Connor FG, Marlowe SS. Low back pain in military basic trainees: a pilot study. Spine 1993; 18: 1351–1354.

9   Volinn E, van Koevering D, Loeser JD. Back sprain in industry: the role of socioeconomic factors in chronicity. Spine 1991; 16: 542–548.

10   Main CJ, Wood PL, Hollis S, Spanswick CC, Waddell G. The distress and risk assessment method: a simple patient classification to identify distress and evaluate the risk of poor outcome. Spine 1992; 17: 42–52.

11   Bigos SJ, Battie MC, Spengler DM, Fisher L, Fordyce WE, Hansson TH, Nachemson AL, Wortley MD. A prospective study of work perceptions and psychosocial factors affecting the report of back injury. Spine 1991; 16: 1–6.

12   Coste J, Delecoeuillerie G, Cohen de Lara C, Le Parc JM, Paolaggi JB. Clinical course and prognostic factors in acute low back pain: an inception cohort study in primary care practice. Br Med J 1994; 308: 577–580.

13   Deyo RA, Diehl AK. Psychosocial predictors of disability in patients with low back pain. J Rheumatol 1988; 15: 1557–1564.

14   Dionne C, Koepsell TD, von Korff M, Deyo RA, Barlow WE, Checkoway H. Formal education and back-related disability: in search of an explanation. Spine 1995; 20: 2721–2730.

15   Fordyce WE, Bigos SJ, Battie MC, Fiser LD. MMPI scale 3 as a predictor of back injury report: what does it tell us? Clin J Pain 1992; 8: 222–226.

16   Gatchel RJ, Polatin PB, Mayer TG. The dominant role of psychosocial risk factors in the development of chronic low back pain disability. Spine 1995; 24: 2702–2709.

17   Klenerman L, Slade PD, Stanley IM, Pennie B, Reilly JP, Atchison LE, Troup JDG, Rose MJ. The prediction of chronicity in patients with an acute attack of low back pain in a general practice setting. Spine 1995; 20: 478–484.

18   Rossignol M, Lortie M, LeDoux E. Comparison of spinal health indicators in predicting spinal status in a 1-year longitudinal study. Spine 1993; 18: 54–60.

19   Troup JDG, Foreman TK, Baxter CE, Brown D. The perception of back pain and the role of psychophysical tests of lifting capacity. Spine 1987; 12: 645–657.

20   Von Korff M, Deyo RA, Cherkin D, Barlow W. Back pain in primary care: outcomes at 1 year. Spine 1993; 18: 855–862.

21   Thomas E, Silman AJ, Croft PR, Papageorgious AC, Jayson MIV, Macfarlane GJ. Predicting who develops chronic low back pain in primary care: a prospective study. Br Med J 1999; 318: 1662–1667.

22   Waddell G, Newton M, Henderson I, Somerville D, Main CJ. A fear–avoidance beliefs questionnaire (FABQ) and the role of fear–avoidance beliefs in chronic low back pain and disability. Pain 1993; 52: 157–168.

23   Waddell G, Main CJ, Morris EW, di Paola M, Gray ICM. Chronic low back pain: psychological distress and illness behaviour. Spine 1984; 9: 209–213.

24   Waddell G. A new clinical model for the treatment of low-back pain. Spine 1987; 12: 632–644.

25   Waddell G, Somerville D, Henderson I, Newton M. Objective clinical evaluation of physical impairment in chronic low back pain. Spine 1992; 17: 617–628.

26   Main CJ, Waddell G. A comparison of cognitive measures in low back pain: statistical structure and clinical validity at initial assessment. Pain 1991; 46: 287–298.

27   Lathem J, Slade PD, Troup JDG, Bentley G. Outline of a fear avoidance model of exaggerated pain perception. J Behav Res Ther 1983; 21: 401–408.

28   Slade PD, Troup JDG, Lathem J, Bentley G. The fear–avoidance model of exaggerated pain perception, II: preliminary studies of coping strategies for pain. Behav Res Ther 1983; 21: 409–416.

29   Philips HC, Jahanshahi M. The components of pain behaviour report. Behav Res Ther 1986; 24: 117–125.

30   Philips HC. Avoidance behaviour and its role in sustaining chronic pain. Behav Res Ther 1987; 25: 273–279.

Medical Management of Acute and Chronic Low Back Pain. An Evidence-Based Approach
Pain Research and Clinical Management, Vol. 13
Nikolai Bogduk and Brian McGuirk
© *2002 Elsevier Science B.V. All rights reserved*

CHAPTER 6

History

1. Introduction

Taking a detailed and appropriate history is the most critical component in the assessment of a patient with low back pain. In detecting clues to red flag conditions, history is more practical and more efficient than clinical examination and investigations. However, there is no evidence-base concerning what is the best or optimal manner of taking a history. Such studies as have been conducted have determined the diagnostic value of certain items of history, but no one has looked at different methods of obtaining a history. What follows in the next section of this chapter, therefore, is not derived from evidence. Others may have or may prefer a different system, but they should consider if their system offers the same face validity and content validity for efficiency and rigour.

The protocol described in this chapter deals explicitly with what might be called the biomedical history, assessing the patients with respect to what might be causing their pain. No less important is the assessment of how the patients are reacting and coping with their pain. That is addressed separately in Chapter 10.

2. A protocol

A systematic approach to obtaining a history of low back pain ensures that practitioners do not forget or neglect features that could be important, but which, in the heat of busy practice, might be overlooked. A system that lends itself to this purpose is one that was developed for headache [1]. It invites obtaining a history in the categories listed in Table I.

TABLE I

Categories under which history can be obtained systematically about any pain problem

Presenting complaint
Length of illness
Site of pain
Location and extent of spread
Quality
Severity
Frequency
Duration
Time of onset
Mode of onset
Precipitating factors
Aggravating factors
Relieving factors
Associated features

The protocol is one that is appropriate for any presenting complaint of pain. By adopting this protocol, practitioners will be equipped to take a comprehensive history of any sort of pain, and do not need to remember a protocol unique to, or special for, back pain.

Several of the categories will not be particularly relevant or contributory for the assessment of back pain. However, practitioners should not assume that a particular category will be irrelevant. Using the generic protocol reinforces discipline and habit, and militates against forgetting categories of enquiry that, every now and then, will unexpectedly become relevant. At other times, it takes little time and effort simply to enter a null response or 'not applicable'. Yet doing so ensures that every history is systematically recorded, and ensures that no category is ever omitted or neglected because the practitioner forgot to ask.

This virtue becomes more pertinent for medicolegal purposes. If a practitioner is accused of missing a diagnosis or a cue to a diagnosis, a record of 'null' under the relevant point may constitute valuable evidence that the practitioner was not negligent when taking the history.

2.1. Presenting complaint

When a patient presents with a complaint of low back pain, it is imperative to establish before anything else that they do, indeed, have back pain. In that regard, the definitions provided in Chapter 2 are pertinent. The patient should have lumbar spinal pain, sacral spinal pain, or lumbosacral spinal pain. These should be distinguished from loin pain and gluteal pain, which have a different differential diagnosis, and attract a different system of assessment and investigation.

If the patient has more than one pain, each of which is ostensibly primary and presumably separate in origin, a separate history should be taken of each. Each might have a different cause and mechanism requiring different investigations and management. If subsequently it proves that the patient has multiple complaints attributable to the one source, it is an easy matter to recombine the separate histories. However, assuming in the first instance that they have only one complaint can cause difficulties if a separate pain, that deserves separate management, is mistaken as part of another complaint.

2.2. Length of illness

It is critical to establish if the patient has acute, subacute or chronic low back pain, for the management options for each, and the evidence-base for each, are quite different. For example, imaging is rarely indicated in acute low back pain but may be more pertinent for chronic back pain (see Chapter 15); intensive multidisciplinary therapy may be appropriate for subacute or chronic low back pain, but has been shown to be inefficient for acute low back pain [2].

2.3. Site

That a patient does, indeed, have back pain will have been established under 'Presenting complaint'. The present category of enquiry asks only that the actual site of pain be recorded, in terms of its topographical location. To do so serves to record what appears to be the primary site of pain, in preparation for a description of to where the pain may radiate or spread.

2.4. Location and extent of spread

Low back pain may be referred to the lower limb girdle, the lower limb, and into the groin or perineum (Chapter 2). The patient will feel pain in the back as well as in any of these regions, but they will not know if they have referred pain. The cardinal cue is that their pain is principally in the back. In order to establish this, enquiry should be directed to asking:

> "Where is your main pain? Where is the pain worst? Where do you feel pain most often, most consistently?"

and reciprocally:

> "Where do you feel the pain only sometimes?"

Patients will be describing referred pain when they indicate low back pain as the consistent site, with pain in the limb occurring only sometimes, when the back pain is worse than the limb pain, or when the back pain clearly appears to spread into the lower limb. A patient who describes equal pain in the back and the limbs, or in other regions, may be describing a problem that is not spinal referred pain. Such patients require a more perspicacious assessment, lest they have multiple pain problems, or a problem that, in common, causes referred pain to the back as well as to the limbs or other regions.

It is critical to establish if pain in the lower limb associated with low back pain is *somatic referred pain* or *radicular pain*. There is no absolute rule by which this distinction can be made, nor is there a good body of evidence that relates clinical features and proven sources and mechanisms of pain. How-

TABLE II

Distinguishing features between somatic referred pain and radicular pain in the lower limb

Feature	Explanation
Pain in the buttock or proximal thigh is unlikely to be radicular pain.	Somatic referred pain stemming from the lumbar zygapophysial joints is most commonly perceived in the gluteal region and proximal thigh [3–5]. In contrast, when produced experimentally, radicular pain is perceived travelling distally into the lower limb [6].
Pain extending below the knee is not necessarily radicular pain.	Although radicular pain characteristically extends into the leg, somatic referred pain can also be perceived below the knee, even into the foot [3,4].
Pain extending across a relatively wide region, and felt deeply, in a relatively constant or fixed location is somatic referred pain. Its boundaries may be hard to define, but its centroid is clearly perceived by the patient.	These are characteristic features of somatic referred pain that have been produced experimentally [7,8], and relieved by anaesthetising somatic structures in the lumbar spine [3–5].
Pain that travels along the length of the lower limb, along a narrow band, will be radicular pain.	This is the distinguishing topographic feature of radicular pain that has been evoked in volunteers by stimulating nerve roots [6]. Distribution along a narrow band has not been produced by stimulating somatic structures nor shown to be relieved by anaesthetising somatic structures.
A patient does not necessarily have to exhibit neurological features to be suffering from radicular pain, but the presence of neurological features favours radicular pain, provided that the preceding features are satisfied.	Neurological features imply radiculopathy but are not themselves diagnostic of radicular pain [9]. However, pain of a radicular nature combined with neurological features implies a common origin of both sets of features.
Deep aching pain indicates somatic referred pain. Lancinating or shooting pain is radicular.	Dull aching pain is the characteristic quality of somatic referred pain produced experimentally [7,8]. Shooting pain is characteristic of pain produced experimentally by stimulating nerve roots [3].

ever, there is sufficient evidence from experiments on normal volunteers and some clinical studies (Chapter 2) that allows the guidelines shown in Table II to be formulated.

Two possible dilemmas arise. A patient may have both radicular pain and somatic referred pain, or a patient may have 'early' radicular pain.

It is possible for a disorder of the lumbar spine to produce both somatic referred pain and radicular pain. A disrupted disc may cause spinal pain and referred pain, but an associated prolapse may add radicular pain to the clinical picture. Alternatively, an inflammatory response to prolapsed disc material may irritate the dural sleeve of a nerve root as well as the roots themselves. The dural inflammation may cause spinal pain and referred pain, while the root inflammation may cause radicular pain. In both

instances the distinction is made by perceiving that the patient has the features of somatic referred pain upon which are superimposed the features of radicular pain. The error that can be made is to assume that all the pain in the lower limb is radicular, instead of recognising the combined state. The distinction is critical because whereas investigations might reveal the cause of the radicular component, the same investigations will not necessarily reveal the cause of the somatic referred pain. Nor will treatment of the radicular component necessarily relieve the somatic component.

'Early' radicular pain is a phenomenon that, anecdotally, some experienced clinicians believe that they can identify. Their confidence stems from recall of previous patients who presented in a particular way and who subsequently proved to have radicular pain.

Unfortunately, this wisdom has not been formally documented or validated. Putative cues include stabbing pain that seems to extend into the buttock but not yet into the entire length of the lower limb. Physicians seeking to make this diagnosis should recognise its lack of validity and reliability. At most they should record their diagnosis as a suspected diagnosis, and one that requires monitoring and possible revision, when further evidence is to hand.

2.5. Quality

Somatic pain is characteristically perceived as a deep, dull ache, or pressure-like in quality[10]. It spreads into the lower limb as if the muscle or bones are expanding. When established it may have a gnawing quality.

In contrast, radicular pain is shooting or lancinating in quality[10]. It may be perceived deeply but usually also with a superficial or cutaneous component. The latter is brought into greater relief if the patient also has neurological symptoms and signs.

Difficult to interpret may be the description of burning pain, which is often a feature of neurogenic pain (i.e. pain resulting from a disease or injury to a nerve, as opposed to pain from musculoskeletal tissues). Some patients with deep pain may use this adjective. Care should be taken to determine if they do, indeed, literally mean burning, or if they are using this word as the best that they can think of to describe a severely irritating pain. Deep, burning pain, in the absence of any other feature, distribution or quality, is not necessarily neurogenic pain. At best, the nature of this pain is indeterminate. On the other hand, burning sensations in the skin strongly implicate a neurogenic mechanism that may be radicular, or some other neurogenic process.

2.6. Severity

The severity of back pain carries little diagnostic weight. Patients may describe their pain as severe, but that does not necessarily implicate a serious or threatening condition. There are no valid guidelines by which to assess the clinical significance of reportedly very severe pain. At most, severity should be considered as one parameter in the context of other features, notably 'Associated features' (see below), in influencing management.

What is helpful is to record the severity of the pain, at baseline and subsequently, using a quantitative measure such as a visual analog scale[11–13]. This provides a measure of whether or not the pain is improving that is more reliable than the patient's or practitioner's memory of the severity over time.

2.7. Frequency

Back pain may wax and wane in severity, but does not exhibit any periodicity that is of diagnostic significance. Frequency is more likely to be a function of aggravating factors than an index of the cause or mechanism of pain. The record, however, should at least, show how often the patient suffers pain.

2.8. Duration

Other than with respect to length of illness (see above) the duration of back pain carries no diagnostic significance. At best, episodes of limited duration imply a lesser problem in terms of disability, but not necessarily lesser pathology.

2.9. Time of onset

No particular cause of low back pain has a characteristic time of onset. Morning stiffness is said to be a feature of ankylosing spondylitis, but while this feature has a high to moderate sensitivity, its specificity is moderate to low, and its positive likelihood ratio is only 1.5[14] or 1.6[15].

On the other hand, alerting, but not diagnostic, is pain that persists at night or wakes the patient from sleep. Under those circumstances, a red flag condition should be considered (see below).

2.10. Mode of onset

Most cases of acute low back pain will be spontaneous in onset or related to some perceived injury, such as twisting or lifting. Neither of these modes of onset are contributory in a diagnostic sense.

Alarming should be spontaneous pain of an explosive onset. The validity of this feature has not been studied, but should raise concerns on the basis of traditional, clinical wisdom. It may be the first cue of a spontaneous fracture, or an infection.

2.11. Precipitating factors

A patient who has pain-free intervals might identify activities that can bring on their pain. However, there are no data to substantiate a relationship between particular precipitating factors and particular causes of back pain. At best, a record of precipitating factors provides only a description of the patient and his problem.

2.12. Aggravating factors

Back pain will commonly be aggravated by particular movements or activities. These carry no diagnostic significance. Virtually any cause of low back pain is likely to be aggravated by movement and activities of daily living.

At best, listing aggravating factors provides a description of the patient and his problem, and foreshadows the assessment of disability. What will be difficult to distil is the extent to which aggravation is due to an actual increase in painful sensations from the back or to fear of aggravation and resultant avoidance of activity (see Chapter 5).

Perhaps more significant is the absence of aggravating factors. A patient with back pain that is not aggravated by spinal movement warrants assessment for a cause of pain that refers pain to the spine. Abdominal aortic aneurysms can present in this way, and misrepresentation of the back pain as musculoskeletal has been recorded as one of the reasons for delay in diagnosis of dissecting aneurysm [16].

2.13. Relieving factors

Patients might identify factors that relieve their pain. These could include medications and quasi-

therapeutic interventions such as ice packs or hot baths, but also may include certain postures or activities. Although worthwhile as a record of the patient's description of their problem, these factors carry no valid diagnostic significance. It is virtually expectable that patients with a painful joint will feel better in postures that do not load that joint, e.g. lying down.

However, vexatious in this regard is the interpretation of unrelenting back pain: pain that is not relieved by rest, and which is constantly causing the patient anguish. Although this could be interpreted as lack of tolerance by the patient, it could also be a sign of a severe and serious disorder. There are no validated guidelines for the interpretation of this feature. On the one hand, the physician risks over-investigating every patient who claims to be distressed by their pain. On the other hand, they risk missing a serious condition. In the absence of guiding data, this judgement must be taken intuitively; but a critical contribution can be made by associated features. Associated features suggestive of a serious disorder are more reliable than persistence of pain.

2.14. Associated features

Associated features offer the most fruitful realm of interrogation of a patient with back pain. It is in this context that systemic and visceral disorders are most likely to be distinguished from spinal pain of unknown origin. Exploration of associated features can be intercalated, for convenience, with a systems review and a general medical history.

General A fever, or a history of sweats or night sweats, requires consideration of osteomyelitis, discitis and epidural abscess, as does a history of recent surgical procedures, catherisation, and venepuncture.

Occupational exposure or recent travel may offer a clue to exotic infections, such as hydatid disease.

Weight loss and a history of cancer are important cues of neoplastic disorders presenting with spinal pain (see below).

Skin Cutaneous infections may be the source of spinal infection.

Psoriatic and similar rashes offer a cue towards the seronegative spondylarthropathies.

Gastrointestinal Symptoms, or a history of diarrhoea, may be a cue towards the seronegative spondylarthropathies.

Cardiovascular A history of vascular disease or the presence of cardiovascular risk factors warrants assessment for aortic aneurysm.

Respiratory A history of cough may warrant consideration of lung cancer as a risk factor for spinal metastases.

Urinary Features, or a history of urinary tract infection, or haematuria warrant an assessment of the renal tract as a source of referred pain to the spine.

Urinary retention or poor stream warrants assessment for prostate cancer.

Reproductive Back pain associated with menstrual periods, with abnormal uterine bleeding, or abnormal menstruation warrants gynaecological assessment.

Haemopoietic Haemopoietic disorders related to back pain are unlikely to be evident on history, but myeloma is an important consideration for back pain in the elderly.

Endocrine Endocrine disorders that erode bone or stretch periosteum may present with spinal pain, but offer few, if any clues on history alone. Hyperparathyroidism and Paget's disease should be recalled as possible occult causes of spinal pain.

Risk factors for osteoporosis such as age and corticosteroid use warrant a consideration of pathological fracture.

Musculoskeletal Pain elsewhere warrants consideration of systemic rheumatic diseases.

Neurological Neurological symptoms are not indicative of any particular cause of spinal pain.

They are features that should be assessed and investigated in their own right, quite apart from any complaint of spinal pain.

3. Circumstances of onset

Given a patient who ascribes the onset of his back pain to an injury, it is worthwhile to record the circumstances of injury both for descriptive and for medicolegal purposes. However, although it is tempting to infer from the circumstances of injury what the possible nature of the injury is, this is a specious exercise.

As a clinically applicable science, biomechanics is still in its infancy concerning back injuries. Essentially, similar external circumstances could produce any number of different injuries to the vertebral column. There is no unique or dependable relationship between external circumstances and internal responses. At worst, such an exercise constitutes diagnosis by imagination. It may be attractive for a practitioner to imagine what happened inside the patient's back during the precipitating episode that they describe, but there is no proven validity to this exercise. A physician's imagination may be limited to what they have been taught, which is not necessarily that which has happened in a patient, or everything that could happen. However, although diagnosis by imagination is neither reliable nor valid, certain general inferences can be drawn from the circumstances of injury, given certain epidemiological and biomechanical data.

It has been shown that twisting in a flexed position, moving external loads of greater than 11.5 kg, constitutes a risk factor for back pain [17]. Furthermore, it has been shown that, under torsion, a variety of lesions can occur in the lumbar spine [18]. These range from tears of the anulus fibrosus, through tears of the zygapophysial joint capsules, to impaction and avulsion fractures of the articular processes, and fractures of the pars interarticularis. Coupling these data provides a basis for suspecting that a patient with a history of twisting may well have suffered a torsion injury; but what that injury is, in specific anatomical terms, cannot be inferred with validity.

Similarly, biomechanical studies have shown that sudden axial loading, as in a fall into a seated position, or repetitive compression loading, as in repeated lifting, can cause acute or fatigue failure, respectively, of the vertebral endplates, resulting ultimately in internal disc disruption [18]. Given a history of lifting under load, one might conceive that the patient possibly has a compression injury, but the specific nature of that injury cannot be inferred validly from the history alone.

At best, imagining a possible diagnosis on the basis of circumstances of onset might raise a diagnostic hypothesis that is worthy of pursuing, but whether or not that diagnosis should be pursued needs to be considered in context. Whereas it might be legitimate and useful to pursue such a diagnosis in a patient with chronic pain that has defied diagnosis, it is not practical to do so for a patient with acute low back pain. The investigations required to confirm a compression injury or a torsion injury, such as discography and anulography, are invasive and uncomfortable. In a patient with acute low back pain, the pre-test likelihoods of such conditions are unknown and are arguably low. The natural history of acute low back pain favours relying on passage of time instead of invasive investigations (Chapter 4). There is no point subjecting to investigation patients who are destined to recover anyway in a matter of days or weeks. In the meantime, failure to institute investigations for subtle injuries will not greatly affect immediate management. Under these conditions, any biomechanical formulation about the patient is best reserved as a plausible hypothesis, perhaps worthy of pursuit once and only if the patient's pain persists despite other immediate and short-term measures.

One possible exception relates to pars interarticularis fractures in sportspeople. Pars fractures are common in sportspeople, and the imperative is to identify individuals who have a stressed pars that has not yet fractured in order that preservative therapy can be instituted (see Chapter 8). For that reason there is justification in considering stress of the pars interarticularis in sportspeople who present with acute low back pain.

4. Red flag conditions

Of paramount concern in the assessment of a patient with acute low back pain is the detection or exclusion of red flag conditions, such as fractures, infections, or tumours. In the past this has led some practitioners to investigate patients intensely, 'just in case', or just to be safe. Such actions are not justified. Not only are red flag conditions uncommon, they can be adequately screened by a meticulous history and physical examination. Moreover, many of the commonly used tests, e.g. X-ray and ESR, lack sensitivity and specificity, and may be false-negative. A negative result, therefore, may create a false sense of security.

Fortunately, many of the practices used to detect red flag conditions have been subjected to scientific scrutiny, and data on their validity are available.

4.1. General remarks

The literature, clinical experience and formal research has shown that:

(1) the red flag conditions are mercifully rare; therefore, the pre-test odds are in favour of the condition not being present, which should be reassuring both to the patient and to the practitioner;

(2) cases of red flag conditions are typically suspected, not on the basis of results of special investigations, but on the basis of history or examination;

(3) when serious conditions have been missed it is not for lack of special investigations but for lack of adequate and thorough attention to clues in the history;

(4) certain conditions will be missed even with special investigations, because the condition is early in its evolution and defies resolution;

(5) missing certain conditions makes no difference to the outcome, because nothing could have

been done to avert the progress of the condition in any case.

Once a red-flag condition has been identified or strongly implicated, conventional algorithms should be implemented for the confirmation and management of that condition.

4.2. Fractures

With respect to fractures, the cardinal indicators are trauma and age (Table III). In the general population, significant fractures, presenting as back pain, occur only in patients with a history of major trauma [19]. Minor trauma is not a risk factor for fractures unless the patient has osteoporosis. In this regard, the patient's age (>50 years) is the cardinal guideline although the literature suggests that patients with osteoporotic fractures following minor trauma tend to be substantially older than this limit [19]. Consumption of corticosteroids is another risk factor for osteoporosis.

4.3. Cancer

The pre-test probability of a patient in general practice who presents with acute low back pain having cancer as the cause is less than 0.7% [20]. The majority of patients who prove to have cancer as the cause of their back pain are elderly [20]. Consequently, in patients older than 50 years of age, the probability of cancer as a cause is 0.56%; in patients under 50, the probability is 0.14%.

Of the various clinical features that have been formally tested (Table IV), relief of pain by bed rest is a relative negative predictor of cancer. Features which, individually, raise the suspicion of cancer are weight loss, age, past history of cancer, failure to

improve with therapy and prolonged pain. A past history of cancer is by far the single strongest indicator. Note that because 'failure to improve', and 'prolonged pain' are indicators, the diagnosis of cancer is unlikely to be made on the first visit, unless other indicators obtain.

The strongest negative predictors are age less than 50, no past history of cancer, no weight loss, and no failure to improve with therapy (Table IV). Patients with this combination of features are extremely unlikely to have cancer as the basis of their back pain.

4.4. Infection

The pre-test probability in general practice of a patient who presents with acute low back pain having an infection as the cause of the pain is said to be less than 0.01% [22]. This figure, however, is not derived from population studies. The literature cited by Deyo et al. [22] derives the figure from personal communications provided to the authors of a cost-effectiveness study of radiographs for low back pain [23]. The figure, therefore, may not be valid. Its order of magnitude, however, indicates nevertheless that spinal infections are a rare cause of acute low back pain.

The cardinal indicator for infection is fever; the cardinal risk factor is the answer to the question: "why should or why could this patient have an infection?". The specific risk factors are penetration of the body by needles, catheters or other instruments, which includes surgical procedures. Statistical data on the validity of clinical signs as indicators of infection being the cause of low back pain are provided in Table V.

4.5. Ankylosing spondylitis

The pre-test probability in general practice of a patient who presents with acute low back pain having ankylosing spondylitis as the cause of their pain is of the order of 0.3% [22] to 0.9% [15]. However, this condition is virtually impossible to diagnose early in its evolution, and failure to do so makes no significant difference to its management. The final diagnosis relies on a combination of family history,

TABLE III

Risk factors and indicators for fractures of the lumbar spine

Major trauma	
Minor truauma associated with:	osteoporosis
	age > 50
	use of corticosteroids

TABLE IV

Statistical data on the validity of clinical features for the diagnosis of cancer of the lumbar spine

Category of enquiry	Response	SENS	SPEC	+LR	−LR	Ref
Length of illness	Longer than 1 month	0.50	0.81	2.6	1.6	19
Relieving features	Not relieved by bed rest	1.00	0.46	1.9	-	19
Spinal tenderness	Primary care patients	0.15	0.60	0.4	0.7	19
	Hospital patients	0.60	0.70	2.0	1.8	20
		0.80	0.78	3.6	3.9	20
Weight	Weight loss	0.15	0.94	2.5	1.1	19
Age	≥50	0.77	0.71	2.7	2.4	19
Past history of illness:						
Respiratory	Lung cancer					
Urinary	Prostate cancer	0.31	0.98	15.5	1.4	19
Breast	Breast cancer					
Treatment	Failure to improve	0.31	0.90	3.1	1.3	19
Haematocrit	<30%	0.09	0.994	15	1.1	19
ESR	>20 mm/h	0.78	0.67	2.4	3.0	
	>50 mm/h	0.56	0.97	15.3	2.2	19
	>100 mm/h	0.22	0.99	55.0	1.3	19
SnNout	<50	1.00				21
	No past history of illness					
	No weight loss					
	No failure to improve					

SENS: sensitivity. SPEC: specificity. +LR: positive likelihood ratio. −LR: negative likelihood ratio. Ref: references. SnNout: if these features, which have a high sensitivity (Sn) are negative (N) they rule the condition out.

TABLE V

Statistical data on the validity of clinical features for the diagnosis of infection of the lumbar spine

Enquiry	Feature	SENS	SPEC	+LR	−LR	Ref
Tenderness		0.86	0.60	2.2	4.3	21
Fever	TB	0.27	0.98	13.5	1.3	21 [a]
	Pyogenic	0.50	0.98	25.0	2.0	21 [a]
	Epidural abscess	0.83	0.98	41.5	5.8	21 [a]
	Epidural abscess	0.32				23
ESR	Elevated	0.92				24
WCC	>10,000	0.42				24
Personal profile:						
Occupation	? farmer, hydatid					
Prescription drugs	? steroids					
Illicit drugs	IV use					24,25
Past history of illness:						
Infections	Skin	0.40				21,26,27
Procedures	IV catheters	0.40				24,26
Urinary	UTI of catheter	0.40				24,27

[a] Although these are the figures provided in the publication cited, it is difficult to determine from that publication from where and how those figures were derived. The sources cited are either wrong, or do not contain the figures cited. Accordingly these figures may not be accurate.

SENS: sensitivity. SPEC: specificity. +LR: positive likelihood ratio. −LR: negative likelihood ratio. Ref: references.

TABLE VI

Statistical data on the validity of clinical features for the diagnosis of ankylosing spondylitis of the lumbar spine

Enquiry	Feature	SENS	SPEC	+LR	−LR	Ref
Length of illness	Age of onset ≤ 35	0.92	0.30	1.3	3.8	14,20
	Age of onset ≤ 40	1.00	0.07	1.1	-	14,21
	Duration > 3 months	0.71	0.54	1.5	1.9	14,21
Relieving features	Not relieved by bed rest	0.80	0.49	1.6	2.5	14,21
Morning stiffness	> 30 min	0.64	0.59	1.6	1.6	14,21
Chest expansion	< 2.5 cm	0.09	0.99	9.0	1.1	14,21
ESR		0.69	0.68	2.2	2.2	20
4 out of 5 of	morning stiffness improved with exercise onset < 40 slow onset duration > 3 months	0.95	0.85	6.3	17.0	21,27

Sacroiliac joint signs are not diagnostic or indicative of AS.

Diagnostic would be the onset of ocular, cardiac, GIT signs and appendicular involvement.

The diagnosis is clinical and does not require or invite an HLAB27.

SENS: sensitivity. SPEC: specificity. +LR: positive likelihood ratio. −LR: negative likelihood ratio. Ref: references.

associated features, and progression of the disease both in extent and in severity.

The earliest warning hallmarks are morning stiffness, a slow onset at an age less than 30, and improvement with exercise (Table VI). These raise the suspicion of ankylosing spondylitis but alone are not diagnostic. The chances of radiographic changes establishing the diagnosis early in the illness are virtually nil because of the insensitivity of plain films to early changes and the poor reliability of readers to grade early changes of ankylosing spondylitis. The HLA B27 serum test is of no diagnostic value because the presence of this antigen in the asymptomatic population is between 50 and 200 times greater than the prevalence of the disease [29].

Table VI is not designed as a guide for the positive diagnosis of ankylosing spondylitis. Rather, it serves to highlight warning signs that alert the physician to consider ankylosing spondylitis instead of lumbar spinal pain of unknown origin. The likelihood ratios are small and are insufficient to make an affirmative diagnosis of a disease that is so rare. Indeed, even the '4 out of 5' criterion results in high false positive rates [30]. For a more comprehensive discussion of how to establish a diagnosis of ankylosing spondylitis see Gran [15].

5. Checklist

The various data and recommendations outlined above can be used to construct a convenient checklist (Fig. 1). The checklist can be adapted to a form suitable for use by practitioners, such that it can be incorporated into any medical record. A positive response to any entry in the checklist does not necessarily implicate the presence of a red flag condition. Rather, it serves only to alert the practitioner to the possibility of a red flag condition, and calls for greater attention to the feature. On the other hand, if all items are checked and all responses are negative, the practitioner can be assured that the possibility of a red flag condition is extremely unlikely, and that further investigation for red flag conditions is not indicated.

Sinister conditions may not be evident early in the history of a patient, but they could manifest in due course. For that reason the red flag checklist is only a temporising measure. It does not excuse the practitioner from continuing vigilance. For that purpose the red flag checklist can be re-administered whenever the patient is again seen, in order not only to maintain, but also to record, responsible vigilance.

Name:				Low Back Pain		
D.O.B.		M.R.N.				
Presence of		*Cardiovascular*		*Endocrine*		
Trauma	Y N	Risk factors?	Y N	Corticosteroids?	Y	N
Night Sweats	Y N	*Respiratory*		*Musculoskeletal*		
Recent Surgery	Y N	Cough?	Y N	Pain elsewhere?	Y	N
Catheterisation	Y N	*Urinary*		*Neurological*		
Venipuncture	Y N	Haematuria?	Y N	Symptoms/signs	Y	N
Occupational exposure	Y N	Retention?	Y N	*Skin*		
Hobby exposure	Y N	Stream problems?	Y N	Infections?	Y	N
Sporting exposure	Y N	*Reproductive*		Rashes?	Y	N
(Overseas) travel	Y N	Menstrual problems?	Y N	*G.I.T.*		
Illicit drug use	Y N	*Haemopoietic*		Diarrhoea?	Y	N
Weight loss	Y N	Problems?	Y N			
History of Cancer	Y N					
Comments			*Signature:*			
			Date:			

Fig. 1. A checklist for red flag clinical indicators, suitable for inclusion in medical records used in general practice, developed by the author, for the Australian National Musculoskeletal Medicine Initiative

6. Investigations

If a red flag condition is suspected, appropriate further investigations should be undertaken. Recommended investigations are shown in Table VIII. In this regard, the investigations listed are not indicated for the routine investigation of low back pain; nor should they be construed as screening tests for patients with back pain. They are tests explicitly indicated only if the patient's history suggests the corresponding red flag condition.

Since these tests are not designed for the investigation of back pain per se, their validity and utility are not considered as part of this text. Rather, they constitute part of the general armamentarium of medical practice, and are subject to the evidence-base of other disciplines.

In Table VIII, imaging is prescribed rather than X-ray, on the grounds that plain radiographs may not be the appropriate investigation for certain conditions. For screening purposes it may be more appropriate to use bone scan because of its greater sensitivity, or MRI because of its combined sensitivity and specificity (see Chapter 8).

An explicit protocol has been advocated for the investigation of patients in whom cancer is suspected[20]. It recommends the following.

Patients with a *past history of cancer* should be considered '*high risk*'. In these patients an immediate ESR and imaging is warranted, and a positive result on either test mandates further work-up. (Deyo and Diehl[20] stipulated 'X-ray' rather than imaging; but it may be more appropriate to use more sensitive or more specific imaging

TABLE VIII

The cardinal red flag conditions and the appropriate investigations for their confirmation

Condition		Investigations
Primary tumours (rare; 0.04% of all tumours)	myeloma	IEPG, imaging, biopsy
	tumours of bone	imaging
	tumours of cartilage	imaging
Secondary tumours	prostate	serum calcium, alkaline phosphatase, acid phosphatase, prostate specific antigen, imaging
	breast, lung, thyroid, kidney, GIT, melanoma	Imaging
Infection	osteomyelitis, epidural abscess	FBC, ESR, imaging
Metabolic bone disease	Paget's disease	serum calcium
	hyperparathyroidism	alkaline phosphatase, acid phosphatase, bone scan
Visceral disease	aortic aneurysm	abdominal exam, ultrasound
	retroperitoneal disease	abdominal exam, ultrasound
	pelvic disease	pelvic examination, rectal examination

modalities according to the nature of the cancer suspected.)

Patients under the age of 50, with no history of cancer, no weight loss, no signs of systemic illness, and who do not fail to improve, are considered '*low risk*'. For these patients no laboratory tests or imaging are warranted.

Patients *over 50*, or those who *fail to respond* to treatment, or who have unexplained *weight loss* or signs of *systemic illness* constitute 'intermediate risk' risk. For these patients, an ESR is appropriate. If the ESR is <20 mm/h, no further investigation is warranted. If the ESR is >20 mm/h, imaging should be undertaken. If the imaging is normal, these patients should be closely monitored.

This protocol secures the detection of cancer without the use of unnecessary imaging. It has,

however, been amended in the light of a recent, theoretical modelling study.

Joines et al. [31] assessed the costs, risks, sensitivity and specificity of a variety of strategies aimed at detecting cancer in patients with back pain. They found that raising the threshold of the ESR to 50 mm/h instead of 20 mm/h reduced sensitivity but increased specificity, and thereby resulted in lower costs and fewer unnecessary biopsies. They found the optimal strategies to include undertaking imaging if the patient has a *history of cancer, age greater than 50, weight loss*, or *failure to improve* with treatment, or an *ESR* greater than 50. In the face of these features, the imaging that should be undertaken is an MRI for most cases. However, for some conditions serial bone scanning and MRI provides greater specificity. The exact choice of imaging requires clinical judgement in the light of the possible nature of the malignancy suspected.

Key points

- A comprehensive history can be obtained by enquiring about:

presenting complaint	ensure that it is back pain
length of illness	establish if it is acute, subacute, or chronic
site of pain	record the primary site of pain
radiation	distinguish somatic referred pain from radicular pain
quality	distinguish somatic pain from radicular pain
severity	record baseline VAS
frequency	(not of diagnostic value)
duration	(not of diagnostic value)
time of onset	beware of night pain
mode of onset	beware of sudden, severe pain
precipitating factors	(not of diagnostic value)
aggravating factors	beware of absence of mechanical aggravating factors
relieving factors	(not of valid diagnostic significance)
associated features	the source of most significant diagnostic features

- The most important and valid alerting features are:
  - past history of cancer
  - age greater than 50
  - prolonged illness
  - failure to improve with treatment
  - unexplained weight loss.

- The alerting features for fracture are:
  - major trauma
  - minor trauma in patients over 50, with osteoporosis, or taking corticosteroids.

- Alerting features for spinal infection are:
  - fever
  - history of body penetration.

- Imaging with MRI is indicated if the patient has the alerting clinical features for cancer or an ESR greater than 50.

References

1 Lance JW. Mechanism and Management of Headache, 5th edn. Butterworth Heinemann, Oxford, 1993.

2 Sinclair SJ, Hogg-Johnson S, Mondloch MV, Shields SA. The effectiveness of an early active intervention program for workers with soft-tissue injuries: the early claimant cohort study. Spine 1997; 22: 2919–2931.

3 Mooney V, Robertson J. The facet syndrome. Clin Orthop 1976; 115: 149–156.

4 Fairbank JCT, Park WM, McCall IW, O'Brien JP. Apophysial injections of local anaesthetic as a diagnostic aid in primary low-back pain syndromes. Spine 1981; 6: 598–605.

5 Fukui S, Ohseto K, Shiotani M, Ohno K, Karasawa H, Naganuma Y. Distribution of referred pain from the lumbar zygapophyseal joints and dorsal rami. Clin J Pain 1997; 13: 303–307.

6 Smyth MJ, Wright V. Sciatica and the intervertebral disc. An experimental study. J Bone Joint Surg 1959; 40A: 1401–1418.

7 Kellgren JH. On the distribution of pain arising from deep somatic structures with charts of segmental pain areas. Clin Sci 1939; 4: 35–46.

8 Feinstein B, Langton JNK, Jameson RM, Schiller F. Experiments on pain referred from deep somatic tissues. J Bone Joint Surg 1954; 35A: 981–987.

9 Bogduk N, Govind J. Medical Management of Acute Lum-

bar Radicular Pain. An Evidence-Based Approach. Newcastle Bone and Joint Institute, Newcastle, 1999.

10 Merskey H, Bogduk N (eds). Classification of Chronic Pain. Descriptions of Chronic pain Syndromes and Definitions of Pain Terms, 2nd edn. IASP Press, Seattle, WA, 1994.

11 Carlsson AM. Assessment of chronic pain, I. Aspects of the reliability and validity of the visual analogue scale. Pain 1983; 16: 87–101.

12 Chapman CR, Casey KL, Dubner R, Foley KM, Gracely RH, Reading AE. Pain measurement: an overview. Pain 1985; 22: 1–31.

13 Strong J, Ashton R, Chant D. Pain intensity measurement in chronic low back pain. Clin J Pain 1991; 7: 209–218.

14 Calin A, Porta J, Fries JF, Schurman DJ. Clinical history as a screening test for ankylosing spondylitis. JAMA 1977; 237: 2613–2614.

15 Gran JT. An epidemiological survey of the signs and symptoms of ankylosing spondylitis. Clin Rheumatol 1985; 4: 161–169.

16 El-Farhan N, Busuttil A. Sudden unexpected deaths from ruptured abdominal aortic aneurysms. J Clin Forensic Med 1997; 4: 111–116.

17 Kelsey JL, Githens PB, White AA, Holford TR, Walter WD, O'Connor T, Ostfeld AM, Weil U, Southwick WO, Calogero JA. An epidemiologic study of lifting and twisting on the job and risk for acute prolapsed lumbar intervertebral disc. J Orthop Res 1984; 2: 61–66.

18 Bogduk N. Clinical Anatomy of the Lumbar Spine and Sacrum, 3rd edn. Churchill Livingstone, Edinburgh, 1997, pp. 187–213.

19 Scavone JG, Latshaw RF, Rohrer V. Use of lumbar spine films: statistical evaluation at a university teaching hospital. JAMA 1981; 246: 1105–1108.

20 Deyo RA, Diehl AK. Cancer as a cause of back pain: frequency, clinical presentation and diagnostic strategies. J Gen Intern Med 1988; 3: 230–238.

21 van den Hoogen MM, Koes BW, Eijk JTM, Bouter LM. On the accuracy of history, physical examination, and erythrocyte sedimentation rate in diagnosing low back pain in general practice: a criteria-based review of the literature. Spine 1995; 20: 318–327.

22 Deyo RA, Rainville J, Kent DL. What can the history and physical examination tell us about low back pain? JAMA 1992; 268: 760–765.

23 Liang M, Komaroff AL. Roentgenograms in primary care patients with acute low back pain: a cost-effectiveness analysis. Arch Int Med 1982; 142: 1108–1112.

24 Sampath P, Rigamonti D. Spinal epidural abscess: a review of epidemiology, diagnosis, and treatment. J Spinal Disorders 1999; 12: 89–93.

25 Sapico FL, Montgomerie JZ. Pyogenic vertebral osteomyelitis: report of nine cases and review of the literature. Rev Inf Dis 1979; 1: 754–776.

26 Chandrasekar PH. Low back pain and intravenous drug abusers. Arch Int Med 1990; 150: 1125–1128.

27 Baker AS, Ojemann RG, Swartz MN, Richardson EP. Spinal epidural abscess. N Engl J Med 1975; 293: 463–468.

28 Waldvogel FA, Vasey H. Osteomyelitis: the past decade. N Engl J Med 1980; 303: 360–370.

29 Hawkins BR, Dawkins RL, Chrisiansen FT, Zilko PJ. Use of the B27 test in the diagnosis of ankylosing spondylitis: a statistical evaluation. Arthritis Rheum 1981; 24: 743–746.

30 Calin A, Kaye B, Sternberg M, Antell B, Chan M. The prevalence and nature of back pain in an industrial complex. A questionnaire and radiographic and HLA analysis. Spine 1980; 5: 201–205.

31 Joines JD, McNuff RA, Carey TS, Deyo RA, Rouhane R. Finding cancer in primary care outpatients with low back pain. A comparison of diagnostic strategies. J Gen Intern Med 2001; 16: 14–23.

Medical Management of Acute and Chronic Low Back Pain. An Evidence-Based Approach
Pain Research and Clinical Management, Vol. 13
Nikolai Bogduk and Brian McGuirk
© *2002 Elsevier Science B.V. All rights reserved*

CHAPTER 7

Physical examination

1. Introduction

Traditional wisdom would maintain that a patient with back pain should be examined. Along standard orthopaedic lines, the lumbar spine should be inspected, palpated and moved. In some circles, even passive intervertebral motion is tested.

Although this process may be conventional and whereas it serves to *provide a description* of the patient, the existing evidence base shows that no particular clinical sign, or combination of signs, found by this process, allows a valid or reliable diagnosis of back pain to be made in anatomical or pathological terms.

2. Inspection

Inspection may reveal minor aberrations of shape or posture of the lumbar spine, such as a loss of lordosis or a list. In some studies, the reliability of detecting gross examples of such aberrations has been found to be good, with kappa scores of the order of 0.5–0.7 [1], but in other studies agreement is worse [2] (Table I). Notwithstanding this agreement, there are no data to show that such features have any construct validity for diagnosis or any predictive validity concerning treatment.

Identifying major postural deformities such as scoliosis is important for the diagnosis of such deformities in their own right, but it has no bearing on making a diagnosis of the cause of back pain. There is no direct relationship between major deformity

TABLE I

The reliability of inspection and palpation in the examination of the lumbar spine

TEST	Kappa score	Source
Inspection		
lordosis	0.50–0.70	1
lordosis (PT)	–	2
lordosis (MD)	0.32	2
list (PT)	0.39	2
list (MD)	0.13	2
asymmetries	0.34–0.84	3
Palpation		
tenderness:		
anywhere	1.0	1
at specific sites	0.11–0.38	1, 4
paravertebral (PT)	0.27	2
paravertebral (MD)	0.22	2
intersegmental	0.40–0.78	3
intersegmental L5–S1 (PT)	0.55	2
intersegmental L5–S1 (MD)	0.40	2
intersegmental L4–L5 (PT)	0.56	2
intersegmental L4–L5 (MD)	0.40	2
spinous process	0.55–0.90	3
iliac crest	0.66	5
trigger points	<0.40	6, 7

PT, physical therapists; MD, medical practitioners.

and any known source or cause of lumbar spinal pain.

Similarly, identifying pigmentation, dimples, or patches of hair at the base of the spine is of significance for the recognition of congenital defects of the spine and spinal cord, but it has no direct bearing on the diagnosis of back pain.

3. Palpation

Palpation can be used to identify hyperaesthesia of the skin over the back. In some studies this has been found to be a common feature amongst patients with back pain[8]; but this feature is nonspecific, for it offers no insight as to the cause or source of pain.

Identifying numbness or hyperaesthesia over the buttocks may draw attention to entrapment neuropathies of the superior clunial nerves in patients with thoracolumbar pain[9].

Otherwise, the cardinal application of palpation has traditionally been to identify tenderness, i.e. a point or points which, when pressed, reproduce the patient's pain. This pursuit, however, is confounded both by lack of reliability and lack of validity.

Studies have shown that two observers can agree on finding tenderness somewhere in the lumbar spine in patients with back pain, with kappa scores equal to 1.00[1], but when the location of tenderness is specified, agreement falls and varies from site to site (Table I). Agreement is poor for paravertebral tenderness defined as tenderness anywhere from the midline to the midaxillary line[2]. In one study, agreement about tenderness at specific sites was poor[4]. In others[2,3], agreement on paramedian, intersegmental tenderness was fair to good.

One site where kappa scores for tenderness are good is over the iliac crest superomedial to the posterior superior iliac spine[5]. The presence of this sign has been invoked as diagnostic of 'iliac crest syndrome'[5,10], but the patho-anatomic basis of this syndrome and, hence, the validity of the sign is unknown. Various interpretations include sprain of the lumbar intermuscular aponeurosis[11], sprain of the iliolumbar ligament[12–14], sprain of the multifidus muscle[15,16], sprain of the gluteus maximus muscle[17], trigger point activity in quadratus lumborum[18,19], muscle imbalance[20], and entrapment of the lateral branches of the lateral branches of the lumbar dorsal rami in the fascia attached to iliac crest[9]. However, no study has validated any of these conjectures. Consequently, this purported syndrome constitutes no more than a single, clinical sign. Although the sign may be reliably de-

tected, it does not constitute a legitimate diagnosis.

The diagnostic validity of muscle tenderness has not been determined. No one knows what tenderness means. There is no evidence that it is a sign of primary pathology in the muscle. It may be no more than a feature of hyperalgesia. Thus, finding tenderness, although perhaps of interest, is not of any diagnostic significance.

Bone tenderness over the lumbar spinous processes has been held to be an alerting sign of osseous disorders such as infection or neoplasm. The reliability of palpation for bony tenderness over the spinous processes has been shown to be good to very good, depending on the segment involved and the examiners (Table I). This sign, however, has poor specificity and offers a positive likelihood ratio of only 2.2 for infection[21].

As a diagnosis, 'trigger point syndrome' lacks validity for there is no objective criterion standard for the entity or its purported pathology. Moreover, in the lumbar spine, the detection of trigger points in the erector spinae or quadratus lumborum has poor reliability, with kappa scores less than 0.4[6,7]. If the diagnostic criteria for a trigger point are relaxed to consist only of tenderness, the kappa scores increase[7], but this increase in reliability occurs at the expense of validity of the diagnosis, for tenderness alone does not constitute a diagnosis of a trigger point syndrome, or any other condition; it is simply tenderness.

The entity of 'muscle spasm' has no validity for there is no known neurophysiological correlate of this clinical sign[22,23]. Moreover, in formal studies, the reliability of finding muscle spasm has been so poor as to defy reporting in terms of kappa scores[1].

4. Range of motion

Gross limitations of range of motion of the lumbar spine can be reliably detected by inspection, although the kappa scores for limited flexion are better than for limited lateral flexion (Table II). Agreement is good on whether movement aggravates pain or

TABLE II

The reliability of selected tests of motion used in the examination of the lumbar spine

Test	Kappa	Source
Motion		
gross range:		
lateral (PT)	0.43	2
lateral (MD)	0.11	2
lateral	0.41	1
extension (PT)	0.74	2
extension (MD)	0.35	2
flexion	0.81	1
pain on:		
lateral flexion (PT)	0.51	
lateral flexion (MD)	0.06	2
extension (PT)	0.76	2
extension (MD)	0.71	2
flexion (PT)	0.63	2
flexion (MD)	0.71	2
mobility:		
L5–S1 (PT)	0.54	2
L5–S1 (MD)	−0.08	2
L4–L5 (PT)	0.75	2
L4–L5 (MD)	–	2
PPIVM:		
flexion	−0.11–0.32	25
extension	−0.02–0.23	25
PAIVM:		
transverse	−0.15–0.23	25
central	−0.14–0.24	25
unilateral	−0.10–0.11	25

PT, physical therapists; MD, medical practitioners; PPIVM, passive physiological intervertebral motion; PAIVM, passive accessory intervertebral motion.

not (Table II). Using a goniometer ostensibly offers greater precision in measuring range of motion, but the probability of an inter-examiner difference of 5° is 0.59, the probability of a difference of 10° is 0.28, and the probability of a 15° difference is as high as 0.11 [24]. Consequently, inter-examiner variation erodes any precision in measurement offered by a goniometer.

Regardless of agreement or otherwise, range of motion offers no diagnostic insight. Limited range of motion is a nonspecific feature that can be expected as a result of any form of low back pain. There is no evidence that any particular pattern of limitation of

movement implicates a particular cause or source of back pain.

Guarded movements carry no specificity. Putatively they might occur as a result of any cause of back pain. Moreover, the reliability of detecting guarded movements is very poor [1].

5. Intervertebral motion

Manual therapists contend that they can identify symptomatic lumbar spinal segments by careful examination of intersegmental motion. For the lumbar spine, the validity of this contention is elusive. One study [25] claimed a good correlation between the findings on manual examination and the results of diagnostic spinal blocks, but the nature of the blocks or their results were not described. Furthermore, the reliability of examination was poor, with kappa scores ranging from *minus* 0.15 to only 0.32 [25].

Other studies have indicated that physiotherapists are able to agree as to whether an L5–S1 or an L4–L5 segment is hypomobile, but that doctors are unable to agree on this feature [2] (Table II). However, when estimates of intersegmental stiffness are compared, agreement is poor [26].

6. McKenzie

The McKenzie school of spinal assessment maintains that discogenic pain can be diagnosed on the basis of whether or not the patient's pain 'centralises' upon certain movements of the lumbar spine, i.e. the extent of radiation of pain into the lower limb retracts [27]. The reliability of McKenzie examination differs amongst observers. Some have found poor reliability [28] but others have found good reliability [27] and have argued that expert training is critical.

The validity of McKenzie examination has been tested against discography as a criterion standard, and the correlation between findings is statistically significant, but as a diagnostic test McKenzie examination is only marginally effective. It offers only modest likelihood ratios [29] (Table III).

TABLE III

Contingency table for the validity of McKenzie tests in the diagnosis of discogenic pain and painful lumbar disc with a competent anulus

	Discogenic pain with competent anulus				
	Yes	No	Sens	Spec	LR
Centralisers	21	10	0.72	0.70	2.4
All others	8	24			
Centralisers	21	10	0.78	0.50	1.6
Peripheralisers	6	10			
Change ±	27	20	0.93	0.41	1.6
No change	2	14			

Based on the data of Donelson et al.[27].
Sens, sensitivity; Spec, specificity; LR, likelihood ratio.

7. Sacro-iliac joint

The sacro-iliac joint has been promoted as an important, if not common, source of back pain, and a number of physical tests have been developed to diagnose so-called sacro-iliac dysfunction. Those tests considered by an international panel of experts to be the most useful have been subjected to scientific scrutiny. It transpires that these tests are highly reliable, with kappa scores of the order of 0.8[30], but as indicators of pain stemming from the sacro-iliac joint, they lack validity, with positive likelihood ratios barely greater than 1.0, and less than 1.0 in some instances[30]. Furthermore, they are positive in some 25% of individuals who have no pain[31].

8. Normal findings

Although physical examination of the lumbar spine may lack reliability or validity when a positive diagnosis is being pursued, there is at least concept validity for the opposite. It should be strange to find no abnormalities on palpation and movement of a patient presenting with lumbar spinal pain. Such a finding should alert the examiner to reconsider referred pain to the lumbar spine from visceral disorders or a red flag condition. Arguably, this possibility

is the singular most important reason for examining the lumbar spine. Finding positive features on examination does not lead to a valid, particular musculoskeletal diagnosis but finding no abnormalities is conspicuous and should be alerting.

9. Neurological examination

Perhaps the most difficult concept to explain in spine medicine is the lack of relevance of neurological examination in a patient with back pain. The tradition and habit of performing a neurological examination stems from an era when it was believed that disc prolapse was the cardinal, if not the only, legitimate, cause of common back pain. Because disc prolapse caused radiculopathy a neurological examination was mandatory, but the misconception arose that, therefore, a neurological examination was mandatory for all patients with back pain. This line of reasoning is false on epidemiological, clinical and neurophysiological grounds.

Disc prolapse accounts for fewer than 5%[32,33] or 12%[34] of lumbar spine presentations. Therefore, the majority of patients do not present with disc prolapse and, therefore, would not be expected to exhibit neurological signs of disc prolapse.

If disc prolapse causes pain, it is radicular pain, which is felt in the lower limb, not in the back. Therefore, although a patient presenting with lower limb pain might warrant a neurological examination, a patient presenting with back pain only, by definition, does not have radicular pain, and does not warrant a neurological examination as does a patient with radicular pain.

Neurological signs are produced by conduction block in motor or sensory nerves, but conduction block does not cause pain. Thus, even in a patient with back pain and neurological signs, whatever causes the neurological signs is not causing the back pain by the same mechanism. Therefore, finding the cause of the neurological signs does not implicitly identify the cause of pain. Conditions such as radiculitis may cause both pain and neurological signs, but in that event the pain occurs in the lower limb, not in the back. If root inflammation also happens to involve the nerve root sleeve, back pain might also arise, but in that event the patient will have three problems, each with a different mechanism: neurological signs due to conduction block, radicular pain due to nerve-root inflammation, and back pain due to inflammation of the dura.

Given these arguments it is informative to consider the place of neurological examination in each of five contexts.

9.1. The patient with back pain only

In patients with back pain only, and who, upon enquiry, deny neurological symptoms, there is no reason axiomatically to suspect a neurological disorder and, therefore, no indication for a neurological examination.

9.2. The patient with somatic referred pain

In patients with back pain and somatic referred pain in the lower limb, particularly if it is focused over the buttock and thigh, there is no reason, prima facie, to suspect a neurological condition or to expect neurological signs. However, if the physician is not certain that the patient's pain is in indeed somatic and referred, and the possibility obtains that the pain is radicular, that patient should be considered under the following category.

9.3. The patient with radicular pain

Patients with radicular pain warrant a neurological examination, but in this context it should be clear that the presenting feature that attracts a neurological examination is not back pain but the radicular pain. Radicular pain invites an assessment parallel but separate to the assessment of back pain for, although in some patients the one condition may cause both symptoms, in others the causes may be different, if not remote, from one another.

9.4. The patient with neurological symptoms

If patients volunteer or acknowledge neurological symptoms, a neurological examination is mandatory, but in that event the patient is not presenting with back pain but with a neurological disorder.

9.5. Insecurity

It may transpire that out of habit, out of respect for traditional practice, or because of uncertainty, a physician feels compelled to perform a neurological examination in patients presenting with back pain. In that event, unless the patient acknowledges neurological symptoms, a screening examination should suffice.

> Integrity of the L5 and S1 myotomes can be rapidly assessed by having the patients walk on their heels and on their toes. Integrity of the sensory roots of L1 to S2 can be assessed by touch in the centres of the respective dermatomes. In this context, studies have shown that neurological examination in patients with and without radiculopathy is quite reliable, with kappa scores in excess of 0.6 [1,4]. Testing reflexes is superfluous if there are no motor or sensory abnormalities in a patient who otherwise complains of no neurological symptoms.

If no neurological abnormalities are found on screening examination, the pursuit of neurological signs can be terminated and the physical examination reverted to the assessment of back pain. However, if at any time a neurological abnormality is encountered it should be assessed in detail with respect to nature, extent and severity, looking also for convergent associated abnormalities, such as motor signs that correlate with sensory signs. In that event, the patients' neurological disorder should be assessed in parallel with, or even ahead of, their back pain, but in either case, as a separate entity lest a potentially false inference be drawn that the cause of the neurological signs is also the cause of their back pain.

10. To examine or not

A nihilistic interpretation of the evidence would be that because it is both not reliable and not valid, physical examination should not be performed. That is not what the data say. The data simply indicate that physical examination of the back lacks reliability and lacks validity. That means that no legitimate diagnostic inferences can be drawn from a physical examination, but it does not mean that a physical examination should not be performed. There are good theoretical reasons for performing a physical examination, but none of them bear on making a diagnosis.

Foremost, patients expect an examination. Performing an examination establishes a bond between the practitioner and the patient. Laying on of hands may be symbolic to the patients, indicating that the practitioner is interested in their problem and knows what they are doing. Accordingly, the opportunity to bond with the patient, show interest, and inspire confidence should not be squandered. But the practitioner should realise that this is why they are performing the examination. It is not to make a diagnosis.

Physical examination also constitutes an opportunity to commence operant conditioning. Instead of focussing on abnormalities, the practitioner can take the opportunity to celebrate normality with the patient; commenting on what they find as good, intact, and strong. Such positive reinforcement can be the first step in reducing the patient's fears and promoting return to activity (see Chapter 11).

The only diagnostic virtues of physical examination are that it provides the opportunity to detect unrecognised features of concurrent abnormalities unrelated to the back pain, and the opportunity to find nothing intrinsically wrong with the back. The latter calls for an assessment of sources of pain not located in the back.

Key points

- Physical examination of the lumbar spine does not provide for a diagnosis of back pain.
- The commonly used tests, and several, more esoteric tests lack reliability, validity or both.
- Apart, perhaps, from a simple screening examination, neurological examination is not indicated in a patient who presents simply with back pain and no neurological symptoms.

References

1   Waddell G, Main CJ, Morris EW, Venner RM, Rae P, Sharmy SH, Galloway H. Normality and reliability in the clinical assessment of backache. Br Med J 1982; 284: 1519–1523.

2   Strender LE, Sjoblom A, Sundell K, Ludwig R, Taube A. Interexaminer reliability in physical examination of patients with low back pain. Spine 1997; 22: 814–820.

3   Boline PD, Haas M, Meyer JJ, Kassak K, Nelson C, Keating JC. Interexaminer reliability of eight evaluative dimensions of lumbar segmental abnormality: Part II. J Manip Physiol Ther 1993; 16: 363–374.

4   McCombe PF, Fairbank JCT, Cockersole BC, Punsent PB. Reproducibility of physical signs in low-back pain. Spine 1989; 14: 908–918.

5   Njoo KH, van der Does E, Stam HJ. Interobserver agreement on iliac crest pain syndrome in general practice. J Rheumatol 1995; 22: 1532–1535.

6   Nice DA, Riddle DL, Lamb RL, Mayhew TP, Ruckler K. Intertester reliability of judgements of the presence of trigger points in patients with low back pain. Arch Phys Med Rehabil 1992; 73: 893–898.

7   Njoo KH, Van der Does E. The occurrence and inter-rater reliability of myofascial trigger points in the quadratus lumborum and gluteus medius: a prospective study in nonspecific low back pain patients and controls in general practice. Pain 1994; 58: 317–323.

8   Glover JR. Back pain and hyperaesthesia. Lancet 1960; 1: 1165–1168.

9   Maigne JY, Doursounian L. Entrapment neuropathy of the medial superior cluneal nerve. Nineteen cases surgically treated, with a minimum of 2 years' follow-up. Spine 1997; 22: 1156–1159.

10 Collee G, Dijkmans AC, Vandenbroucke JP, Cats A. Iliac crest syndrome in low back pain: frequency and features. J

Rheumatol 1991; 18: 1064–1067.

11 Bogduk N. A reappraisal of the anatomy of the human lumbar erector spinae. J Anat 1980; 131: 525–540.

12 Hackett GS. Referred pain from low back ligament disability. AMA Arch Surg 1956; 73: 878–883.

13 Ingpen ML, Burry HC. A lumbo-sacral strain syndrome. Ann Phys Med 1970; 10: 270–274.

14 Hirschberg GG, Froetscher L, Naeim F. Iliolumbar syndrome as a common cause of low back pain: diagnosis and prognosis. Arch Phys Med Rehabil 1979; 60: 415–419.

15 Livingstone WK. Back disabilities due to strain of the multifidus muscle. West J Surg 1941; 49: 259–263.

16 Bauwens P, Coyer AB. The 'multifidus triangle' syndrome as a cause of recurrent low-back pain. BMJ 1955; 2: 1306–1307.

17 Fairbank JCT, O'Brien JP. The iliac crest syndrome. A treatable cause of low-back pain. Spine 1983; 8: 220–224.

18 Sola AE, Kuitert JH. Quadratus lumborum myofasciitis. Northwest Med 1954; 53: 1003–1005.

19 Travell JG, Simons DG. Myofascial Pain and Dysfunction. The Trigger Point Manual. Vol. 2. The Lower Extremities. Williams and Wilkins, Baltimore, MD, 1992: 23–88.

20 Janda V, Jull GA. Muscles and motor control in low back pain: assessment and management. In: Twomey LT, Taylor JR (eds) Physical Therapy of the Low Back. Churchill-Livingstone, New York, NY, 1987: 253–278.

21 Deyo RA, Rainville J, Kent DL. What can the history and physical examination tell us about low back pain? JAMA 1992; 268: 760–765.

22 Andersson G, Bogduk N et al. Muscle: clinical perspectives. In: Frymoyer JW, Gordon SL (eds) New Perspectives on Low Back Pain. American Academy of Orthopaedic Surgeons, Park Ridge, IL, 1989: 293–334.

23 Roland MO. A critical review of the evidence for a pain–spasm–pain cycle in spinal disorders. Clin Biomech 1986; 1: 102–109.

24 Mayer RS, Chen IH, Lavender SA, Trafinow JH, Andersson GBJ. Variance in the measurement of sagittal lumbar spine range of motion among examiners, subjects, and instruments. Spine 1995; 20: 1489–1493.

25 Phillips DR, Twomey LT. A comparison of manual diagnosis with a diagnosis established by a uni-level lumbar spinal block procedure. Man Ther 1996; 2: 82–87.

26 Maher C, Adams R. Reliability of pain and stiffness assessments in clinical manual lumbar spine examination. Phys Ther 1994; 74: 801–811.

27 Donelson R, Aprill C, Medcalf R, Grant W. A prospective study of centralization of lumbar and referred pain. Spine 1997; 33: 1115–1122.

28 Riddle DL, Rothstein JM. Intertester reliability of McKenzie's classifications of the syndrome types present in patients with low back pain. Spine 1993; 18: 1333–1344.

29 Bogduk N, Lord SM. Commentary on: A prospective study of centralization of lumbar and referred pain: a predictor of symptomatic discs and anular competence. Pain Med J Club J 1997; 3: 246–248.

30 Dreyfuss P, Michaelsen M, Pauza K, McLarty J, Bogduk N. The value of history and physical examination in diagnosing sacroiliac joint pain. Spine 1996; 21: 2594–2602.

31 Dreyfuss P, Dreyer S, Griffin J, Hoffman J, Walsh N. Positive sacroiliac screening tests in asymptomatic adults. Spine 1994; 19: 1138–1143.

32 Friberg S. Lumbar disc degeneration in the problem of lumbago sciatica. Bull Hosp Joint Dis 1954; 15: 1–20.

33 Mooney V. Where is the pain coming from? Spine 1987; 12: 754–759.

34 Deyo RA, Tsui-Wu YJ. Descriptive epidemiology of low-back pain and its related medical care in the United States. Spine 1987; 12: 264–268.

35 Merskey H, Bogduk N (eds). Classification of Chronic Pain. Descriptions of Chronic pain Syndromes and Definitions of Pain Terms, 2nd edn. IASP Press, Seattle, WA, 1994.

Medical Management of Acute and Chronic Low Back Pain. An Evidence-Based Approach
Pain Research and Clinical Management, Vol. 13
Nikolai Bogduk and Brian McGuirk
© *2002 Elsevier Science B.V. All rights reserved*

CHAPTER 8

Imaging

1. Introduction

X-rays and low back pain go hand-in-hand. So has been the nature of conventional practice in the past. Physicians request radiographs of the lumbar spine, and patients with back pain expect radiographs to be taken.

Physicians request radiographs of the lumbar spine for a variety of reasons. Perhaps they believe that a radiograph will show something that has escaped diagnosis by history and physical examination, but often they request them for fear of malpractice litigation [1–3], or because they wish to reassure the patient [1,3–6] or themselves [5,6] (that there is nothing seriously wrong), or simply to comply with the patient's wish (to have an X-ray) [1].

Patients expect radiographs for a variety of other reasons. Often the reason is axiomatic: "because my back hurts"; or because their physician recommended it; or because their physiotherapist, chiropractor, or homeopath "had suggested that they should have radiographs because further treatment would otherwise be risky or difficult" (sic) [1]. Some patients view radiographs as important so that they can "stop worrying", "get some answers", "put a name to it", or "to rule out serious disease" [1].

Both on the part of the physicians and on the part of the patients, these reasons are dissonant with the available evidence. In the vast majority of cases, radiographs do not detect valid explanations for the patient's pain, and serve poorly to protect the physician against accusations of malpractice. And there are safer and more direct ways of reassuring patients.

2. Plain radiography

The utility of plain radiographs can be considered in terms of the following questions, which should underlie any request for X-ray examination:

What *can* they show?

What *do* they show?

Are they reliable?

Are they valid?

What are the hazards?

2.1. Lesions demonstrable

A fundamental realisation is that X-rays do not show pain. X-rays reveal bone, and may provide a crude image of some soft tissues. When a practitioner requests a plain radiograph, therefore, they are asking for picture of the patient's vertebrae. If they are looking for a cause of pain, they are looking for a lesion that affects bone and is associated with pain. Other causes of pain will not be demonstrated.

The conditions that plain radiographs might demonstrate in a patient with acute low back pain fall into four categories:

Normal: when no abnormality is detected.

Abnormal but of no clinical significance: when radiographs reveal abnormalities *not related* to pain, such as spondylosis, spina bifida occulta, transitional vertebrae, spondylolysis and spondylolisthesis.

Abnormal but of questionable clinical significance: when radiographs reveal abnormalities that may or may not be related to pain, and whose detection makes little or no difference to management, e.g. diffuse idiopathic skeletal hyperostosis.

Incidental abnormalities: when radiographs reveal conditions that may or may not be related to the patient's pain, but which, in their own right, warrant treatment, e.g. Paget's disease, osteoporosis.

Red flag conditions: osteomyelitis, discitis, paraspinal infections, tumours, fractures.

2.2. Yield

In patients with acute low back pain, lumbar radiographs are typically normal or show only spondylosis. In the published literature, the incidence of normal radiographs ranges from 21% in medical centre settings [7,8], to 38% in emergency departments [9], and 37% [10] or 43% in primary care [11]. Spondylosis or degenerative joint disease accounts for between 26% and 48% of cases [7–11].

Minor congenital abnormalities are found in 5–10% of cases [7], and old fractures in a further 5–10% [7,9]. Spondylolisthesis occurs in 2–5% of cases [7,8,11], and spondylolysis in some 5% [1]. The prevalence of osteoporosis is determined by the age of the population surveyed, but ranges from 2–4% [7,8] to 10% [11] in reported studies.

Incidental and red flag conditions are rare in primary care populations.

2.3. Reliability

Few studies have been reported concerning the reliability of reading plain radiographs of the lumbar spine. Such data as have been published, indicate that the reliability of reading various features on plain films ranges from very good to poor [12] (Table I). Good to very good agreement obtains for osteophytes at all segmental levels, and for disc space narrowing and vertebral sclerosis at lower lumbar

TABLE I

Reliability of plain films, based on Coste et al. [12]

Feature	Kappa score				
	L1–L2	L2–L3	L3–L4	L4–L5	L5–S1
Narrowing	0.3	0.5	0.6	0.6	0.6
Sclerosis	0.5	0.3	0.6	0.5	0.4
Osteophytes	0.8	0.6	0.5	0.6	0.6
Facet sclerosis	0.3	0.3	0.3	0.3	0.2
Schmorl's nodes	0.4	0.3	0.5	0.4	0.4

levels. The agreement for facet sclerosis is poor. The latter means that diagnoses of facet sclerosis are inadmissible. Reliability data are not available for the recognition of other conditions.

2.4. Validity

Other than in the context of red flag conditions, plain radiographs lack validity in establishing the source of back pain (Table II).

2.4.1. Spondylosis

Spondylosis, disc degeneration, facet degeneration or osteoarthritis does not constitute a legitimate diagnosis of the cause of back pain. These conditions occur too frequently in asymptomatic individuals to permit them to be diagnostic of the cause of back pain. The correlation between pain and the presence of these conditions on radiographs is low.

According to a systematic review [13], studies with low methodologic scores show essentially no correlation between pain and the features of spondylosis or disc degeneration [14–18]. More highly ranked studies show a positive, but weak correlation, with odds ratios ranging between 1 and 3 [19–28]. The data show that for the diagnosis of low back pain, finding degenerative changes on a plain film has a poor sensitivity, a poor specificity, and positive likelihood ratio barely greater than 1.0 (Table II), which renders the finding non-diagnostic.

2.4.2. Congenital anomalies

Congenital anomalies such as transitional vertebrae, non-dysjunction (congenital fusion), and spina bifida

TABLE II

The validity of finding degenerative changes on plain radiographs as a diagnosis of low back pain

Ref.	Degenerative changes	Back pain		Sensitivity	Specificity	LR
		Present	Absent			
19,20	Present	130	92	0.55	0.61	1.4
	Absent	106	142			
19,20	Present	170	135	0.72	0.44	1.3
	Absent	66	106			
21	Present	90	61	0.46	0.68	1.4
	Absent	105	127			
22	Present	45	19	0.23	0.80	1.2
	Absent	151	77			
23	Present	115	71	0.32	0.77	1.4
	Absent	243	237			
24	Present	39	42	0.58	0.70	1.9
	Absent	28	100			
25	Present	462	360	0.59	0.52	1.1
	Absent	320	390			
26	Present	55	77	0.75	0.37	1.2
	Absent	18	45			
27	Present	139	51	0.80	0.45	1.5
	Absent	35	41			
28	Present	177	35	0.81	0.36	1.3
	Absent	41	20			
Pooled	Present	1422	943	0.56	0.58	1.3
	Absent	1113	1285			

LR, positive likelihood ratio.

occulta, occur equally commonly in symptomatic and asymptomatic individuals [16,17,21,23,29,30], and bear no correlation with back pain [13].

2.4.3. Spondylolysis

Spondylolysis is a term pertaining to a defect in the pars interarticularis of a vertebra (typically of L4 or L5), passing obliquely from the superior border to the lateral border of the lamina, filled with fibrous tissue [31]. The defect typically undercuts the capsules of the zygapophysial joints above and below [31]. This means that on arthrography, the defect may appear to communicate with the joint spaces of either or both of these joints [32]. The fibrous tissue filling the defect contains nerve fibres and free nerve endings [33] which contain neuropeptides [34]. Therefore, the defect is, in principle, capable of intrinsically being a source of pain.

The pars is the thinnest part of the vertebra. In many individuals it is endowed with only enough bone to tolerate average activities of daily living [35]. Larger forces will fracture the pars. The pars interarticularis transmits forces from the inferior articular process and spinous process to the pedicle and thence to the vertebral body, and is involved in resisting anterior translation, torsion and flexion of the intervertebral joint [36–38]. In flexion, the pars bends forwards, not backwards, ostensibly because of tension on the inferior articular process exerted by the zygapophysial joint capsule [38]. Consequently, the pars is susceptible to fatigue fracture in repeated loading in compression with flexion [36]. It can also be fractured by axial rotation [39].

In 32,600 asymptomatic adults, the prevalence of a pars defect was found to be 7.2% [40]. It is equally prevalent in symptomatic and asymptomatic adults [41,42] (Table III).

TABLE III

The prevalence of spondylolysis in symptomatic and asymptomatic individuals, based on Libson[41]

Pars defect	Asymptomatic		Symptomatic	
Unilateral	26	3%	2	0.3%
Bilateral	65	7%	62	9%
All	91	10%	64	9%
N	936		662	

TABLE IV

The prevalence of spondylolysis in sportspeople

Category	Prevalence	Ref.
Contact sports	>20%	44
Gymnasts	11%	45
Various sports	>20%	46
Football	13%	47
Fast bowlers (cricket)	50%	48

There are no proven risk factors, but anthropological surveys implicate arduous activities involving bending and twisting. Pars defects are particularly prevalent amongst Eskimos but the prevalence is not racially based or genetically based; rather, the prevalence differs amongst different tribes whose activities of daily living differ[43]. Pars fractures appear to be more prevalent amongst sports people involved with twisting movements alone or in combination with flexion or extension (Table IV).

Previous beliefs that pars defects were due to nonunion of two ossification centres in the lamina are not true. Evidence against this belief includes:

- the lamina has only one ossification centre[49]
- pars defects do not occur in infants[49]
- pars defects do not occur in non-ambulatory individuals[50]
- the prevalence increases with age[51]
- the prevalence is related to repeated activities that involve hyperextension, rotation or flexion or a combination of both[51].

The biomechanical and epidemiological evidence points to pars defects being an acquired fracture,

either as a result of single, severe trauma or as a result of fatigue failure[36,38,50,52,53]. The fibrous tissue that fills the defect may contain osseous debris which is evidence of its traumatic origin[34].

Pain is the only alleged clinical feature, but the relationship may be specious. *Presumably*, pain can arise from either or both of at least two mechanisms:

(1) movement of the lamina may strain the innervated fibrous tissue of the defect;
(2) in cases of bilateral pars defects, movement of the flail lamina and spinous process may distort the zygapophysial joint to which the flail segment is still attached.

Pain aggravated by activity is said to be the cardinal clinical feature of pars fracture[50], although this feature alone cannot discriminate spondylolysis from other mechanical causes of back pain. In children, symptoms reportedly occur in only 13% of individuals who exhibit a pars defect, usually at growth spurts[50]. However, it is not evident whether this pain arises from the defect or as a result of the onset or progression of isthmic spondylolisthesis. Tight hamstrings resulting in an abnormal gait are considered to be a clinical feature of pars defects[50], but it is not clear whether this is due to the defect or to the development of isthmic spondylolisthesis.

In the absence of diagnostic clinical features, radiography has been the cardinal means of identifying pars fractures. However, finding a pars defect on a plain film does not constitute establishing a diagnosis of the patient's pain. Because of the high prevalence of this condition in the asymptomatic population, the likelihood ratio of plain radiography is too close to 1.0 to allow the diagnosis to be established on this basis (Table V).

The definitive test of whether a pars defect is symptomatic is to anaesthetise the defect[54]. Pars blocks are the only means available by which to determine whether or not a radiographically evident defect is a symptomatic or an asymptomatic one. Such a test is imperative in view of the high prevalence of defects in asymptomatic individuals. Relief of pain implies that the defect is actually the source of pain, and predicts surgical success[54]. Patients

TABLE V

The validity of plain radiography in the diagnosis of painful spondylolysis, based on Libson[41]

Pars fracture	Pain	No pain	Sensitivity	Specificity	+LR
Unilateral	2	26	0.03	0.97	1.08
None	660	910			
Bilateral	62	65	0.09	0.93	1.3
None	600	871			
Any	64	91	0.097	0.90	1.0
None	598	845			

LR, positive likelihood ratio.

who do not respond to blocks pre-operatively are less likely to respond to fusion of the defect, even if the fusion is technically satisfactory[54].

However, pars blocks are not indicated in the investigation of patients with acute low back pain. They are a procedure reserved for the investigation of patients with persisting, if not chronic, symptoms. For the assessment of patients with a high risk of pars fractures, bone scan rather than plain radiography, is the better investigation (see below).

2.4.4. Spondylolisthesis

Spondylolisthesis has a prevalence of 8% in men and 5% in women, and may be totally asymptomatic[21,23,27,28,42,55,56]. In men with spondylolisthesis back pain is not significantly more common than in the general population[13], although women with spondylolisthesis are slightly more likely to suffer back pain[55]. Overall, the odds ratios for spondylolisthesis being a cause of back pain are not significantly different from 1.0[13].

2.5. Hazards

Plain radiographs of the lumbar spine are not without hazard. These need to be balanced against requesting radiographs gratuitously, 'just in case' or in the hope of finding something not suspected from history or clinical examination.

It has been estimated that

the radiation dose of a lumbar spine series delivers 40 times the radiation dose received from a chest X-ray[8,57];

a single lumbar spine series delivers to the gonads a radiation dose equivalent to that from having a daily chest radiograph for 6 years[8,9,58,59];

the absorbed radiation from lumbar spine films is 2 mSv; the risk of fatal cancer is one in 80,000 per mSv[10];

one million lumbar spine radiographs can result in 20 excess deaths from leukaemia, and 400 excess cases of genetic disease[8,10,58].

Notwithstanding these biological hazards, practical hazards obtain. Normal films may create a false sense of security. Lumbar spine radiographs may be false-negative in up to 41% of patients with known vertebral cancer[8]. Radiological evidence of vertebral osteomyelitis does not appear before 2–8 weeks of evolution of the disease; wherefore, a normal radiologic picture does not exclude the diagnosis of spinal infection[60]. Since degenerative joint disease does not equate to back pain, attributing the back pain to these findings is misleading.

3. Patients expect X-rays

Patients often harbour misconceptions about the utility and need for lumbar spine films[8,61,62]; they may believe that an X-ray will establish the diagnosis, or that a normal film will exclude serious pathology, and that X-rays are safe. Rather than indulge these misconceptions, practitioners have the opportunity of dissuading patients from their misconceptions, and explaining to them what evidence-based, quality care involves.

Practitioners concerned that patients' expectations can only be met by conceding to 'order an X-ray' can be reassured that this is not the case. A controlled study[62] assessed the impact of a brief (5 min) educational intervention for patients eligible for lumbar spine films. At follow-up, the proportion of patients in the educational group who believed that

X-rays were necessary fell only slightly, but was substantially and significantly less (44% vs 73%) than in the control group. Fewer educated patients underwent radiography after the study, but there were no significant differences in patient satisfaction, and no serious diagnoses were missed.

Other controlled studies have denied any psychosocial utility to obtaining radiographs. One showed that providing or withholding the results of plain radiographs made little difference to outcomes at 6 weeks or 1 year [63]. Another showed that patients randomised to undergo radiography were actually more disabled and more likely to still be in pain at 3 months after inception [6]. Finding an abnormality in those patients who had radiographs taken made no difference to outcome.

4. Red flag conditions

It is perhaps for fear of missing a red flag condition that most practitioners, who do so, request plain films. Epidemiologically, this fear is not justified, and several studies have provided sobering, objective evidence against the unbridled use of plain films.

In a utilisation review covering 871 patients, Scavone et al. [65] found that one in four lumbar films were normal, and that only one in eight were diagnostic. Most of those ostensibly diagnostic films, however, were of degenerative joint disease and spondylolysis, which are not diagnostic of either the source or cause of pain. The next largest group were 'fractures', but major fractures occurred only in patients with a history of major trauma, and minor fractures occurred only in elderly patients with osteoporosis. In ten patients (1%) metastases were revealed, but only two (0.2%) were new findings; the rest had a history indicative of cancer. There were four cases of osteomyelitis, but no data were provided as to whether, prior to radiography, these patients had signs or history indicative of infection.

In the light of these findings, Scavone et al. [65] concluded that radiation exposure and the cost of noncontributory studies could be substantially reduced by the judicious consideration of the potential

TABLE VI

Indications for the use of plain films of the lumbar spine, as studied by Deyo and Diehl [11]

1. Age more than 50 years
2. Significant trauma
3. Neurological deficit
4. Weight loss
5. Suspicion of ankylosing spondylitis
6. Drug or alcohol abuse
7. History of cancer
8. Use of corticosteroids
9. Temperature $> 37.8°C$
10. No improvement over one month
11. Seeking compensation

diagnostic yield of the examination. In the same vein, Liang and Komaroff [64] showed that the risks of radiation exposure and additional cost did not justify taking plain films on the first visit, compared to reserving radiographic studies until the eighth week for patients with continuing symptoms.

In an earlier study, Scavone et al. [7] established that AP and lateral lumbar spine films were an adequate study; there was no need to include oblique films. This echoes other reports on the same issue [66].

Deyo and Diehl [11] assessed the merits of a list of criteria for the use of plain films in primary care to screen for red flag conditions. Based on the literature, they tested a list of criteria that could apply to ordering plain films of the lumbar spine (Table VI). They compared 227 patients who satisfied one or more of the criteria with 84 who did not.

In no patient who did not satisfy the criteria did radiography reveal any unexpected or diagnostic findings. In the 227 patients who satisfied the criteria, findings on X-ray related to malignancy or fracture were identified in 15 (6.6%). There were no patients detected with osteomyelitis or spondylarthropathy.

All four patients with malignancy had indications for radiography: three were aged over 50, and one had not responded to conservative therapy; two had unexplained weight loss. The final diagnoses were lymphoma (2), metastatic prostate cancer (1) and retroperitoneal liposarcoma (1). However, only two of these four patients had lytic or blastic lesions; the other two had normal lumbar spine films. Thus, the criteria, but not the films, were 100% sensitive for the detection of cancer.

Of the 14 patients with fracture, 13 satisfied the criteria for radiography. Eleven were aged over 50, five had recent trauma, and three were seeking compensation. The one patient with a fracture who did not satisfy the criteria had an old transverse process fracture.

The results of this study vindicate reserving plain films for explicit criteria. Patients who do not satisfy the criteria do not need plain films of the lumbar spine. The chances of detecting a red flag condition under those conditions are essentially nil, which means that the chances of missing an important diagnosis are nil in patients who do not satisfy the criteria.

The criteria, therefore, constitute a proven guideline for reserving plain films. Following the guideline allows practitioners confidently, on the basis of evidence, to reduce the indiscriminate use of plain films, for fear of missing an important diagnosis.

On the other hand, the criteria *do not* guarantee finding an important diagnosis. Even under the criteria, the yield of an important diagnosis is only 6%. There is nonetheless a 94% wastage.

In the study of Deyo and Diehl[11] the proportion of patients who satisfied the criteria was 390/621 (58%). This indicates that, on the average, only about half of all patients presenting with back pain warrant an X-ray. However, subsequent studies have challenged the utility of the Deyo and Diehl criteria, reporting that if followed, they actually result in higher utilisation of lumbar spine radiology than do intuitive protocols of responsible physicians[8,67]. In particular, they found that the age criterion had low specificity, and that in the absence of other red flags, this criterion could be relaxed without compromising sensitivity.

Other studies[9] and, indeed, Deyo and Diehl's own study[11] found the 'seeking compensation' criterion to be neither specific nor sensitive. In no patient X-rayed for this reason was a significant finding detected[9,11]. Some 95% or more of patients exhibited normal findings or spondylosis. The remainder showed old fractures.

TABLE VII

Operational criteria for the use of plain films in low back pain

---

For low back pain of unknown origin
Plain films of the lumbar spine should not be used as screening test for patients presenting with acute low back pain, unless a 'red flag' condition is suspected.

Plain films may be used as a screening test for 'red flag' conditions if a patient presents with any of the following features.
1. History of cancer
2. Significant trauma
3. Weight loss
4. Temperature > 37.8°C
5. Risk factors for infection
6. Neurological deficit
7. Minor trauma in patients
   – over the age of 50 years, or
   – known to have osteoporosis, or
   – taking corticosteroids
8. No improvement over 1 month

A study from an Emergency Department[9] found that in 482 patients presenting with back pain, radiographs were normal or showed only spondylosis in 86% of cases. Fractures were detected in 11% but the majority (9%) were chronic or of indeterminate age. None of the patients had major trauma. All the acute fractures occurred in patients with osteoporosis or in patients over the age of 64 who had suffered a fall. The seven cases of neoplasm occurred in patients with a known history of cancer, and all of who were at least 60 years old.

In the light of these studies, the criteria of Deyo Diehl[11] can be modified without loss of security. In the pursuit of red flag conditions, plain radiographs should be reserved for:

- patients with a history of trauma;
- patients with a history of cancer;
- older patients with minimal trauma;
- failure to respond to treatment.

The previous criterion of 'drug and alcohol abuse' is probably idiosyncratic of the American population that Deyo and Diehl[11] studied. The conditions sought for by this criterion can be covered by the criterion 'risk factors for infection', viz. surgical procedures, body penetration, etc. (Chapter 6).

Although 'neurological deficit' remains a putative indication for imaging, a patient with neurological signs should be investigated in accordance with the neurological deficit, and not because they have back pain.

Accordingly the criteria of Deyo and Diehl [11] can be re-cast as shown in Table VII.

References

1 Espeland A, Baarheim A, Albrektsen G, Korsbrekke K, Larsen JL. Patients' views on importance and usefulness of plain radiography for low back pain. Spine 2001; 26: 1356–1363.

2 Dewar MA. Defensive medicine. It may not be what you think. Fam Med 1994; 26: 36–38.

3 Van-Boven K, Dijksterhuis O, Lambert H. Defensive testing in Dutch family practice: is the grass greener on the other side of the ocean? J Fam Pract 1997; 44: 468–472.

4 Veldhuis M. Defensive behaviour of Dutch family physicians: widening the concept. Fam Med 1994; 26: 27–29.

5 Owen JP, Rutt G, Keir MJ, Spencer H, Richardson D, Richardson A, Barclay C. Survey of general practitioners' opinions on the role of radiology in patients with low back pain. Br J Gen Pract 1990; 40: 98–101.

6 Kendrick D, Fielding K, Bentley E, Kerslake R, Miller P, Pringle M. Radiography of the lumbar spine in primary care patients with low back pain: randomized controlled trial. Br Med J 2001; 322: 400–405.

7 Scavone JG, Latshaw RF, Weidner WA. AP and lateral radiographs: an adequate lumbar spine examination. AJR 1981; 136: 715–717.

8 Frazier LM, Carey TS, Lyles MF, Khayrallah MA, Mc-Gaghie WC. Selective criteria may increase lumbosacral spine roentgenogram use in acute low-back pain. Arch Int Med 1989; 149: 47–50.

9 Reinus WR, Strome G, Zwemer F. Use of lumbosacral spine radiographs in a level II emergency department. AJR 1998; 170: 443–447.

10 Halpin SFS, Yeoman L, Dundas DD. Radiographic examination of the lumbar spine in a community hospital: an audit of current practice. Br Med J 1991; 303: 813–815.

11 Deyo RA, Diehl AK. Lumbar spine films in primary care: current use and effects of selective ordering criteria. J Gen Intern Med 1986; 1: 20–25.

12 Coste J, Paolaggi JB, Spira A. Reliability of interpretation of plain lumbar spine radiographs in benign, mechanical low-back pain. Spine 1991; 16: 426–428.

13 Van Tulder MW, Assendelft WJJ, Koes BW, Bouter LM. Spinal radiographic findings and nonspecific low back pain. A systematic review of observational studies. Spine 1997; 22: 427–434.

14 Torgerson WR, Dotter WE. Comparative roentgenographic study of the asymptomatic and symptomatic lumbar spine. J Bone Joint Surg 1976; 58A: 850–853.

15 Magora A, Schwartz A. Relation between the low back pain syndrome and x-ray findings. Scand J Rehabil Med 1976; 8: 115–126.

16 Fullenlove TM, Williams AJ. Comparative roentgen findings in symptomatic and asymptomatic backs. Radiology 1957; 68: 572–574.

17 Splithoff CA. Lumbosacral junction: Roentgenographic comparison of patients with and without backaches. JAMA 1953; 152: 1610–1613.

18 Witt I, Vestergaard A, Rosenklint A. A comparative analysis of x-ray findings of the lumbar spine in patients with and without lumbar pain. Spine 1984; 9: 298–300.

19 Symmons DPM, van Hemert AM, Vandenbroucke JP, Valkenburg HA. A longitudinal study of back pain and radiological changes in the lumbar spines of middle aged women: I. clinical findings. Ann Rheum Dis 1991; 50: 158–161.

20 Symmons DPM, van Hemert AM, Vandenbroucke JP, Valkenburg HA. A longitudinal study of back pain and radiological changes in the lumbar spines of middle aged women: II. radiographic findings. Ann Rheum Dis 1991; 50: 162–166.

21 Horal J. The clinical appearance of low back disorders in the city of Gothenburg, Sweden: comparison of incapacitated probands with matched controls. Acta Orthop Scand Suppl 1969; 118: 1–73.

22 Frymoyer JW, Newberg A, Pope MH, Wilder DG, Clements J, MacPherson BJ. Spine radiographs in patients with low-back pain. J Bone Joint Surg 1984; 66A: 1048–1055.

23 Biering-Sorensen F, Hansen FR, Schroll M, Runeborg O. The relation of spinal X-ray to low-back pain and physical activity among 60-year old men and women. Spine 1985; 10: 445–451.

24 Wiikeri M, Nummi J, Riihimaki H, Wickstrom G. Radiologically detectable lumbar disc degeneration in concrete reinforcement workers. Scand J Work Environ Health 1978; 1 (Suppl): 47–53.

25 Lawrence JS. Disc degeneration: its frequency and relationship to symptoms. Ann Rheum Dis 1969; 28: 121–137.

26 Kellgren JH, Lawrence JS. Rheumatism in miners: part II. X-ray study. Br J Ind Med 1952; 9: 197–207.

27 Sairanen E, Brushhaber L, Kaskinen M. Felling work, low back pain and osteoarthritis. Scand J Work Environ Health 1981; 7: 18–30.

28 Hult L. The Munkfors investigation. Acta Orthop Scand Suppl 1954; 16: 1–75.

29 Magora A, Schwartz A. Relation between the low back pain syndrome and X-ray findings: 3. spina bifida occulta. Scand J Rehabil Med 1980; 12: 9–15.

30 Magora A, Schwartz. Relation between the low back

pain syndrome and X-ray findings: 2. transitional verte-bra (mainly sacralization). Scand J Rehabil Med 1978; 10: 135–145.

31 Roche MB. The pathology of neural-arch defects. J Bone Joint Surg 1949; 31A: 529–537.

32 Ghelman B, Doherty JH. Demonstration of spondylolysis by arthrography of the apophyseal joint. Am J Roentgenol 1978; 130: 986–987.

33 Schneiderman GA, McLain RF, Hambly MF, Nielsen SL. The pars defect as a pain source: a histological study. Spine 1995; 20: 1761–1764.

34 Eisenstein SM, Ashton IK, Roberts S, Darby AJ, Kanse P, Menage J, Evans H. Innervation of the spondylolysis 'ligament'. Spine 1994; 19: 912–916.

35 Cyron BM, Hutton WC. Variations in the amount and dis-tribution of cortical bone across the partes interarticulares of L5. A predisposing factor in spondylolysis? Spine 1979; 4: 163–167.

36 Cyron BM, Hutton WC. The fatigue strength of the lumbar neural arch in spondylolysis. J Bone Joint Surg 1978; 60B: 234–238.

37 Farfan HF, Osteria V, Lamy C. The mechanical etiology of spondylolysis and spondylolisthesis. Clin Orthop 1976; 117: 40–55.

38 Green TP, Allvey JC, Adams MA. Spondylolysis: bending of the inferior articular processes of lumbar vertebrae dur-ing simulated spinal movements. Spine 1994; 19: 2683–2691.

39 Farfan HF, Cossette JW, Robertson GH, Wells RV, Kraus H. The effects of torsion on the lumbar intervertebral joints: the role of torsion in the production of disc degen-eration. J Bone Joint Surg 1970; 52A: 468–497.

40 Moreton RD. Spondylolysis. JAMA 1966; 195: 671–674.

41 Libson E, Bloom RA, Dinari G. Symptomatic and asymp-tomatic spondylolysis and spondylolisthesis in young adults. Int Orthop 1982; 6: 259–261.

42 Magora A, Schwartz A. Relation between the low back pain syndrome and X-ray findings: 4. lysis and olisthesis. Scand J Rehabil Med 1980; 12: 47–52.

43 Stewart TD. The age incidence of neural-arch defects in Alaskan natives, considered from the standpoint of etiol-ogy. J Bone Joint Surg 1953; 35A: 937–950.

44 Ichikawa N, Ohara Y, Morishita T, Taniguichi Y, Koshi-lawa A, Matsujura N. An aetiological study on spondylol-ysis from a biomechanical aspect. Br J Sports Med 1982; 16: 135–141.

45 Jackson DE, Wiltse LL, Cirincione RJ. Spondylolysis in the female gymnast. Clin Orthop 1976; 117: 68–73.

46 Hoshina I. Spondylolysis in athletes. The Physician and Sportsmedicine 1980; 8: 75–78.

47 McCarroll JR, Miller JM, Ritter MA. Lumbar spondyloly-sis and spondylolisthesis in college football players. Am J Sports Med 1986; 14: 404–406.

48 Foster D, John D, Elliot B, Ackland T, Fitch K. Back injuries to fast bowlers in cricket: a prospective study. Br J Sports Med 1989; 23: 150–154.

49 Rowe GG, Roche MB. The etiology of separate neural arch. J Bone Joint Surg 1953; 35A: 102–110.

50 Hensinger RN. Spondylolysis and spondylolisthesis in children and adolescents. J Bone Joint Surg 1989; 71A: 1089–1107.

51 Fredrickson BE, Baker D, McHolick WJ, Yuan HA, Lu-bicky JP. The natural history of spondylolysis and spondy-lolisthesis. J Bone Joint Surg 1984; 66A: 699–707.

52 O'Neill DB, Micheli LJ. Postoperative radiographic evi-dence for fatigue fracture as the etiology in spondylolysis. Spine 1989; 14: 1342–1355.

53 Wiltse LL, Widell EH, Jackson DW. Fatigue fracture: the basic lesion in isthmic spondylolisthesis. J Bone Joint Surg 1975; 57A: 17–22.

54 Suh PB, Esses SI, Kostuik JP. Repair of a pars interartic-ularis defect — the prognostic value of pars infiltration. Spine 1991; 16 (Suppl 8): S445–S448.

55 Virta L, Ronnemaa T, Osterman K, Aalto T, Laakso M. Prevalence of isthmic lumbar spondylolisthesis in middle-aged subjects from eastern and western Finland. J Clin Epidemiol 1992; 45: 917–922.

56 Virta L, Ronnemaa T. The association of mild-moderate isthmic lumbar spondylolisthesis and low back pain in middle-aged patients is weak and it only occurs in women. Spine 1993; 18: 1496–1503.

57 Whalen JP, Balter S. Radiation risks associated with diag-nostic radiology. Dis Mon 1982; 28: 73.

58 Hall FM. Back pain and the radiologist. Radiology 1980; 137: 861–863.

59 Ardran GM, Crooks HE. Gonad radiation dose from diag-nostic procedures. Br J Radiol 1957; 30: 295–297.

60 Waldvogel FA, Vasey H. Osteomyelitis: the past decade. N Engl J Med 1980; 303: 360–370.

61 Kaplan DM, Knapp M, Romm FJ, Velez R. Low back pain and x-ray films of the lumbar spine: a prospective study in primary care. South Med J 1986; 79: 811–814.

62 Deyo RA, Diehl AK, Rosenthal M. Reducing roentgenog-raphy use: can patient expectations be altered? Arch Int Med 1987; 147: 141–145.

63 Ferriman A. Early X-ray for low back pain confers little benefit. Br Med J 2000; 321: 1489.

64 Scavone JG, Latshaw RF, Rohrer V. Use of lumbar spine films: statistical evaluation at a university teaching hospi-tal. JAMA 1981; 246: 1105–1108.

65 Liang M, Komaroff AL. Roentgenograms in primary care patients with acute low back pain: a cost-effectiveness analysis. Arch Int Med 1982; 142: 1108–1112.

66 DeLuca S, Rhea JT. Are routine oblique roentgenograms of the lumbar spine of value? J Bone Joint Surg 1981; 63A: 846.

67 Suarez-Almazor ME, Belseck E, Russell AS, Mackel JV. Use of lumbar radiographs for the early diagnosis of low back pain. Proposed guidelines would increase utilization. JAMA 1997; 277: 1782–1786.

TABLE VIII

The prevalence of abnormalities on CAT scan in a population 52 asymptomatic individuals aged between 21 and 80 years, based on Wiesel et al. [1]

	N	Herniated nucleus pulposus		Degenerative joint disease		Spinal stenosis	
Age < 40	21–24	4	20%	0	0%	0	0%
Age > 40	24–27	7	27%	3	10%	1	3%
Reader 1	45 (22 + 23)	7	16%	1	4%	2	9%
Reader 2	49 (24 + 25)	15	31%	4	16%	2	4%
Reader 3	51 (24 + 27)	9	18%	3	12%	1	2%

The percentage figures are as reported in the study (but rounded to integer values). The numbers have been derived from data provided in the paper, but in some instances are not internally consistent. This arises because not all readers reported on exactly the same number of films. Although the total number of films read by each reader was reported, the total read in each age group was not reported.

5. CAT scans

CAT scans have no place in the investigation of low back pain of unknown or unsuspected origin. Even in the context of 'red flag' conditions, their role is restricted to the confirmation of pathology otherwise indicated by history, clinical examination or other imaging tests. They have *no* place as a screening tool.

CAT scans may serve to confirm the diagnosis of disc herniation or other causes of radicular pain but in this context are indicated only if the patient's history and clinical features clearly indicate radicular pain and radiculopathy. These features, however, are distinct from those of low back pain of unknown origin. Back pain alone, or even back pain in association with somatic referred pain is not a sign of disc herniation, and cannot be justified as the basis for ordering a CAT scan.

5.1. Reliability

Formal studies, from which kappa scores might be calculated, of the reliability of reading lumbar CAT scans have not been reported. Such data as do exist, however, suggest substantial differences between observers with respect to recognising various features as worthy of reporting [1]. Some readers report certain abnormalities more frequently than others (Table VIII).

5.2. Validity

The abnormalities most frequently encountered in CAT scans are common in patients with no symptoms [1] (Table VIII). These figures, however, do not prove that there is no clinically or statistically significant relationship between symptoms and the presence of these abnormalities. That would require figures on the prevalence of these abnormalities in patients with symptoms. However, they do warn that finding herniated discs, degenerative joint disease or spinal stenosis on CAT scans does not prove that that abnormality is the cause of symptoms.

References

1   Wiesel SW. A study of computer-assisted tomography. 1. The incidence of positive CAT scans in an asymptomatic group of patients. Spine 1986; 9: 549–551.

6. MRI

Because of its relatively high cost, the use of MRI cannot be justified for the investigation of acute low back pain, even to screen for 'red flag' conditions. Utilisation reviews attest to the relative paucity of 'red flag' conditions rendered evident by MRI. In one review of 169 consecutive lumbar scans taken over a 3-month period, no cases of tumour or infection were recorded [1]. In another, covering 667 scans over

TABLE IX

Observer concordance in the identification and reporting of disc bulges and disc protrusion in MRI scans of 98 asymptomatic individuals, based on Jensen et al. [3]

N	Age	Number of positive cases reported by each of two observers									
		L1–L2		L2–L3		L3–L4		L4–L5		L5–S1	
		Obs 1	Obs 2	Obs 1	Obs 2	Obs 1	Obs 2	Obs 1	Obs 2	Obs 1	Obs 2
Bulge											
20	20–29	0	0	0	0	4	0	5	2	4	2
28	30–39	2	1	1	1	4	1	6	8	4	3
23	40–49	1	0	1	2	3	8	7	10	5	8
17	50–59	3	3	5	4	10	8	9	6	12	9
10	>60	0	1	1	4	4	5	5	6	4	5
Protrusion											
20	20–29	0	0	0	0	0	0	3	2	2	1
28	30–39	1	1	1	1	1	1	5	2	2	2
23	40–49	0	1	0	0	1	0	5	3	4	4
17	50–59	0	0	1	1	2	1	2	4	0	0
10	>60	0	0	2	1	1	0	4	0	3	1

N, number of subjects examined in each age group; Obs, observer.

a 13-month period, 102 neoplasms were reported [2] but 80% were tumours affecting the central nervous system rather than the lumbar vertebrae, and which presumably presented with neurological symptoms. A further 9% were postoperative investigations, and 5% were unspecified. Five cases of lymphoma were reported, but the presenting features of these patients were not described; it was not made evident whether they presented with neurological features or simply with spinal pain.

6.1. Reliability

A study has been published that reported separately the observations of two observers, but insufficient data were reported to allow kappa scores to be determined [3]. Observers are apt to disagree about disc bulges but are less likely to disagree about disc protrusions (Table IX).

6.2. Validity

Two studies have reported the prevalence in asymptomatic individuals of certain abnormalities encountered in MRI scans but which otherwise have sometimes been implicated as diagnostic of back pain [3,4]. Herniated discs, disc bulges, spinal stenosis and disc degeneration all occur in asymptomatic individuals (Tables X–XIII). They occur with increasing frequency with age. Disc degeneration is virtually

TABLE X

The prevalence of abnormalities on MRI scans of 67 asymptomatic individuals, as reported by Boden et al. [4]

	N	Herniated nucleus pulposus		Disc bulge		Spinal stenosis		Disc degeneration	
All ages	67	16	24%			3	4%		
Age 20–39	35	7	20%	19	54%	0		12	34%
Age 40–59	18	4	22%			0			
Age 60–80	14	5	36%	11	79%	3	21%	13	92%

TABLE XI

The prevalence of abnormalities on MRI scans of 67 asymptomatic individuals, as reported by Boden et al.[4]

	N	Herniated nucleus pulposus		Disc bulge		Spinal stenosis		Disc degeneration	
All ages	67	16	24%			3	4%		
Age 20–39	35	7	20%	19	54%	0		12	34%
Age 40–59	18	4	22%			0			
Age 60–80	14	5	36%	11	79%	3	21%	13	92%

TABLE XII

The prevalence of abnormalities on MRI scans of 98 asymptomatic individuals, based on Jensen et al.[2] (ranges of percentages obtain because of differences between observers)

N	Age	Prevalence by segmental level				
		L1–L2	L2–L3	L3–L4	L4–L5	L5–S1
Bulge						
20	20–29	0%	0%	0–20%	10–25%	10–20%
28	30–39	3–7%	4%	4–14%	21–28%	11–14%
23	40–49	0–4%	4–9%	13–34%	30–43%	22–35%
17	50–59	18%	23–29%	47–59%	35–53%	53–71%
10	>60	0–10%	10–40%	40–50%	50–60%	40–50%
Protrusion						
20	20–29	0%	0%	0%	10–15%	5–10%
28	30–39	4%	4%	4%	7–18%	7%
23	40–49	0–4%	0%	0–4%	13–22%	17%
17	50–59	0%	6%	12%	12–24%	0%
10	>60	0%	10–20%	0–10%	0–40%	10–30%

TABLE XIII

The prevalence of other abnormalities evident on MRI in asymptomatic individuals, based on Jensen et al.[2]

Anular defects	14%
Degenerative joint disease	8%
Spondylolysis	7%
Spondylolisthesis	7%
Spinal stenosis	7%

ubiquitous in individuals over the age of 60. Spinal stenosis occurs in asymptomatic individuals only over the age of 60. Disc bulges are more common than disc protrusions. Both are more common at lower lumbar levels.

The prevalence of abnormalities in the MRI scans of asymptomatic individuals has been used to indict the use of MRI scans but, although this nihilism might be justified for abnormalities such as degeneration and disc bulge, it is not justified for disc protrusion. Disc protrusion on MRI correlates positively, although not strongly with back pain (Table XIV). In this regard, MRI has too high a false-positive rate for it to allow disc protrusion to be diagnosed as a cause of back pain.

Notwithstanding the reservations that can be raised concerning the utility of MRI in the investigation of acute low back pain, the circumstances and data are different concerning chronic low back pain. In that context, MRI has utility as a screening test, but also is able to pinpoint certain causes of pain. This matter is resumed in Chapter 15.

TABLE XIV

The correlation between back pain and disc protrusion on MRI, based on Jensen et al.[1]

	Symptomatic	Asymptomatic	Sensitivity	Specificity	LR
Protrusion	14	27	0.52	0.72	1.9
No protrusion	13	72			

LR, positive likelihood ratio.

References

1   Kitchener P, Houang M, Anderson B. Utilisation review of magnetic resonance imaging: the Australian experience. Aust Clin Rev 1986; September: 127–136.
2   Sorby WA. An evaluation of magnetic resonance imaging at The Royal North Shore Hospital of Sydney, 1986–1987. Med J Aust 1989; 151: 8–18.
3   Jensen MC, Bran-Zawadzki MN, Obucjowski N, Modic MT, Malkasian D, Ross JS. Magnetic resonance imaging of the lumbar spine in people without back pain. N Engl J Med 1994; 331: 69–73.
4   Boden SD, Davis DO, Dina TS, Patronas NJ, Wiesel SW. Abnormal magnetic-resonance scans of the lumbar spine in asymptomatic subjects. J Bone Joint Surg 1990; 72A: 403–408.

7. Bone scan

Bone scanning with ^{99}Tc is a very sensitive test for lesions of the lumbar spine that involve hyperaemia. As such it is perhaps the preferred test for screening for possible sites of infection[1]. Only rarely might the test be false-negative, in cases where the infected area has infarcted[1]. However, bone scanning is indicated only if there are clinical grounds for suspecting an infection.

Where bone scanning is perhaps more pertinent in the context of acute low back pain is in the detection of incipient fracture of the pars interarticularis. Detecting a stress reaction prior to fracture optimises the opportunity to avert fracture by instituting rest and avoidance of the activities responsible for the bone fatigue.

Since bone scans show reactive bone, they can show stress reactions, a recent fracture, or a healing fracture[2,3]. Bone scans are of no value if symptoms have been present for longer than 1 year[2].

Once a pars fracture has occurred, the role and utility of bone scan is questionable, for the relationship between pain, radiographic defects and positive bone scans is imperfect. In patients with a radiographically evident pars defect, positive scans are related to history and pain but imperfectly (Table XV). Pars defects are not positive on bone scan in asymptomatic individuals, they may be positive in patients with chronic back pain or patients with a history of repeated minor trauma, and they are more likely to be positive in patients with a history of a traumatic incident, but not reliably so[4].

In athletes with back pain, one study showed that most patients suspected of having a pars fracture were negative to both bone scan and X-ray[5] (Table XVI). Nine patients had a pars defect on X-ray that was negative on bone scan. Four patients had five pars defects that were positive to both tests, and four patients each had one defect that was positive to both tests but another defect that was positive on scan but not X-ray.

Another study of athletes[6,7] showed a spread of relationships (Table XVII). Of the seven patients with positive scans but negative radiographs, all were able to return to sport, and follow-up radiographs revealed no defects. Of the eighteen with both tests positive, five returned to sport and follow-up studies revealed improvement or resolution of the bone scan but persistence of the radiographic defect. Three of eighteen patients did not return to sport; ten were lost to follow-up.

TABLE XV

Relationship between history and bone scan in patients with a radiographically evident pars defect, based on Lowe et al.[4]

History	Bone scan	
	Positive	Negative
Trauma within 1 year	9	4
Repeated minor trauma	9	20
Chronic back pain	5	35
No pain	0	14

TABLE XVI

Correlation between bone scan and X-ray in 33 athletes with suspected spondylolysis, based on Elliot et al.[5]

Bone scan	X-ray	
	Positive	Negative
Positive	9	4
Negative	9	16

TABLE XVII

Correlation between bone scan and X-ray in 37 athletes with back pain, based on Jackson [6,7]

Bone scan	X-ray	
	Positive	Negative
Positive	18	5
Negative	7	7

TABLE XVIII

Correlation between bone scan and X-ray in 66 patients with back pain, based on Van den Oever [8]

Bone scan	X-ray	
	Positive	Negative
Positive	5	1
Negative	22	38

These data suggest the following indications:

(1) In an individual at risk of a stress fracture, a bone scan is the investigation of choice to screen for stress reactions prior to fracture. In principle, this action is likely to be sensitive in that if a patient does have a stress reaction a bone scan will detect it, but it will not be specific because most individuals with back pain will have neither a stress reaction nor a positive scan. In this regard, the study of Elliot [5] is germane in that it showed that most patients suspected of a stress fracture were negative to both scan and X-ray. Therefore, the problem with this indication is that it is likely to yield many negative results. Physicians, therefore, need to be judicious about ordering scans, lest they over-order this investigation. Indeed, in a general population the yield of positive scans is very low and bone scans are of little value for primary diagnosis (Table XVIII). Accordingly, scans are best reserved until after simple conservative therapy has failed.

(2) If the scan is negative, no radiography is indicated, for whatever the radiographs show will be immaterial or invalid. If the radiographs are negative they are redundant for the scan is already negative. If the radiographs show a defect they are irrelevant, for there is nothing to say that the defect, which is present on X-ray but 'cold' on scan, is not just an incidental finding.

(3) If the scan is positive, radiographs should be taken to determine if a fracture has occurred. If the radiographs are normal, rest and avoidance of activities should be instituted in an effort to avert progression to fracture.

(4) If the scan is positive and the radiographs are also positive, the evidence implies a recent fracture that might be presumed, but not guaranteed, to be the source of pain. Rest and avoidance of activities can still be prescribed, as it is still possible for healing to occur.

References

1   Waldvogel FA, Vasey H. Osteomyelitis: the past decade. N Engl J Med 1980; 303: 360–370.
2   Hensinger RN. Spondylolysis and spondylolisthesis in children and adolescents. J Bone Joint Surg 1989; 71A: 1089–1107.
3   Papanicolau N et al. Bone scintigraphy and radiography in young athletes with low back pain. Am J Roentgenol 1985; 145: 1039–1044.
4   Lowe J, Schachner E, Hirschberg E, Shapiro Y, Libson E. Significance of bone scintigraphy in symptomatic spondylolysis. Spine 1984; 9: 654–655.
5   Elliot S, Huitson A, Wastie ML. Bone scintigraphy in the assessment of spondylolysis in patients attending a sports injury clinic. Clin Radiol 1988; 39: 269–272.
6   Jackson DE, Wiltse LL, Cirincione RJ. Spondylolysis in the female gymnast. Clin Orthop 1976; 117: 68–73.
7   Jackson DW, Wiltse LL, Dingeman RD, Hayes M. Stress reactions involving the pars interarticularis in young athletes. Am J Sports Med 1981; 9: 304–312.
8   Van den Oever M, Merrick MV, Scott JHS. Bone scintigraphy in symptomatic spondylolysis. J Bone Joint Surg 1987; 69B: 453–456.

8. SPECT scanning

SPECT scanning offers the advantage of providing better resolution of the anatomical location of hyperaemia evident on technetium bone scanning. Accordingly it has attracted application as a screening test for low back pain. However, its utility has not been established.

A systematic review [1] found the literature to be weak; only 3 of 13 reports provided a reasonable criterion standard against which the validity of SPECT could be determined. The review concluded that there was weak evidence for the utility of SPECT for detecting pseudarthrosis after spinal fusion, and distinguishing benign from malignant lesions in cancer patients. Neither of these applications pertain to acute low back pain.

SPECT does appear to be marginally more sensitive than planar bone scanning for the detection of painful pars defects [2,3], and some authors have argued that a negative SPECT scan essentially rule out a stress fracture. In patients with a high risk of stress fracture, in whom it is critical to exclude a stress reaction, SPECT would be the investigation of choice.

References

1 Littenberg B, Siegel A, Tosteson ANA, Mead T. Clinical efficacy of SPECT bone imaging for low back pain. J Nucl Med 1995; 36: 1707–1713.

2 Collier BD, Johnson RP, Carrera GF et al. Painful spondylolysis or spondylolisthesis studied by radiography and single-photon emission computed tomography. Radiology 1985; 154: 207–211.

3 Mandell G, Harcke T. Scintigraphy of spinal disorders in adolescents. Skeletal Radiol 1993; 22: 393–401.

Key points

- Plain X-rays are not indicated as a routine investigation for acute low back pain.
- Nor are plain X-rays indicated as a screening test to rule out serious or unsuspected conditions.
- Spondylosis is not a cause of back pain and does not constitute a diagnosis.
- Nor does finding spondylolysis, spondylolisthesis or congenital abnormalities in adults provide a diagnosis of the cause of pain.
- Plain films constitute a biological hazard because the radiation exposure involved.
- Patients can be successfully dissuaded from pursuing or demanding unnecessary plain films.
- Medical imaging is indicated only if one or more of the following clinical features is present:

history of cancer	neurological deficit
weight loss	failure to improve
temperature > 37.8°	risk factor for fracture
risk factors for infection	

- CT is not indicated for the investigation of back pain.
- MRI is not indicated for the investigation of acute low back pain.
- If a patient has a high risk of having an impending or acute pars fracture, bone scan is the investigation of choice.

Medical Management of Acute and Chronic Low Back Pain. An Evidence-Based Approach
Pain Research and Clinical Management, Vol. 13
Nikolai Bogduk and Brian McGuirk

CHAPTER 9

Electrodiagnostic studies

1. Introduction

In some quarters, practitioners are accustomed to ordering electromyography (EMG) and related studies for the investigation of back pain. Indeed, when a recent essay on back pain failed to mention EMG as an investigation[1], electromyographers responded stridently in letters to the editor, lamenting the omission[2]. Yet EMG and conduction studies have no place in the investigation of low back pain. This conflict of opinion is so paradoxical as to be almost bizarre. It warrants an explanation.

2. Electromyography

EMG detects electrical activity in muscles; it determines the integrity of alpha motor neurons, and the health of muscles. Conduction studies determine the integrity and health of alpha motor neurons and Ia afferents. Somatosensory evoked potentials determine the integrity of cutaneous afferents.

None of these investigations measure pain. Nor are they applied to the back. They are performed in the lower limb.

In principle, electrodiagnostic studies are appropriate for the investigation of radiculopathy. They can confirm objective neurological signs of numbness and weakness detected clinically; they may have some virtue in detecting subclinical abnormalities. However, even in the context of radiculopathy, they have limited or no utility.

A pragmatic review of electrophysiological tests[3] reported only three studies of the sensitivity and specificity of these tests, one of which was a conference proceeding. That review concluded that:

"Based on available studies, it currently can be concluded that the overall sensitivity and specificity of the neurophysiological assessment is low for patients with lumbar radiculopathy caused by nerve root compression. In the diagnosis of patients with radiculopathy, there are few indications for neurophysiological tests:

- exclusion of a more distal nerve damage (neuropathy, nerve entrapment);
- verification of subjective muscle weakness by needle EMG in patients presenting with pain inhibition or lack of cooperation; and
- recurrent disc operation if difficult surgery is expected to document the preoperative muscle status (medicolegal aspects)."

These conclusions stand in stark contrast to the way in which electrophysiological investigations appear to be applied in conventional practice.

An accompanying consensus statement[4] recorded:

"Although neurophysiological testing is frequently used to diagnose patients with radiculopathy associated with disc herniation, these tests are *not clinically necessary* to confirm the presence of radiculopathy. Neurophysiological testing can determine the chronicity and severity of spinal nerve root lesions, and differentiate the nervous system level of involvement (i.e. cord, peripheral nerve and muscle). Therefore, neurophysiological testing is appropriate when the clinical situation is less clearly delineated, and to differentiate a disc herniation from other neurological disorders such as neuropathy or peripheral nerve entrapment."

- Neurophysiological testing *cannot accurately determine* the precise spinal nerve level associated with disc herniations.
- A patient's *radicular pain cannot be explained by neurophysiological testing.*
- There is no gold standard against which the neurophysiological tests can be compared.

Later, the same statement explained that:

"Electrophysiological testing does not directly evaluate neurologic mechanisms associated with pain generation."

The validity of electrophysiological tests is limited by technical, idiosyncratic and anatomical factors. Pain is mediated by Aδ and C fibres, but EMG examines the effects of Aα fibres. Therefore, EMG is not a direct test of pain. Any diagnostic inference relies on a relationship between activity perceived by the patient in Aδ and C fibres, and a lack of activity in Aα fibres. Such a relationship, in turn, depends on motor roots being consistently affected by lesions that generate radicular pain, and to the same degree, which is often not the case. Similarly, for F waves and H reflexes to be useful, there would have to be a consistent relationship between nociceptive activity and activity in motor neurones and Ia afferents, which is not the case. For electrophysiological tests to be useful in identifying the segmental location of an affected nerve root there has to be a discrete and reliable distribution of segmental nerves to specific muscles or sites in muscles. However, overlap of innervation both in muscles and between segmental nerves confounds this ideal distribution.

Inference. If EMG lacks utility in the investigation of radiculopathy and radicular pain, it is even less useful in patients with just back pain, or back pain with somatic referred pain. Such patients lack neurological symptoms and signs, and have no indication for electrodiagnostic studies. Ordering such tests becomes superfluous. It amounts to looking for something that is not going to be there.

3. The paradox

The confusion concerning electrodiagnostic tests stems from the age-old confusion between back pain and sciatica. While so long as practitioners believed and portrayed that the two conditions were synonymous, or somehow always combined, i.e. back pain and sciatica, the propensity obtained to investigate as for sciatica.

This confusion disappears if and once the two conditions are clearly segregated. Back pain is not sciatica and sciatica is not back pain. What might be appropriate for sciatica is not necessarily appropriate for back pain. This pertains not just to electrodiagnostic studies, but also to other investigations such as CT scanning, and even unto treatment.

The confusion returns when advocates argue: "but what if the patient also has radiculopathy. . . ?". This does not change the argument; it changes the question. Radiculopathy is a separate condition, with a different mechanism, different causes, and an entirely different evidence-base [5]. It is not back pain.

Yet even changing the question does not change the answer. In as much as electrodiagnostic studies are not indicated even for radiculopathy, they have absolutely no place in the investigation of back pain.

Key point

- EMG and electrodiagnostic studies have no place in the investigation of back pain.

References

1   Deyo RA, Weinstein JN. Low back pain. N Engl J Med 2001; 344: 363–370.
2   Haig AJ, Wallbom A. Correspondence. Low back pain. N Engl J Med 2001; 344: 1644–16445.
3   Dvorak J. Neurophysiologic tests in diagnosis of nerve root compression caused by disc herniation. Spine 1996; 21 (Suppl 24S): 39S–44S.
4   Andersson GBJ, Brown MD, Dvorak J, Herzog RJ, Kambin P, Malter A, McCulloch JA, Saal JA, Spratt KF, Weinstein JN. Consensus summary on the diagnosis and treatment of lumbar disc herniation. Spine 1996; 21 (Suppl 24S): 75S–78S.
5   Bogduk N, Govind J. Medical Management of Acute Lumbar Radicular Pain. An Evidence-Based Approach. Newcastle Bone and Joint Institute, Newcastle, 1999.

Medical Management of Acute and Chronic Low Back Pain. An Evidence-Based Approach
Pain Research and Clinical Management, Vol. 13
Nikolai Bogduk and Brian McGuirk
© *2002 Elsevier Science B.V. All rights reserved*

CHAPTER 10

Psychosocial assessment

1. Introduction

Chapter 5 described how psychosocial factors were amongst the potentially remediable prognostic risk factors for chronicity of low back pain. Although these factors correlate only weakly with pain, they correlate strongly with disability attributed to back pain.

Psychosocial factors are not the sole determinant of chronicity. Indeed, they account for something like only 30% of the variance between patients who become chronic and those who do not. However, factors that account for the remainder of the variance have not been determined. They have not been found amongst biomedical factors.

At present, therefore, any prospect of reducing chronic disability resulting from acute back pain lies not in a more accurate patho-anatomic diagnosis, for that is not feasible (Chapters 7 and 8), nor does it lie in more specific biomedical intervention based on such a diagnosis. The leading prospect lies in reducing or eliminating the influence of psychosocial factors; and whereas this may not be the total or complete answer to preventing chronic disability, it offers the prospect of being a substantial contribution.

Consequently, if psychosocial factors are to be addressed in the course of management, they need to be identified during initial assessment. The pursuit of psychosocial factors, therefore, becomes an integral component of assessment; indeed, more pertinent than medical imaging and, perhaps, even physical examination.

2. Yellow flags

In order to highlight the importance of psychosocial factors in the assessment of patients with low back pain, psychologists developed the notion 'yellow flags'. Just as there are 'red flag' indicators to medical conditions that need to be recognised early in the patient's history (Chapter 6), there are psychosocial conditions or behaviours that some authorities believe should be recognised early in the patient's history, and managed. The descriptor 'yellow flags' refers to these factors, with the intention of emphasising that they should be recognised, although not as urgently as the 'red flag' conditions.

Many of the psychosocial factors that constitute yellow flags stem from the fear-avoidance model (Chapter 5). They are the fears and beliefs that patients may express or harbour, that putatively interfere with their rehabilitation by reducing their motivation to stay active or to resume activity, and which thereby compound the patient's disability. The prospect is that by changing these counter-productive beliefs and behaviours, physical and social rehabilitation will be improved and disability will be reduced.

Yellow flags are not a specific condition, but behaviours and beliefs that individually constitute proven or presumed risk factors for chronicity of back pain, and which take on putatively greater significance when present in clusters or in great numbers in a given patient. Without limiting the possibilities [1], the cardinal yellow flags are listed in Table I.

TABLE I

A list of the cardinal yellow flags

Work	Behaviours
belief that all pain must be abolished before attempting to return to work or normal activity	passive attitude to rehabilitation
expectation of increased pain with activity or work	use of extended rest
fear of increased pain with activity or work	reduced activity with significant withdrawal from activities of daily living
belief that work is harmful	avoidance of normal activity
poor work history	impaired sleep because of pain
unsupportive work environment	increased intake of alcohol or similar substances since the onset of pain
Beliefs	**Affective**
belief that pain is harmful, resulting in fear-avoidance behaviour	depression
catastrophising, thinking the worst	feeling useless and not needed
misinterpreting bodily symptoms	irritability
belief that pain is uncontrollable	anxiety about heightened body sensations
poor compliance with exercise	disinterest in social activity
expectation of 'techno-fix' for pain	over-protective partner/spouse
low educational background	socially punitive partner/spouse
	lack of support to talk about problems

3. Evidence

At present there is no published evidence that identifying and managing yellow flag conditions results in reduced disability resulting from acute low back pain. Such belief that it could do so is based on extrapolation from experience with other conditions and experience with chronic low back pain.

At present, any attraction of the yellow flag concept rests on its concept validity. It seems plausible that psychosocial factors may hinder the rehabilitation of some patients. It seems plausible that some of these factors might be remediable. It seems plausible that eliminating or reducing some of these factors might improve rehabilitation and reduce chronicity.

4. Implementation

One advantage of the yellow flag concept is that its implementation does not require or involve a major or costly modification of medical practice with respect to acute low back pain. It does not require special investigations or treatment (in the first instance). Rather, attention to yellow flags constitutes

only good medical practice by ensuring attention to personal and behavioural dimensions of a patient who reports low back pain. This attention can be integrated into the management of patients without interfering with, and without replacing, any biological, medical management. In essence, it is no more than a formal description of what should, in any case, be good medical practice.

The absence of a definitive evidence-base for yellow flags, renders the concept a conjecture in a scientific sense. Therefore, practitioners who implement the yellow flags concept should do so in the knowledge that they are exploring an, as yet, unproven idea. But it is an idea that imposes no risk of harm, yet has the prospect of benefiting the patient, and also providing the treating doctor with an option that may help them cope with what might appear a difficult and complex patient-problem.

Some practitioners may be unfamiliar with, or uncomfortable with, formally recognising and managing behavioural problems. However, the yellow flag concept does not call for consummate expertise. Rather, it seeks to highlight, in the first instance, the need to recognise problems. To do so is no more than good medical practice. Moreover, guidelines have been developed to assist medical practitioners recognise the yellow flag conditions. Furthermore, guidelines have been formulated to assist medical practitioners to manage these conditions if they feel so able. It is only in the event of major or difficult problems that formal referral to experts is indicated [1].

5. Guidelines

5.1. Recognition

The New Zealand Guidelines [1] describe how yellow flag conditions can be recognised, both by way of conventional medical interview, and by way of a simple questionnaire. That questionnaire has not been validated; but it provides a handy, expeditious means of screening (putatively) for yellow flag conditions.

Without resorting to questionnaires, practitioners can include an exploration of yellow flags in the course of usual interactions with patients. The objective is to look for [1]

- beliefs that back pain is harmful or potentially severely disabling
- fear-avoidance behaviours
- tendency to low mood and withdrawal from social interaction
- an expectation that passive treatments rather than active participation will help.

Questions that can be rephrased into the practitioner's own style are [1]

- What do you understand is the cause of your back pain?
- What are you expecting will help you?
- How is your employer responding to your back pain? Your family? Your co-workers?
- What are you doing to cope with your pain?
- Do you think that you will return to work?

The source literature on fear-avoidance behaviour includes short and long questionnaires that have been used to identify patients with yellow flags [2,3]. The administration of these questionnaires could be cumbersome or intrusive. However, the items from these questionnaires that ostensibly signify yellow flag risk factors can be introduced into conventional interactions with patients.

Fear-avoidance behaviour can be suspected if the patient indicates that:

Physical issues
- Physical activity makes their pain worse
- Physical activity might harm their back
- They should not do physical activity which might make their pain worse
- They avoid
    lifting heavy objects
    bending
    walking
    standing
    sitting
    physical exertion
    stairs
    stretching or carrying
    travelling by public transport
    travelling in a car

Domestic issues
- They avoid
    cooking
    housework
    gardening
    cleaning car
    shopping
    odd jobs

Social issues
- They avoid
    spending time with family
    going to restaurants
    going to pub
    sexual activity
    going out
    going to parties
    visitors

Vocational issues
- Their pain was caused by their work

- Their work aggravated their pain
- Their work is too heavy for them
- Their work makes their pain worse
- Their work might harm their back
- They should not do their normal work with their present pain
- They do not think that they will be back to their normal work within 3 months
- They avoid going to work

This list is not intended as a questionnaire. It does not imply that a practitioner should assiduously ask about each and every item. Rather, the list is designed as a reference and prompt. The practitioner should be alert to these issues, and skilfully evoke them in the normal course of interaction. Rather than confront the patient, the practitioner can raise the issues, almost casually, as if it is part of their normal duty of care and concern.

The assessment of yellow flags should be part of any ongoing management of a patient, at any time in the course of their problem. The New Zealand Guidelines[1] recommend the administration of their screening questionnaire at 2–4 weeks after onset of pain. There is no evidence that this is the optimal time. This is early in the natural history of complaints of low back pain, and other interventions may take this long to achieve their effects. Indeed, over this time-frame, practitioners may still be concerned about red flag conditions, and their time with the patient may still be consumed with medical matters such as ensuring compliance with home rehabilitation and analgesics.

At the other extreme, waiting until the patient develops chronic pain (3 months) may be too late; the window of opportunity to prevent chronicity will have passed, by definition. Therefore, in patients with persisting pain, formal exploration of yellow flags should occur no later than 2 months after onset of pain, and possibly by the end of the first month. A less formal approach, however, can commence as soon as possible; indeed, even at the first consultation (Chapter 11).

Key points

- Psychosocial factors should be explored as part of a normal consultation.
- The practitioner should look for beliefs and behaviours that are counter-productive to recovery and which pose a risk for chronic disability.
- Those beliefs and behaviours pertain to physical activity, domestic responsibilities, social interactions, and vocational matters.

References

1 Kendall NAS, Linton SJ, Main CJ. Guide to Assessing Psychosocial Yellow Flags in Acute Low Back Pain: Risk Factors for Long-term Disability and Work Loss. Accident Rehabilitation and Compensation Insurance Corporation of New Zealand an the National Health Committee, Wellington.

2 Philips HC, Jahanshahi M. The components of pain behaviour report. Behav Res Ther 1986; 24: 117–125.
3 Waddell G, Newton M, Henderson I, Somerville D, Main CJ. A fear-avoidance beliefs questionnaire (FABQ) and the role of fear-avoidance beliefs in chronic low back pain and disability. Pain 1993; 52: 157–168.

Medical Management of Acute and Chronic Low Back Pain. An Evidence-Based Approach
Pain Research and Clinical Management, Vol. 13
Nikolai Bogduk and Brian McGuirk

CHAPTER 11

Algorithm for acute low back pain

1. Introduction

Different practitioners may have a preferred method of treating acute low back pain. Often, however, if not frequently, these methods focus on a single technique or intervention, or a collection of similar techniques. Furthermore, these interventions are essentially passive in nature — the practitioner delivers treatment to the patient, be that in the form of drugs, injections, manual therapy, supervised exercises, or the application of devices.

The available evidence, however, does not support such approaches. The evidence testifies to a lack of any significant effectiveness, or no greater effectiveness than simpler methods of management. Moreover, there is evidence in addition that passive interventions are counter-productive, and that the important ingredients of management are:

- empowering the patient to take responsibility for their own rehabilitation;
- avoiding rest and restoring activity;
- providing an explanation for the patient's pain;
- addressing the patient's fears and misconceptions.

In the next chapter the evidence is reviewed against rest, and in favour of explanation, reassurance, self-rehabilitation, and resuming activity as is the evidence for and against specific interventions. This evidence is provided both for reference and in support of the recommendations outlined in the present chapter.

2. An algorithm

The algorithm depicted in Fig. 1 summarises the essential components of a cogent approach to acute low back pain. Not only is it based on the best available evidence, it has been tested and found to be remarkably successful (q.v.).

The algorithm is structured around four phases of intervention:

Triage
the initial phase when the patient is assessed, and during which patients with neurological disorders or red flag conditions are identified.

Management
in which phase treatment is implemented, checked, and reinforced.

Concern
a phase in which the practitioner demonstrates concern for the patients, not only by reviewing their progress when they are not recovering but also to confirm that they have, indeed, recovered.

Vigilance
a recurrent phase, applied whenever the patient is seen subsequently, in order to detect either lack of recovery or the emergence of a red flag condition.

3. Triage

Triage occurs at the initial consultation. At this time the practitioner obtains a history, and records the red flag checklist (Chapter 6). If the patient has a

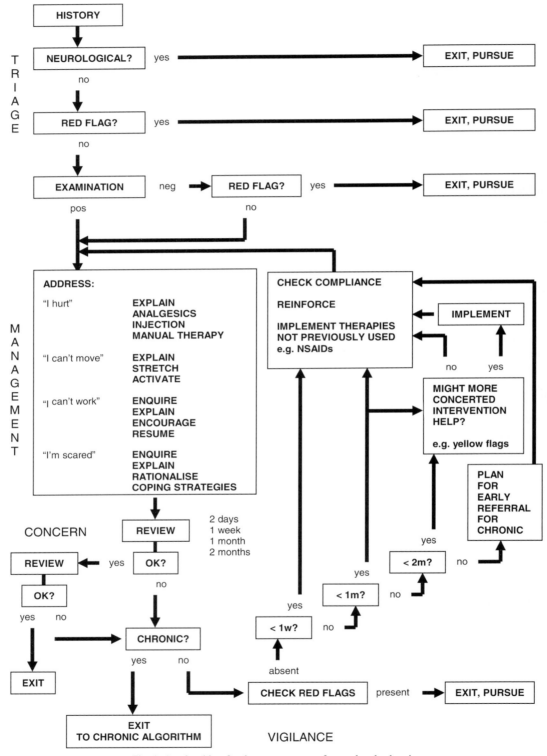

Fig. 1. An algorithm for the management of acute low back pain.

neurological condition or a red flag indicator, their management is no longer covered by this algorithm. They are managed as having another medical condition.

At the first consultation the practitioner should perform a physical examination, recognising, however, the limitations of this examination with respect to formulating a diagnosis (Chapter 7). Most significantly, if physical examination reveals no signs in the back, the possibilities of a red flag condition should be assiduously revisited, particularly with respect to visceral and vascular causes of back pain.

Regardless of the physical findings, and provided that there are no red flag indicators, the patient enters the management phase of the algorithm.

4. Management

The management of the patient is predicated on the patient's presenting problems. These have been encapsulated by an Australian primary care physician [1] as:

"I hurt";

"I can't move";

"I can't work"; and

"I'm scared".

Each of these complaints constitutes a separate domain of the patient's presenting problem. Each requires management; and although there may be some overlap, each domain entails different interventions. Failure to address each domain compromises total management. Even if one intervention eases their pain, the patients may still harbour fears that persist in causing disability; they may still not move properly and behave as if they still have pain, because they anticipate pain with movement; they may be reluctant or afraid to return to work.

Not all of these domains need to be (or necessarily can be) addressed on the occasion of the first consultation. They can be systematically pursued on return visits, if and as necessary. However, they should be identified at the first consultation, and flagged for future attention. Nevertheless, Watson [1] recommends, as a measure of good practice, that no patient should leave the first consultation without showing an improvement in at least one of the domains.

4.1. I hurt

Foremost in the management of a patient's pain is an explanation. The practitioner should provide a cogent, biological explanation of the pain that is credible, convincing, and understood by the patient. It does not matter if this explanation is not academically valid; it simply has to indicate to the patient that the practitioner does know what is going on. In this regard it is not so much what the practitioner says that is important, but the manner in which they say what they do. Providing an explanation is the opposite of appearing uncertain, or alarmed at what the problem might be. Providing an explanation is the opposite of panicking and pursuing unnecessary investigations that alarm the patients and reinforce their fears that something serious is wrong.

Individual practitioners may develop their own patter, in offering an explanation. One that has been tested [2] is to explain to patients, in simple terms, that they have internal disc disruption (see Chapter 14) — that they have a small injury that is presently inflamed and sore, but which will settle [2].

The practitioners also have at their disposal the facts about the natural history of acute low back pain (Chapter 4). Not just an academic piece of background information, these data can be harvested as a legitimate and truthful therapeutic tool. Explain to the patients, in terms that they will understand, that the odds are in their favour; that there is every chance of recovering (even regardless of treatment); but that it will take time. Remember that the median time to recovery is 7 weeks (Chapter 4). In the meantime, there are certain measures that both the practitioner and the patient can take to ease the situation while this recovery takes place.

Explain also that the chances of a serious cause are extremely low (Chapter 6), and are even lower because of their negative responses to the red flag checklist. If pressed, the practitioner can explain why there is no need for any special investigations. If patients ask about X-rays, take the time to explain why they are not indicated:

- they really do not show what is causing the pain;
- if negative, they create a false sense of security;
- they could well show something spurious that is more disconcerting than relevant;
- they constitute a health hazard.

Introduce this information by asking the patient: why do you want an X-ray; what do you think it will show; and what do you know about X-rays? Be conciliatory, if necessary, by venturing that if investigations prove necessary in due course, then proper and better tests can be arranged; but they are not necessary at this stage. Remember that explaining this in 5 min has been tested and proven effective in reducing the mistaken demand for X-rays (Chapter 8). It also constitutes good public health practice.

Having explained the pain to the patient, the practitioner has at their disposal several options for easing the pain. These include analgesics, and perhaps manual therapy, or the judicious use of injections of local anaesthetics. The specifics of these interventions are elaborated in Chapter 12.

4.2. I can't move

Patients with back pain will have movements that aggravate their pain and which they avoid; or they may adopt a global antalgic attitude. As a result their normal movements are impaired and reduced. This is a problem in its own right, and invites intervention quite apart from measures taken specifically for the pain.

Foremost again is explanation. Practitioners may develop their own preferred model. One that has been tested is to explain that, in response to pain, the back muscles tighten; they, in turn, become painful, and compound the problem; whereupon the objective is to reduce the tightness and, therefore, the magnitude of the problem[2]. [Whether or not this is a biologically valid explanation is not at issue; it simply constitutes a means of encouraging activity, which is the cardinal goal.]

The practitioner should instruct the patient in simple stretching exercises. If they are unfamiliar with these, they can consult colleagues who do know them, or various texts in which they are described[3,4]. The critical objective is to arm the patient with exercises that they can do for themselves whenever they need to, and which encourage and achieve mobility.

The exercises need not be formal, in the sense that they are undertaken in a gymnasium or even on an exercise mat. Nor are they intensive, in the sense that patients must exert themselves in order to build up muscle strength. The exercises should be manoeuvres that the patients can undertake in the course of their normal activities of daily living, be that sitting on a chair, standing, or lying on a carpet. Nor is the efficacy of the exercises the issue. They are not designed to be therapeutic in the sense of relieving pain. They are designed to encourage and enable movement.

Beyond simple exercises, the patient should be encouraged to resume normal activities. What they are encouraged to do, and instructions given to them are detailed in Chapter 12. If necessary, reactivation can be approached in a graded fashion. Establish the patient's present limits; set a reasonable goal to improve that limit; monitor progress; and celebrate achievement. What the patient actually does is not important. Each patient will have their own personal requirements, desires, and goals. The essence is that the patient should not do nothing.

Explain how resuming return to activity is evidence-based (Chapter 12); that patients who remain active recover sooner and for longer; those who do not, languish. Rest is out.

4.3. I can't work

This is perhaps the most vexatious domain of the patient's problem. It is here that the issue of yellow flags comes to the fore (Chapter 10).

The foremost intervention is to enquire. Determine what the patients actually mean. Are they afraid of the workplace; are they afraid of being injured again? Or do they simply dislike work? Does work really aggravate their pain? If so, have they tried, or are they simply expecting that it will? If the problems prove difficult, exploration of these issues may need to be adjourned until future consultations when more time can be dedicated to them.

Once the practitioner is aware of what the patient means, they can explore the problem with the patient. They can assess if the reservations and fears are rational and realistic. At their disposal the practitioner has the epidemiological facts about returning to work (Chapter 12). Explain that those who return to work have every chance of remaining at work. Patients who do not return to work have a greater chance of never returning to work.

If there are no real impediments to returning to work, the patients should be encouraged and assisted to do so. Whereupon, their progress should be monitored and reinforced as required. [What is not good practice is simply to dismiss the patient with an insistence that they get back to work. The practitioner needs to engage the patients about their beliefs, expectations and fears.]

A workplace intervention may be required. Often, this need not be a major exercise, especially when the employer is co-operative and accommodating. All that may be required is a discussion between the patient, their supervisor, and the practitioner, to determine what can be done about the patient's concerns, and to implement any minor ergonomic changes that may be required, or to adjust work practices in a manner agreeable to all parties. In order to facilitate and to expedite return to work, restrictions may need to be implemented, but if imposed, they need to be progressively relieved as the patient's condition improves. Other considerations pertaining to workplace intervention are explored in Chapter 12.

If done immediately, or as soon as possible, after the first consultation, such intervention stands to create an environment that welcomes a rapid return to work. There is no reason to expect that postponing such an intervention will make it any easier in the future. Yet doing so accelerates the return to work, and avoids the patient languishing, nurturing fears, and breeding resentment towards the workplace.

4.4. I'm scared

This is perhaps the most important domain of the patient's problem, yet the one that has received least attention under traditional medical management. The patients harbour beliefs and fears about their back pain. These beliefs, more than their pain, produce disability (Chapter 5). Therefore, if disability is to be averted, these beliefs and fears must be addressed. Analgesics and exercises alone do not take them away.

Establish what the patients think about their back pain: what do they think is wrong; what does it mean to them; what do they expect will happen; what are they going to do about it?

If the patient has misapprehensions, engage the patient about them. Rectify any mistaken beliefs. Much of this is achieved when providing a convincing, credible, biological explanation; for with that explanation comes the predictions of progress and recovery. These are complemented by the data on natural history.

Beyond just educating the patients about back pain, assess their beliefs and fears, and provide coping strategies for them. In this regard, if the patients are distraught, fearful, and do not really understand their problem, they may resort to coping in primitive ways, such as catastrophising or avoiding all activity. In contrast, the practitioner is emotionally unaffected and can provide intellectual insights of which the patient is not immediately capable. Think and solve for them. Hence, provide solutions to simple ergonomic problems; work out other ways that the patient can acquit activities of daily living, instead of the unproductive ways to which they may have resorted.

Equip the patients with first-aid measures that constitute strategies for dealing with exacerbations of pain. This may entail the correct use of analgesics in a time-contingent manner, the judicious application of exercises, or the use of ice-packs or heat as domestic interventions. Explain and instruct how they must become responsible for these interventions. Explain the virtues of 'warming up' before taking on an activity that threatens to aggravate their pain.

5. Concern

There is no explicit evidence that showing concern
is in any way therapeutic in its own right. There
is only a theoretical expectation that patients will
appreciate it when their practitioner demonstrates
concern by checking on their progress, even if it is
only to confirm that they have recovered. There is
also a theoretical possibility that patients who are not
checked, and who continue to languish may feel that
their initial treatment has failed and that there is no
point returning to their doctor. Such patients do not
understand the virtues and necessity of follow-up to
check compliance and to amend interventions.

Where the evidence does obtain is with respect
to the practitioner's sense of success. The data show
that patients who do not return have not necessarily
recovered (Chapter 4). They continue to suffer or
go elsewhere. At the very least, these data indicate
that failing to check patients overestimates success.
They imply a duty of care to check progress. Thus,
expressing concern by reviewing patients not only
inherits the theoretical positive virtues of doing so, it
averts abandoning patients who, for reasons of their
own, are reluctant to return for a follow-up.

Accordingly, schedule a follow-up to check
progress. Follow-up visits allow the status of the
patients, and their response to treatment, to be monitored. If they have recovered, all is well; but the
practitioner knows that they have recovered. If they
have not recovered, the opportunity arises to check
compliance with earlier instructions. Perhaps the patients did not understand. Are they taking their medications correctly? Can they demonstrate back to you
the exercises that you showed them? If necessary,
other interventions can be implemented (as shown in
the algorithm, Fig. 1).

Some patients who recover rapidly may consider
a formal, follow-up appointment as an unnecessary
inconvenience, and perhaps an unnecessary cost. In
those circumstances, scheduled appointments may
be cancelled, but the patient's recovery can be confirmed by a telephone call, which serves also to
communicate concern.

6. Vigilance

Vigilance is the second protection for the practitioner
fearful of missing something important. The first was
the initial use of the red flag check list. However,
some patients may present early in the evolution of a
serious disorder, at a time when there are insufficient
clues to warrant concerted investigation.

At each follow-up visit, the practitioner should
repeat the red flag checklist. If new features have
arisen, those new features are pursued outside the
confines of the present algorithm. If there are still no
red flag features, the algorithm continues to operate.

Early in the course of managing acute low back
pain, the practitioners can afford to recycle through
their management plan. They have the opportunity to
check compliance, reinforce previous interventions
if they seem to be working, or to add new interventions.

If the patient is not progressing well, psychosocial
issues should be more vigorously explored (Chapter
10). If the practitioner is able to address these, they
should become the forefront of further intervention.
If the nature of the problems is beyond the expertise
of the practitioner, a more concerted intervention
may be called for. The opportunity should be taken
sooner rather than later to enlist the assistance of a
counsellor, psychologist, or a pain clinic. At stake
may be a limited window of opportunity to redress
psychosocial factors before they become entrenched
and irresurrectable.

In this regard, however, practitioners should note
that early multidisciplinary and behavioural intervention is not indicated, as a rule (Chapter 12). Such
intervention is best tailored for patients who have
entered the subacute phase of back pain.

Similar comments apply to biomedical investigations in patients who do not have red flag indicators.
These investigations are appropriate for patients who
have developed chronic low back pain, but they are
not appropriate for patients with acute pain. However, it may be difficult to obtain services in this
regard promptly when requested. Therefore, it is
perhaps wise to start planning referrals or booking
investigations for patients who, at two months or so,

are not improving and who appear likely to become chronic sufferers of back pain.

7. Efficacy

For many practitioners this recommended algorithm constitutes a cultural shift or even a threat. It defies traditional paradigms in that it shuns specific passive interventions; it does not recommend a particular (and eponymously named) exercise; it does not recommend a particular manual treatment; it does not recommend referral to a particular 'specialist' in 'backs'. What it does do is place a different burden and responsibility on the average practitioner. It asks that the practitioner engages the patients, spends more time with them than it takes to write a referral or a request for an X-ray. It asks that investigations be avoided unless absolutely indicated, and it asks that patients be dissuaded from demanding such futile investigations.

All this takes time, and perhaps a different attitude. But the practitioner is already equipped with the resources. Their cardinal tools are their ears (to listen), their mouth (to explain), and their mind (to analyse and solve the problems of a distressed patient who is unable to do so themselves). The average practitioner does not need to feel underequipped or disenfranchised because they do not know manual therapy, or how to inject trigger points. They have enough skills to be able to engage patients. If they want to know about other interventions, they can learn about them from the next chapter.

Faced with the prospect of having to change the way they do things, practitioners are entitled to ask if it is worth doing, and if there is evidence to this effect. Evidence is to hand.

The National Musculoskeletal Medicine Initiative was established in Australia in 1996. It was designed to develop evidence-based guidelines concerning the medical management of acute musculoskeletal pain, to evaluate the safety, efficacy, and cost-effectiveness of practice according to these guidelines, and to determine how these conditions were managed in usual care. Inter alia, the Initiative addressed neck pain, shoulder pain, elbow pain, hip and knee pain, but acute low back pain was its primary index condition.

A selection of primary care practitioners, and a smaller contingent of rheumatologists, rehabilitation physicians, and occupational physicians agreed to abide by evidence-based guidelines for the management of acute low back pain, and to have their outcomes independently audited. In essence, they followed the algorithm described in this chapter. Collectively they conducted 13 special clinics located variously in teaching hospitals, community health centres, and in conventional primary care practices. Meanwhile, several general practitioner groups agreed to have their practices audited in order to provide an indication of how patients are managed under 'usual care'. The results of the study vindicate the algorithm [5].

Some 430 patients with acute low back pain were managed according to evidence-based guidelines, and 83 were managed under usual care. At the first consultation, using the red flag checklist, six patients in the evidence-based clinics (1.4%) were found to have a red flag condition (two osteoporotic fractures, one crush fracture, and three cases of metastatic carcinoma). This incidence compares exactly with the prevalence figures in the literature (Chapter 6). The fact that no additional red flag conditions were diagnosed in the following 12 months of follow-up attests to the sensitivity of the red-flag checklist.

Moreover, the evidence-based practitioners relied on history and clinical features. They used investigations sparingly. Only 7% of patients underwent medical imaging, compared to 30% under usual care.

The cardinal interventions used by the evidence-based practitioners were as outlined in the algorithm. Critically, they provided explanation, encouragement and reassurance. With respect to other measures, they largely used home rehabilitation, manual therapy, and simple analgesics (Chapter 12). In doing so and in reviewing patients they averaged one initial and three subsequent consultations, lasting 50 min and 20 min each, respectively.

In contrast, usual care involved one initial consultation, and a median number of zero subsequent

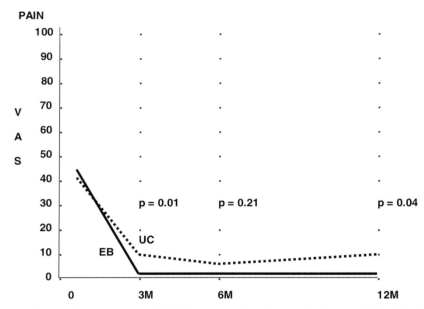

Fig. 2. The median scores for visual analogue scale (VAS) for pain, at inception, 3 months, 6 months, and 12 months, of patients with acute low back pain, treated in the evidence-based (EB) clinics and in usual care (UC). The *p* values pertain to the results of a Mann–Whitney test for differences between the two samples at the times indicated.

consultations. The care provided consisted primarily of simple analgesics, opioids such as dextropropoxyphene, non-steroidal anti-inflammatory drugs, rest, physiotherapy, and hot packs. Strikingly, however, over 20% of patients under usual care resorted to interventions not prescribed by their treating doctor, with 23% using so-called complementary health care. Only 7% of patients under evidence-based care resorted to non-prescribed interventions.

The outcomes were both striking and sobering. Under both types of care the vast majority of patients rapidly recovered. Pain scores plummeted, and disability scores on the SF-36 scales returned to normal and supranormal levels for age, on the average. Certain differences arose, however, that were significant statistically, clinically, and socially.

Improvements in pain were dramatic in both groups, but significantly better under evidence-based care (Fig. 2). At three months, 77% of patients under evidence-based care required no continuing care of any sort, compared with 56% of patients under usual care. At 12 months these figures were 77% and 68%,

respectively. At three months, 67% of patients under evidence-based care had fully recovered, compared with 49% under usual care. (Full recovery was defined as zero pain, or a score of less than 10 on a 100-point visual analogue pain scale.) At 12 months these figures were 71% and 56%, respectively. The recurrence rate at 12 months was only 16% in the evidence-based group, and 27% under usual care. Despite the greater number of consultations required under evidence-based care, the average cost per patient was $AUS 276. The average cost for usual care was $AUS 472. The greater cost of consultations under evidence-based care was more than offset by the greater cost of physiotherapy, investigations, drug treatment, and complementary care, under usual care.

In essence, these results showed that evidence-based care, following the algorithm outlined in this chapter, achieved outcomes that were at least equal to those obtained under good usual care, but included relatively greater relief of pain, less need for continuing care, and greater rates of full recovery.

Moreover, evidence-based care was safe, in that it did not miss any serious conditions; it was efficient, in that it did not use unnecessary investigations, and it was cost-effective.

Furthermore, consumers approved of evidence-based care. Whereas 43% of patients under usual care rated their treatment as extremely helpful, 82% of those under evidence-based care so rated their treatment. In unsolicited responses, the patients highlighted the value of having had their problem explained, and having been empowered and assisted to take charge of their own rehabilitation.

These results stand in contrast to figures stemming from previous, epidemiological studies. Under evidence-based care, the recurrence rates and chronicity rates were substantially lower than those previously reported (Chapter 4). Yet, no special interventions were employed. The recovery rates echoed those reported by Indahl et al.[2], upon whose work the algorithm was largely based (Chapter 12).

References

1   Watson P. The MSM quartet. Australas Musculoskeletal Med 1999; 4(2): 8–9.
2   Indahl A, Velund L, Reikeraas O. Good prognosis for low back pain when left untampered: a randomized clinical trial. Spine 1995; 20: 473–477.
3   McKenzie R. Treat Your Own Back, 5th edn. Spinal Publications, Lower Hutt, 1997.
4   McKenzie R. A physical therapy perspective on acute spinal disorders. In: Mayer TG, Mooney V, Gatchel RJ (eds) Contemporary Conservative Care for Painful Spinal Disorders. Lea and Febiger, Philadelphia, PA, 1991: 211–220.
5   McGuirk B, King W, Govind J, Lowry J, Bogduk N. The safety, efficacy, and cost-effectiveness of evidence-based guidelines for the management of acute low back pain in primary care. Spine 2001; 26: 2615–2622.

Medical Management of Acute and Chronic Low Back Pain. An Evidence-Based Approach
Pain Research and Clinical Management, Vol. 13
Nikolai Bogduk and Brian McGuirk
© *2002 Elsevier Science B.V. All rights reserved*

CHAPTER 12

The evidence

1. Introduction

To a greater or lesser extent, every conventional, or traditional, treatment for acute low back pain has been tested. All have been subjected to some form of controlled trial. Some have been subjected to systematic reviews. For some interventions, the evidence is either strongly supportive or strongly negative. For others, the evidence is mixed or contentious.

The measures outlined in Chapter 11 are based on a distillation of this evidence, harvesting the proven and worthwhile interventions while avoiding the disproven and contentious. The present chapter provides a summary of that evidence, and a retrospective justification of the algorithm provided in Chapter 11.

2. Activity vs bed rest

For no other treatment of acute low back pain are the results of studies as consistent and uniform as they are for bed rest and activity. Two systematic reviews [1,2] have reached the same conclusions.

The first review [1] was published in 1994, and covered five studies of bed rest. The second review [2] identified a further three studies published since that time, or not included in the first review. All eight acceptable trials found bed rest to be *ineffective*. Two trials showed that bed rest for 7 days is no better than bed rest for 2–3 days. Five trials showed that rest for 2–4 days was no different or worse than no bed rest. Bed rest is no different or less effective than alternative treatments in terms of rate of recovery, relief of pain, return to daily activities, and time lost from work.

Eight trials of advice to stay active showed consistent findings [2]. Three trials showed faster return to work, and reduced time off work in the following year. All trials showed reduced use of health care, and reduced chronic disability. Conspicuously, no trials found that early activity had any harmful effects. Two trials that compared bed rest with advice to stay active showed that ordinary activity produced faster recovery.

On the strength of this evidence, bed rest has no place in the management of acute low back pain. Rather, patients should be advised to remain active. Specifically how this might be achieved is pursued in the following section.

Key points

- Bed rest should not be prescribed as a treatment for acute low back pain.
- Patients with acute low back pain should be encouraged to stay active and resume their normal activities of daily living.
- The lack of benefit of bed rest should be explained to patients, and the alternatives explained, justified and promoted.

References

1   Koes BW, van den Hoogen HMM. Efficacy of bed rest and orthoses of low back pain. A review of randomized clinical trials. Eur J Phys Med Rehabil 1994; 4: 96–99.

2   Waddell G, Feder G, Lewis M. Systematic reviews of bed rest and advice to stay active for acute low back pain. Br J Gen Pract 1997; 47: 647–652.

3. Home rehabilitation

Fear is a predictor of poor outcome in patients with acute low back pain (Chapter 5). Patients may not understand what is causing their pain, and fear that it is a serious and threatening disease. They may be afraid that movement, activity, or work may worsen the pathology. They fear aggravation of their pain if they move or maintain normal activities.

Since fear is a determinant of chronicity of low back pain, reassurance should be effective in minimising chronicity. This has been demonstrated in a seminal controlled trial.

Indahl et al.[1] studied patients who had been suffering from back pain for at least 8 weeks but not more than 12 weeks. They randomly allocated 512 patients to undergo control therapy which consisted of no active intervention from the research team, but freedom to undertake whatever therapy was offered to them by their own medical officers. The active treatment group of 463 patients received a programme of intervention:

(1) Patients were provided with a biological model of their pain. They were told how a possible crack in a disc could cause inflammation in innervated parts of the disc and that this could cause reflex contraction of the paraspinal muscles; that this activation would diminish circulation in the muscles and lead to stiffness and pain; that pain and anticipation of pain could add to the binding and guarding of the back which would lead to increased muscle contraction and increased pain.

(2) Patients were assured that light activity would not further injure the disc or any other structure that could be involved in the process, and that, rather, it was more likely that it would enhance the repair process. They were told that low back pain should be thought of as a sign that the circulation in the muscles was inadequate and that their response should be to alleviate this condition.

(3) The link between emotions and low back pain was explained as a muscular response and that increased tension in muscles for whatever reason would increase the pain and thereby add to the problem. It was explained how long-standing pain could create vicious circles and chronic pain as a result. The point that the worst thing they could do to their backs was to be careful, was strongly emphasised.

(4) All patients, regardless of clinical and radiographic findings, were told to mobilise their lumbar spine by light activity. No fixed exercise goals were set, but patients were given guidelines and encouraged to set their own goals. Great emphasis was put on the effort to remove fear about low back pain and focus on sickness behaviour.

(5) Misunderstandings about back pain were dealt with.

(6) The principal recommendation was to normalise gait, as well as to try to walk as flexibly as possible. Activities involving static work for the back muscles were discouraged.

(7) Acute attacks of back pain were to be treated as an acute muscle spasm with stretching and light activity.

(8) With respect to lifting:
twisting when bending was to be avoided;
for heavy objects, patients were to use the thighs with a vertical back;
at other times, they were to use the back and flex it;
patients were not to be afraid.

Instruction was reinforced at 3 months and at 1 year. Patients were free to call the investigators if they felt any need for to do so.

Fig. 1 summarises the results. The actively treated

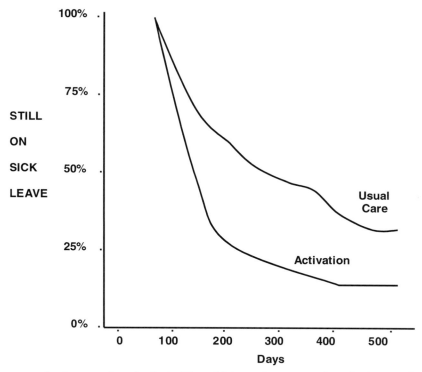

Fig. 1. Survival curves comparing the proportion of patients still on sick-leave after treatment by activation or under usual care. Based on Indahl et al. [1].

patients exhibited a clinically and statistically significant difference from the control group with respect to decrease in sickness-leave. At 200 days, 60% in the control group, but only 30% in the intervention group, were still on sickness-leave. At the end of the study, 64 patients from the control group, but only 24 from the intervention group were still on sickness-leave.

This study demonstrated, under controlled conditions, that a simple programme of reassurance and elementary rehabilitation instruction is more successful at reducing sickness-leave than conventional therapies, for patients who had been on sickness-leave for more than 8 weeks but not more than 12 weeks. A five-year follow-up demonstrated that these differences were maintained [2]. Only 19% of the intervention group were still on sick-leave at 5 years, compared with 34% in the control group.

Although this intervention was applied to patients with subacute back pain, there is nothing, in principle, logistically, or financially, that prevents it from being applied earlier to patients with acute low back pain.

Key points

- Provide patients confidently with a sound biological model of their pain.
- Confidently assure patients that light activity will not further injure any structure that could be involved in their pain.

Key points (continued)

- Explain that:
  increased tension in muscles will increase the pain and thereby add to the problem;
  the worst thing they can do to their backs is to be careful.
- Stipulate that all patients must mobilise their lumbar spine by light activity.
- It is not necessary to set exercise goals, but provide patients with guidelines and encourage them to set their own goals.
- Make every effort to remove fear about low back pain and avoid sickness behaviour.
- Enquire about and redress any misunderstandings about back pain.
- Encourage and help patients to try to walk as flexibly as possible.
- Discourage activities involving static work for the back muscles.
- Treat acute attacks of back pain as an acute muscle spasm with stretching and light activity.
- Instruct patients to avoid twisting with bending, but not to be afraid to lift.
- Remain available to see the patient at their request.

References

1   Indahl A, Velund L, Reikeraas O. Good prognosis for low back pain when left untampered: a randomized clinical trial. Spine 1995; 20: 473–477.

2   Indahl A, Haldorsen EH, Holm S, Reikeras O, Ursin H. Five-year follow-up study of a controlled clinical trial using light mobilization and an informative approach to low back pain. Spine 1998; 23: 2625–2630.

4. Workplace intervention

Not every patient who presents with acute low back pain will have a problem with work. Once they have been properly assessed, have had their condition explained, and have been empowered with a plan of management, some patients can resume their normal work. Others may do so tentatively and be surprised, yet relieved, that they can successfully resume work.

For other patients, matters pertaining to work may be important factors in delaying or preventing rehabilitation. The possible problems can range from inappropriate beliefs and fears on the part of the patient to outrightly unsafe and even outrageous work practices that oppressively are imposed on the patient. Whether or not serious workplace issues obtain in a particular case is a matter of judgment on the part of the practitioner and the patient; but

can only be determined if work is examined in a concerted manner during the consultations with the patient.

In assessing work matters, a practitioner may be at a significant disadvantage if they do not really understand what is involved in a particular job. Not only will they be unable to offer any sensible and realistic ergonomic advice, they may appear foolish or elitist to the patient, and therefore, unconvincing, e.g. "what would you know?".

In such cases, the practitioner could ask what the job involves, and learn from the patient. With the patient they could reconstruct the work station, and mimic the worker's activities. It would be better still if the practitioner was actually familiar with the work practices, by having visited the workplace, if not having experienced the work practices.

Rural practitioners may well be able to do this. If they are faced with large or regular numbers of patients with back pain, it would be profitable for them to become familiar with the various work sites of their patients. Not only does this provide them with familiarity with the sites and their practices, they can establish social contact with management, which can be of advantage should the need arise, in the future, for the practitioner to intervene on behalf of a patient. When advocacy is required, it is potentially impressive and reassuring to the patient when it emerges, in the course of a consultation, that the practitioners not only knows what the job entails but knows also the key personnel.

For urban practitioners, this may not be practicable. Their patients may work far afield, and the practitioner may not be able to have visited and experienced all the possible work sites of their patients. Beyond learning what they can about the job from the patient, the urban practitioner may need to collaborate with a colleague or specialist practitioner trained in occupational health, if concerted workplace intervention is required.

The present text does not pretend to be a textbook on Occupational Medicine. Workplaces and work practices vary enormously, as do laws and regulations. The permutations and possibilities are too numerous to allow examples of practical solutions to be enunciated for every possible situation. What this present chapter does focus on, however, is the importance of doing something at the workplace, in cases where this becomes necessary.

4.1. Principles

The importance of workplace intervention has increasingly been recognised in the literature on back pain rehabilitation. This intervention should not be misrepresented or misconstrued as an adversarial occupational health and safety visit. Rather, it involves several, overt and subtle, dimensions.

Foremost, the patient's practitioner, or a surrogate representative (e.g. rehabilitation provider, occupational therapist), should become familiar with the patient's work and work environment, so that they can help the patient return to work in an informed and insightful manner.

Secondly, on behalf of the worker, they can negotiate with the employer:

any amendments to the workplace specifically to prevent recurrences of accidents of the type in which the worker may have been injured;

modifications to the workplace otherwise to prevent or avoid recurrences of back pain problems;

mutually acceptable modified duties that allow the worker to return to work and therein feel welcome.

Thirdly, the practitioner can be seen to have been the patient's advocate. In this regard, it is not so much what the practitioner does in terms of actual ergonomic changes, but that they are seen to have done something. While the full implications of this dimension have never been evaluated, its power should not be underestimated, given the extent to which fear of work, and dissatisfaction with the workplace are prognostic of poor outcome (Chapter 5).

4.2. Efficacy

In some studies [1,2], a workplace visit seems to be an integral component of successful multidimensional rehabilitation programs. However, in these studies, the effect of the workplace visit cannot be dissected from the effect of graded activity.

One study, however, directly compared the efficacy of usual care only, clinical intervention only, occupational intervention alone, and both clinical and occupational intervention combined [3]. Adding occupational intervention resulted in reduced absence from work, faster return to work, less disability, less sickness impact, and reduced pain. The effects were greater, and statistically significant when clinical intervention was combined with occupational intervention, than when occupational intervention or clinical intervention were used in isolation.

The occupational intervention was undertaken after the worker had been absent from work for 6 weeks, and consisted of a visit by an occupational physician and an ergonomist. The physician would recommend investigations or treatment, or could try to set up light duties that enabled the patient to return to work. The ergonomic intervention involved union and employer representatives in determining the need for job modifications. For each patient, a group was formed that included the ergonomist, the injured worker, the worker's supervisor, and representatives of management and unions. After observation of the worker's task, a meeting of the group allowed for a specific ergonomic diagnosis, and precise solutions to improve the worksite were submitted to the employer. These were designed to enable the stable return of the worker to the worksite.

The literature on what constitutes optimal workplace intervention is varied in quality, but abundant. A pragmatic review [4] emphasised the virtue and importance of modified duties (as opposed to so-called light duties). Such duties consist of appropriately modified work according to the injured worker's physical capacity, developed in the context of sympathetic communication with the worker, and non-

adversarial handling of the worker's compensation claim. A critical issue in this regard is to return the worker to their pre-injury job, as far as possible, with restrictions if required, rather than allotting them to different and usually more menial duties. Moreover, it is recommended that a supportive workplace response to injury needs to start when the pain is first reported, and that an individualised and accommodative approach to return to work should follow promptly [4]. Such measures can reduce both the incidence and the duration of disability resulting in time lost from work by up to 50% [4].

Key points

- Not every patient with acute low back pain will necessarily need workplace assessment and intervention, but
- for those patients for whom it is indicated, a workplace visit and appropriate intervention may be indicated as an integral part of medical management.
- Workplace intervention should involve the worker, their medical and union representative (if available), and the employer; and be designed to accommodate a prompt return to work.
- Workplace intervention has been shown to achieve substantial improvements disability and time lost from work.

References

1 Lindstrom I, Ohlund C, Eek C, Wallin L, Peterson LE, Nachemson A. Mobility, strength, and fitness after a graded activity program for patients with subacute low-back pain. A randomized prospective clinical study with a behavioural therapy approach. Spine 1992; 17: 641–649.
2 Lindstrom I, Ohlund C, Nachemson A. Physical performance, pain, pain behavior and subjective disability in patients with subacute low back pain. Scand J Rehab Med 1995; 27: 153–160.
3 Loisel P, Abenhaim L, Durand P, Esdaile JM, Suissa S, Gosselin L, Simard R, Turcotte J, Lemaire J. A population-based, randomized clinical trial on back pain management. Spine 1997; 22: 2911–2918.
4 Frank J, Sinclair S, Hogg-Johnson S, Shannon H, Bombardier C, Beaton D, Cole D. Preventing disability from work-related low-back pain: new evidence gives new hope — if we can just get all the players onside. Can Med Ass J 1998; 158: 1625–1631.

5. Drugs

Drugs are probably the single most common intervention that medical practitioners in primary care provide for patients with acute low back pain. Yet, the evidence for their efficacy is scanty or lacking. Indeed, some studies have highlighted the lack of efficacy of some drugs that are used. Also, much of the literature is consumed with studies that compare one drug with another, without either having been compared with natural history.

5.1. Analgesics

Drugs that might be used or have been used to relieve acute low back pain are:

(1) simple analgesics
(2) compound analgesics
(3) non-steroidal anti-inflammatory drugs

(NSAIDs)
(4) opioids
(5) antidepressants.

5.1.1. Simple analgesics

The use of simple analgesics presumes no particular cause or mechanism for back pain. These drugs are used for their central, analgesic effects. The drug of choice is paracetamol.

Various groups that have developed guidelines for the treatment of acute low back pain have recommended paracetamol as the first drug of choice, on the grounds that it is the safest, effective medication[1-4]. These recommendations, however, seem to have been made on the basis of either the reputation of paracetamol as a generic analgesic, or indirect evidence of efficacy, in that paracetamol is no less effective than non-steroidal anti-inflammatory agents for acute low back pain (q.v.). There have been no controlled trials comparing paracetamol with placebo for back pain.

One study[5] used paracetamol as the control for diflunisal in acute low back pain. Four of 12 patients treated with paracetamol considered the efficacy of therapy to be good or excellent, but 10 of 16 patients treated with diflunisal found it to be good or excellent. This result reflects common clinical experience that, despite recommendations to use paracetamol for acute low back pain, few patients find it satisfying, and prefer something 'stronger'.

5.1.2. Compound analgesics

Compound analgesics were designed to be 'stronger', i.e. more potent, than paracetamol, by combining a small quantity of codeine with paracetamol into the one tablet. A meta-analysis, however (based largely on literature on oral surgery and postoperative pain), showed that codeine added only a 5% increase in pain relief to that afforded by paracetamol alone[6]. The addition of codeine significantly increased the risk of side effects, particularly with repeated use.

The few studies that have expressly investigated the efficacy of compound analgesics for low back pain compared them with non-steroidal anti-inflammatory drugs[7-9]. They found that compound analgesics were not more effective, but did produce more side effects. Similarly, studies of compound analgesics containing dextropropoxyphene have found them to be no more effective than paracetamol with caffeine[10], or either non-steroidal anti-inflammatory drugs or paracetamol alone[11].

Accordingly, despite their reputation as being 'stronger' analgesics, the data show that these agents are not demonstrably more effective than simple analgesics or non-steroidal anti-inflammatory agents, for the relief of back pain. Although these agents appear to reduce pain by some 50%[7-11], that effect has not been controlled for the natural recovery of acute low back pain.

5.2. NSAIDs

NSAIDs are designed to act peripherally on sources of pain that involve inflammation. However, there is no evidence that any of the common causes of back pain involve inflammation. Therefore, NSAIDs are not indicated in the treatment of low back pain for their anti-inflammatory properties. They are indicated only for their central analgesic effects.

An earlier systematic review[12] of the efficacy of NSAIDs for back pain, did not discriminate between acute and chronic low back pain, but has been superseded by subsequent systematic reviews. One review that specifically addressed acute low back pain[13] has been updated by the same authors[14]. The more recent review found that:

- there is strong evidence that NSAIDs prescribed at regular intervals provide effective pain relief for simple acute low back pain, but they do not affect return to work, natural history, or chronicity;
- there is strong evidence that different types of NSAIDs are equally effective.

What these conclusions do not reveal is how weak and limited the efficacy of NSAIDs is. Most studies that were reviewed assessed efficacy for periods of only 1 or 2 weeks[13,14]. In studies that did not control for natural history, NSAIDs appeared to reduce pain by 50% or more[13,14]. However, when compared to placebo, NSAIDs are slightly more effective at 3 days, but not at 7 days [15]; and are more effective only for patients with moderate to severe pain at inception [16]. Most of the apparent effect of NSAIDs, therefore can be accounted for by natural history. The only advantage of NSAIDs lies in reducing initially severe pain to tolerable levels while natural recovery occurs, or perhaps as other interventions are applied.

Serious side effects are unlikely to be a problem if NSAIDs are used for a brief period for acute low back pain that is destined to improve through natural history. Nevertheless, between 10% and 20% of patients are likely to report side effects, even during a 10-day course [17]. COX-2 inhibitors have been promoted on the grounds that they have a much lower incidence of serious side effects than classical NSAIDs, but in the context of acute low back pain, they do not have significantly fewer minor side effects; nor are they demonstrably more effective in providing pain relief [17].

5.3. Opioids

Opioids are a tempting option for doctors treating patients whose back pain remains reportedly severe despite treatment with simple analgesics, NSAIDs, compound analgesics, and other measures. Their undisciplined use, however, invites serious problems associated with the side effects and properties of these drugs.

There have been no controlled trials of the use of opioids for severe, acute low back pain. Consequently, there is no evidence upon which guidelines might be based. However, from time to time, practitioners might encounter patients for whom they might consider opioids appropriate. For that purpose, the National Health and Medical Research Council of Australia has prepared guidelines on the management of acute pain, that contain a section on the use of opioids [18]. The Working Party was not able to provide evidence of efficacy of opioids in the management of acute pain of musculoskeletal origin, but provided a consensus view that for severe pain, for which there was no other sensible option, opioids could be used judiciously.

The assistance of an expert unit is invaluable in terms of determining appropriate doses and routes of administration, and varying agents in order to minimise tolerance and habituation. Such assistance would seem wise in the course of any long term use of opioids.

5.4. Antidepressants

Antidepressants have been used as primary agents and as co-analgesics in the treatment of a variety of pain problems, most commonly, headache, post-herpetic neuralgia, and a variety of 'rheumatic' conditions. Their apparent success in general pain management spawned their use for low back pain. However, the available literature does not support their perceived or alleged value.

A systematic review [19] found the literature on antidepressants and low back pain to be poor and uncompelling for their favour. The controlled studies that have been published suffer from various deficiencies such as incomplete data and less than rigorous evaluation and follow-up of outcome; all have addressed chronic low back pain.

One study indicated a superiority of imipramine over placebo, but only with respect to "number of days had to lie down" and "number of days with at least some restriction of normal activity"; there were no differences with respect to pain intensity, depression, feeling miserable, overall evaluation of symptoms and physical findings [20]. Another study showed amitriptyline to be superior to placebo, but only with respect to use of analgesics [21]. Trazadone showed no superiority over placebo [22]; nor did tofranil [23].

In the absence of any studies of their use for acute low back pain, and in the face of consistently negative results when used for chronic back pain, there would seem to be no rational basis for prescribing antidepressants for the treatment of acute low back pain.

5.5. Muscle relaxants

The rationale for the use of muscle relaxants is purported to be to relieve painful muscle spasm.

However, there is no evidence that spasm of the back muscles is painful or contributes to the patient's pain. There is no evidence that so-called muscle spasm can be reliably diagnosed. There is no correlation between clinical muscle spasm and any biological parameter, such as EMG. Indeed, eminent authorities have decried the wisdom of belief in muscle spasm [24] or lamented its lack of validity [25]. Nevertheless, the use of muscle relaxants in back pain has from time to time been explored, and remains a temptation for physicians to do something for their patients in need.

Two systematic reviews by the same authors [13,14] have concluded that there is strong evidence that muscle relaxants effectively reduce acute low back pain and that the different types of muscle relaxants are equally effective. In both respects, inspection of the original studies suggests that this conclusion may have been overly generous.

The data are conflicting for orphenadrine. One study [26] found only that nine out of 20 patients treated with orphenadrine had reduced pain at 48 hr after treatment, compared to four out of 20 patients treated with placebo. No other, or better measure of outcome was reported. In contrast, another study found no superiority over placebo [27]. Diazepam is no more effective than placebo for the relief of acute low back pain [28].

Dantrolene was considered more effective than placebo on the grounds that it reduced pain during maximum voluntary movement to a greater extent [29]. Carisoprodol was considered effective because it reduced pain to a greater extent than placebo at 4 days [30]. Methocarbamol was as effective as chlormezanone [31], but chlormezanone was as effective as an NSAID [32].

Conflicting data concerning tizanidine have been reported by the same investigators in two separate studies. One found no differences in outcome at 3 and at 7 days between patients treated with tizanidine and those treated with placebo [33]. The other study compared tizanidine plus ibuprofen with tizanidine plus placebo [34]. It found no differences in pain scores between the two groups at 3 and at 7 days. The success attributed to tizanidine was based on a larger proportion of patients having no pain or only mild pain at night, at 3 days but not at 7 days; and a larger proportion of patients having no pain or only mild pain at rest, both at 3 and at 7 days. The respective proportions in the latter instance were 90% vs 72% at 3 days, and 93% vs 77% at 7 days.

Baclofen is significantly more effective than placebo in reducing pain, but the magnitude of the difference is about 10% in absolute terms, and 20% in relative terms, but applies to assessment at 10 days after treatment [35]. Cyclobenzaprine is more effective than placebo in so far as it achieved a reduction in pain, 9 days after treatment, of 5.5 points on a 10-point scale, compared with 4 points for placebo [36]. However, cyclobenzaprine is not more effective than NSAIDs [37].

These data indicate that whereas some muscle relaxants may be equipotent not all are effective. Some are no more effective than placebo. Even those that are more effective than placebo have been studied for only 3, 7 or 10 days. Their attributable effect, however, is small. Yet muscle relaxants have consistently been associated with a greater incidence of central nervous system side effects [13,14]. This factor, balanced against their limited attributable effect, gives cause to question the propriety of their use for acute low back pain, especially when other interventions are no less effective, or even more effective, with far less risk of troublesome side effects.

Key points

- Although paracetamol is widely recommend as an analgesic for acute low back pain, there is little direct evidence for its efficacy.
- NSAIDs are minimally more effective than placebo, if at all, for acute low back pain.
- Compound analgesics are not more effective than NSAIDS.

Key points (continued)

- No studies have evaluated the efficacy of opioids for acute low back pain.
- If opioids are indicated because of the severity of the patient's pain, they should be used carefully, perhaps with expert assistance.
- Antidepressants do not provide analgesia for acute low back pain.
- Some muscle relaxants provide slightly more relief of pain than placebo, when used over a short period, but their utility is marred by a high incidence of side effects.

References

1   American Academy of Orthopaedic Surgeons and North American Spine Society. Draft Clinical Algorithm on Low back Pain. American Academy of Orthopaedic Surgeons and North American Spine Society, April 1996.

2   American Academy of Orthopaedic Surgeons. Evidence-based recommendations for patients with acute activity intolerance due to low back symptoms. Orthopaedic Update 1995; 5: 625–632.

3   National Advisory Committee on Core Health and Disability Services, Accident Rehabilitation and Compensation Insurance Corporation. Clinical Practice Guidelines. Acute Low Back Problems in Adults: Assessment and Treatment. Wellington: Core Services Committee, Ministry of Health (New Zealand), 1995.

4   Agency for Health Care Policy and Research. Acute Low Back Pain in Adults: Assessment and Treatment. US Department of Health and Human Services, Rockville, MD, 1994.

5   Hickey RFJ. Chronic low back pain: a comparison of diflunisal with paracetamol. NZ Med J 1982; 95: 312–314.

6   de Craen AJM, Di Giulio G, Lampe-Schoenmaeckers AJEM, Kessels AGH, Kleijnen J. Analgesic efficacy and safety of paracetamol–codeine combinations versus paracetamol alone: a systematic review. Br Med J 1996; 313: 321–325.

7   Brown FL, Bodison S, Dixon J, Davis W, Nowoslawski J. Comparison of diflunisal and acetaminophen with codeine in the treatment of initial or recurrent acute low back pain. Clin Ther 1986; 9 (Suppl C): 52–58.

8   Innes GD, Croskerry P, Worthington J, Beveridge R, Jones D. Ketorolac versus acetaminophen-codeine in the emergency department treatment of acute low back pain. J Emerg Med 1998; 16: 549–556.

9   Muncie HL, King DE, DeForge B. Treatment of mild to moderate pain of acute soft tissue injury: diflunisal vs acetaminophen with codeine. J Fam Pract 1986; 23: 125–127.

10 Kuntz D, Brossel R. Action antalgique et tolerance clinique de l'association paracetamol 500 mg–caffeine 50 mg versus paracetamol 400 mg dextropropoxyphene 30 mg dans les rachialgies. Presse Med 1996; 25: 1171–1174.

11 Evans DP, Burke MS, Newcombe RG. Medicines of choice in low back pain. Curr Med Res Opin 1980; 6: 540–547.

12 Koes BW, Scholten RJPM, Mens LMA, Bouter LM. Efficacy of non-steroidal anti-inflammatory drugs for low back pain: a systematic review of randomised clinical trials. Ann Rheum Dis 1997; 56: 214–223.

13 van Tulder MW, Koes BW, Bouter LM. Conservative treatment of acute and chronic nonspecific low back pain. A systematic review of randomized controlled trials of the most common interventions. Spine 1997; 22: 2128–2156.

14 van Tulder MW, Waddell G. Conservative treatment of acute and subacute low back pain. In: Nachemson A, Jonsson E (eds) Neck and Back Pain: The Scientific Evidence of Causes, Diagnosis, and Treatment. Lippincott, Williams and Wilkins, Philadelphia, PA, 2000: 241–269.

15 Amlie E, Weber H, Holme I. Treatment of acute low back pain with piroxicam: results of a double-blind placebo-controlled trial. Spine 1987; 12: 473–476.

16 Lacey PH, Dodd GD, Shannon DJ. A double-blind placebo controlled study of piroxicam in the management of acute musculoskeletal disorders. Eur J Rheumatol Inflamm 1984; 7: 95–104.

17 Pohjolainen T, Jekunen A, Autio L, Vuorela H. Treatment of acute low back pain with COX-2-selective anti-inflammatory drug nimesulide. Results of a randomised, double-blind comparative trial versus ibuprofen. Spine 2000; 25: 1579–1585.

18 National Health and Medical Research Council. Acute pain management: scientific evidence. NHMRC publication CP57, cat no: 9810211. Commonwealth of Australia, Canberra, 1998.

19 Turner JA, Denny MC. Do antidepressant medications relieve chronic low back pain? J Fam Pract 1993; 37: 545–553.

20 Alcoff J, Jones E, Rust P, Newman R. Controlled trial of imipramine for chronic low back pain. J Fam Pract 1982; 14: 841–846.

21 Pheasant H, Bursk A, Goldfarb J, Azen SP, Weiss JN, Borelli L. Amitriptyline and chronic low back pain. Spine 1983; 8: 552–557.

22 Goodkin K, Gullion CM, Agras W. A randomized, double-blind, placebo-controlled trial of trazodone hydrochloride in chronic low back pain syndrome. J Clin Psychopharmacol 1990; 10: 269–278.

23 Jenkins DG, Ebbutt AF, Evans CD. Tofranil in the treat-

ment of low back pain. J Int Med Res 1976; 4 (Suppl 2): 28–40.

24 Johnson EW. Editorial: The myth of skeletal muscle spasm. Am J Phys Med 1989; 68: 1.

25 Andersson G, Bogduk N et al. Muscle: clinical perspectives. In: Frymoyer JW, Gordon SL (eds) New Perspectives on Low Back Pain. American Academy of Orthopaedic Surgeons, Park Ridge, IL, 1989: 293–334.

26 Gold RH. Orphenadrine citrate: sedative or muscle relaxant? Clin Ther 1978; 1: 451–453.

27 Tervo T, Petaja L, Lepisto P. A controlled clinical trial of a muscle relaxant analgesic combination in the treatment of acute lumbago. Br J Clin Pract 1976; 30: 62–64.

28 Hingorani K. Diazepam in backache: a double-blind controlled trial. Ann Phys Med 1966; 8: 303–306.

29 Casale R. Acute low back pain: symptomatic treatment with a muscle relaxant drug. Clin J Pain 1988; 4: 81–88.

30 Hindle TH. Comparison of carisoprodol, butabarbital, and placebo in treatment of the law back syndrome. Calif Med 1972; 117: 7–11.

31 Middleton RSW. A comparison of two analgesic muscle relaxant combinations in acute back pain. Br J Gen Pract 1984; 38: 107–109.

32 Sweetman BJ, Baig A, Parsons DL. Mefenamic acid, chlormezanone–paracetamol, ethoheptazine–aspirin–meprobamate: a comparative study in acute low back pain. Br J Clin Pract 1987; 41: 619–624.

33 Berry H, Hutchinson DR. A multicentre placebo-controlled study in general practice to evaluate the efficacy and safety of tizanidine in acute low-back pain. J Int Med Res 1988; 16: 75–82.

34 Berry H, Hutchinson DR. Tizanidine and ibuprofen in acute low-back pain: results of a double-blind multicentre study in general practice. J Int Med Res 1988; 16: 83–91.

35 Dapas F, Hartman SF, Martinez L, Northrup BE, Nussdorf RT, Silberman HM, Gross H. Baclofen for the treatment of acute low-back syndrome: a double-blind comparison with placebo. Spine 1985; 10: 345–349.

36 Barratta RR. A double-blind study of cyclobenzaprine and placebo in the treatment of acute musculoskeletal conditions of the low back. Curr Ther Res 1982; 32: 646–652.

37 Borenstein DG, Lacks S, Wiesel SW. Cyclobenzaprine and naproxen versus naproxen alone in the treatment of acute low back pain and muscle spasm. Clin Ther 1990; 12: 125–131.

6. Exercise

Exercises have long been a mainstay of treatment for back pain, both acute and chronic. Their nature varies, and includes isometric exercises, endurance exercises, intensive exercises, graded exercises, flexion exercises, extension exercises, and exercises specific to certain presumed diagnoses. In the context of acute low back pain, however, the preoccupation with exercises is not supported by the evidence.

6.1. Rationale

An explicit rationale for exercises for back pain is hard to find in the literature. A convenient summary, however, is that of Jackson and Brown [1]. They maintain that exercises may be beneficial to decrease pain; strengthen weak muscles; decrease mechanical stress by stretching tight muscles; improve fitness; improve trunk mobility; and provide conditioning. These objectives fall into two groups — symptomatic and mechanical.

Quite clearly, but not overtly, exercises are prescribed if and because patients present with pain. Implicitly, exercises are supposed to benefit that pain, as if exercises are a form of analgesic. However, how exercises are supposed to decrease pain has never been explained; nor has it been unequivocally demonstrated that exercises per se do relieve pain (as opposed to other factors operant in an exercise programme).

This lack of relationship, and the failure of studies to show consistent or clinically significant relief of pain has generated a paradigm shift — that, whether or not exercises relieve pain, they at least can be shown to achieve mechanical changes.

Strengthening muscles, stretching tight muscles and improving fitness all seem laudable objectives, but their relationship to back pain is either unclear or elusive. Rather, the mechanical rationale for exercises is loosely based on observations from epidemiologic studies that show that, on average, patients with back pain tend to have weaker muscles and be less fit; but these relationships are far from absolute; the distributions of muscle strength and fitness in patients with and without back pain are great and overlap considerably. Furthermore, there are no compelling data that show that muscle weakness produces pain or that restoring strength relieves pain. There are no data that show that an examiner can reliably detect abnormally tight muscles. There are no data that show that lack of fitness causes pain, or that restoring fitness relieves pain.

There is no clear relationship between mobility and pain, other than patients with back pain are usually prevented by their pain from exhibiting an expected full range of motion. It has not been shown that lack of mobility causes pain and that, therefore, restoring mobility should relieve pain. Nevertheless, it is commonly believed that immobility is somehow deleterious for the back. This belief is based on the assumption that back pain implies some sort of injury, and that this injury must be allowed to heal, but by analogy with disorders of the appendicular skeleton, this healing must not be allowed in a position of rest for fear of developing painful stiffness; therefore, painful backs must be mobilised[2]. However, while so long as the causative lesion of back pain remains unknown, this principle is no more than a generic principle of musculoskeletal medicine that has been applied to the back without any concrete link to spinal pathophysiology.

At best, the available data allow that if muscles are strengthened and stretched, if mobility is restored and if fitness is improved, patients may also obtain relief of pain. However, the operant factor in this expected relationship is not known, and it is not entirely evident that exercises do benefit pain. In acute back pain, the passage of time and natural history may be the operant factor. These factors have bedevilled the empirical evaluation of the efficacy of exercises for back pain.

6.2. Efficacy

There have been four systematic reviews of exercises for back pain: one surveyed the literature from 1966 to 1990[3], a second completed the period 1991–1995[4]. The third review[5] covered 1975–1993. The most recent review covered the literature from 1966 to 1995[6].

The first review found four studies on acute back pain, one on subacute back pain, and seven on chronic back pain, and lamented the poor quality of research on this topic[3]. It concluded that:

"Despite its frequent application, exercise therapy has not been shown to be more efficacious than any other treatment modalities, nor has it been shown to be ineffective. There is little evidence in favour of a specific exercise regime."[3]

The second review found an additional 11 studies (four on acute back pain, one on subacute back pain, and six on chronic back pain)[4]. Studies with a better methodological score reported negative results. The few studies that reported positive results had low methodological scores. The review concluded that:

"In patients with acute back pain, exercise therapy is ineffective. The graded activity program with exercises in patients with subacute back pain and intensive extension exercises or fitness exercises in patients (with) chronic back pain deserves attention. There is a need for more research to clarify the efficacy of the McKenzie therapy and that of the different components of the graded activity program with exercises. Also, additional trials in patients with chronic back pain are needed in which fitness exercises are compared with intensive training."[4]

The third review[5] echoed the conclusions of the other reviews. It found that:

"For sudden, nonneurologic mild backache in a general population, there appears to be little benefit from an acute exercise program, particularly if patients can be guided to (return to work) on their own within 2 weeks."[5]

In the context of acute low back pain, the fourth review[6] found ten randomised controlled trials, two of high quality and eight of low quality. Seven trials, including the two high-quality studies, reported negative results. The review concluded that:

"There is strong evidence that exercise therapy is not more effective than other conservative treatments, including no intervention for acute low back pain."[6]

Contemporary authorities recommend exercises in order to maintain mobility and functional activity despite pain, while other interventions or natural history address the patient's pain[7]. In this regard, exercises are used not for muscle-specific reasons, but rather as the antithesis to bed rest or immobilisation[7–9].

Proponents of exercise therapy have criticised negative studies on the grounds that they did not specifically tailor the exercises used to the patients concerned or that the exercises were trivial [10–12]; but these proponents have not furnished evidence to justify their faith to others, and their criticisms have been answered [13].

Recent studies not covered by previous systematic reviews provide additional information concerning the efficacy of exercises.

One study compared McKenzie therapy with chiropractic manipulation and with an educational booklet [14]. The outcome measures used were pain score, the Roland Disability Scale, use of health care, and time lost from work. At 4 weeks and at 12 weeks after treatment, there were no significant differences in outcome between each of the groups, in any of the outcome measures. This study answers the call of the second systematic review above [4], which asked for more research to clarify the efficacy of McKenzie therapy.

The second study compared a programme of exercises with usual care [15]. The usual care consisted of treatment by a general practitioner, and referral to a physiotherapist in some cases. The index treatment consisted of eight, 1-hr sessions of stretching exercises, low impact aerobic exercises, and strengthening exercises aimed at all the main muscle groups. The overall aim was to encourage normal movement of the spine. Moreover, the exercises were undertaken according to cognitive–behavioural principles, encouraging self-reliance, and viewing the exercise classes as steps to increasing their own levels of activity. At 6 months and 1 year after treatment, improvement in the exercise group was some 80% greater with respect to disability scores, and some 25–50% greater with respect to pain scores.

Reservations that might be raised about this study are that the patients treated were not greatly disabled (a mean score of 6 on the 24 point Roland Disability Scale), and their mean improvement was 3 on this scale. Moreover, the patients did not specifically have acute back pain, but pain that had persisted for more than 4 weeks but less than 6 months. Nevertheless, the authors were modest in their recommendations, that their programme would suit patients who are not improving at 6 weeks after onset of back pain. Of note, is that the programme was not one of specific 'therapeutic' exercises, but general exercises conducted in a cognitive–behavioural manner to encourage activity.

Key points

- Therapeutic exercises are not effective and not indicated for acute low back pain.
- There may be grounds for using exercise as a means of maintaining mobility and avoiding a sick-role for patients, while natural history takes its course or other treatment is implemented.
- A supervised programme of general stretching, strengthening, and aerobic exercises, conducting in a cognitive–behavioural manner to encourage activity may be beneficial for patients who are not improving after 6 weeks of onset of low back pain.

References

1 Jackson CP, Brown MD. Is there a role for exercise in the treatment of patients with low back pain? Clin Orthop 1983; 179: 39–45.
2 Troup JDG, Videman T. Inactivity and the aetiopathogenesis of musculoskeletal disorders. Clin Biomech 1989; 4: 173–178.
3 Koes BW, Bouter LM, Beckerman H, van der Heijden GJMG, Knipschild PG. Physiotherapy exercises and back pain: a blinded review. Br Med J 1991; 302: 1572–1576.
4 Faas A. Exercises: which ones are worth trying, for which patients, and when? Spine 1996; 21: 2874–2879.
5 Scheer SJ, Radack KL, O'Brien DR. Randomized Controlled Trials in Industrial Low Back Pain Relating to return to Work. Part 1. Acute Interventions. Arch Phys

Med Rehabil 1995; 76: 966–973.

6   van Tulder MW, Koes BW, Bouter LM. Conservative treatment of acute and chronic nonspecific low back pain. A systematic review of randomized controlled trials of the most common interventions. Spine 1997; 22: 2128–2156.

7   Royal College of General Practitioners, Chartered Society of Physiotherapy, Osteopathic Association of Great Britain, British Chiropractic Association, National Back Pain Association. Clinical Guidelines for the Management of Acute Low Back Pain. Royal College of General Practitioners, London, 1996.

8   Lindstrom I, Ohlund C, Eek C, Wallin L, Peterson LE, Nachemson A. Mobility, strength, and fitness after a graded activity program for patients with subacute low back pain. Spine 1992; 17: 641–649.

9   Twomey L, Taylor J. Spine update: exercises and spinal manipulation in the treatment of low back pain. Spine 1995; 20: 615–619.

10   Mooney V. Letter to the Editor. Spine 1994; 19: 1101.

11   Van Dyke M. Letter to the Editor. Spine 1994; 19: 1101.

12   Bunch RW. Letter to the Editor. Spine 1994; 19: 1101–1103.

13   Faas A, Chavannes AW, van Eijk JThM, Gubbles JW. Spine 1994; 19: 1103–1104.

14   Cherkin DC, Deyo RA, Battie M, Street J, Barlow W. A comparison of physical therapy, chiropractic manipulation, and provision of an educational booklet for the treatment of patients with low back pain. New Engl J Med 1998; 339: 1021–1029.

15   Klaber Moffett J, Torgerson D, Bell-Syer S, Jackson D, Llewlyn-Phillips H, Farrin A, Barber J. Randomised controlled trial of exercise for low back pain: clinical outcomes, costs, and preferences. Br Med J 1999; 319: 279–283.

7. Manual therapy

Manual therapy is perhaps the most contentious and most bitterly contested treatment for low back pain. This arises because manual therapy is the principal therapeutic tool of several craft-groups. Manipulation is the hallmark of chiropractic therapy; it is the hallmark of certain groups within Physiotherapy and in Musculoskeletal Medicine. Within each group, there is a strong tradition of using manual therapy, and of belief in its efficacy. Each group is, therefore, sensitive to any suggestion that manual therapy may not work as well as it is professed to do.

Although manual therapy may include a variety of techniques and procedures, the two cardinal categories are manipulation and mobilisation, and these have been the ones most commonly and most extensively evaluated in the literature. Even so, the definition of each type of therapy lacks consensus. In essence, however,

> manipulation involves the sudden application of a single, forceful thrust to a region of the spine, ostensibly to a selected joint or joints in that region;

whereas

> mobilisation involves the systematic application of forces of progressively increasing magnitude, to a region of the spine, ostensibly to a selected joint or joints in that region.

These definitions describe, and are based on, what the therapist does. Other definitions based on what they believe they achieve — such "taking the joint beyond its physiological range of movement", or "within the joint's normal range of movement", cannot be objectively verified. These may be the intentions or the perceptions of the manipulative therapist, but there is no evidence on what constitutes the normal range of passive movement of spinal joints, and whether particular techniques exceed these or not.

Various expert panels have recommended that manual therapy be included in guidelines for the management of acute low back pain [1,2], but these recommendations seem to be based on a favourable interpretation of the literature, and possibly reflect how popular manual therapy is rather than how effective it actually is. Other guidelines have not recommended manual therapy for acute low back pain [3].

7.1. Efficacy

It has been found that the number of reviews of manipulation for back pain now exceed the number of original controlled trials [4]. Moreover, it has been found that the conclusions of pragmatic reviews are a function of the discipline of the author of the review [4].

Over the last 10 years, several systematic reviews have progressively modified their conclusions as new studies have appeared, and as older literature has been reappraised. The first major systematic review, published in 1991[5], commented on the generally poor quality of the literature, and concluded that: "so far the efficacy of manipulation has not been convincingly shown"[5]. The second systematic review, published in 1992[6], offered a statistical pooling of available results, and was more liberal in its conclusions. It found that, on the average, lumbar spinal manipulation for acute low back pain offered a 17% greater chance of more rapid recovery than usual. Thus, whereas manipulation did offer a benefit, its attributable effect was very modest. The third review, which appeared in 1996[7], reported that it could not find evidence in favour of manipulation in patients with acute low back pain. The authors explained their difference in conclusion from that of Shekelle et al.[6] on the basis of having included a greater number of trials.

A fourth review[8] concluded that:

"There is limited evidence that manipulation is more effective than a placebo treatment",

but

"There is no evidence that manipulation is more effective than (other) physiotherapeutic applications (massage, shortwave diathermy, exercises) or drug therapy (analgesics, NSAIDs) for acute low back pain, because of the contradictory results."[8]

The most recent review[9], published by the same team that produced the fourth review[8], offered a slightly modified conclusion that:

"There is moderate evidence that manipulation is more effective than a placebo treatment for short-term relief of acute low back pain",

but

"Because of inconsistent findings, it is not possible to judge whether manipulation is more effective than (other) physiotherapeutic applications (massage, short-wave diathermy, exercises) or drug therapy (analgesics, NSAIDs) for acute low back pain."[8]

None of these conclusions by systematic reviews can be construed as particularly complimentary or enthusiastic about manual therapy for acute low back pain, and the evidence seems to be dissonant with the enthusiasm and vigour with which manual therapy has been promoted in clinical practice.

A closer examination of the literature reveals how limited the evidence is for manual therapy. Table I lists all the literature covered by the most recent systematic reviews[10–28], but includes as well studies that those reviews did not cover[29], or that have been published since those reviews were prepared[30,31].

The table shows a polarisation. Successful outcomes have been reported largely by studies that assessed outcomes only at 5 or 7 days. So, there would appear to be immediate benefits of manual therapy. However, three of the four studies that reported benefits at this time, found them to apply only to certain subgroups of patients: those with pain that had been persistent for 2–4 weeks, in two studies[11,12]; and those with restricted straight leg-raising[13]. In other patients, those same studies found no superiority of manipulation over control.

Of studies that followed their patients for 2–4 weeks, six[16–20,29], found no benefit greater than control with respect to pain, range of motion, or general symptoms. The one positive study reported benefit only with respect to improved range of motion[21].

Four studies that followed patients for longer than 1 month found largely no greater benefit than control treatment[22,23,30,31]. The one exception found greater reduction in pain when manipulative therapy was compared with placebo, but this difference applied only at the 3-week follow-up, and was extinguished by the 2- and 4-month follow-up[23]. In that study, manipulative therapy was not found to be superior to other non-placebo controls, including bed rest[23].

Only one study that provided a long-term follow-up has shown a positive outcome. It compared manipulative therapy delivered by a medical practitioner with usual care[24–28]. At all follow-up periods, manipulative therapy was found to be superior to usual care in all outcome measures. Indeed, this is the only study that reported change in pain, proportion of patients completely relieved, sick-leave, use of other

TABLE I

The studies of manual therapy for acute low back pain, indicating the control used, the outcome measure used, and whether or not manual therapy was shown to be better than control at the follow-up time indicated

Study	Control used	Outcome measure	Follow-up											Comment
			Days		Weeks					Months				
			3	5	1	2	3	4	6	2	3	4	6	
DeLitto et al. [10]	exercise	disability	yes											
MacDonald and Bell [11]	exercise	recovery			yes									pain 2–4 weeks
Hadler et al. [12]	exercise	recovery			yes									pain 2–4 weeks
Matthews et al. [13]	heat	recovery			yes									SLR positive
Rasmussen [14]	SWD	recovery				yes								
MacDonald and Bell [11]	exercise	recovery			no									
Hadler et al. [12]	exercise	recovery			no									
Glover et al. [15]	detuned SWD	pain			no									
Matthews et al. [13]	heat	recovery			no									
Waterworth and Hunter [16]	SWD	pain				no								
Godfrey et al. [17]	massage	general				no								
Wreje et al. [18]	massage	pain					no							faster recovery
Farrell and Twomey [19]	exercise	pain, ROM					no							faster recovery
Pope et al. [29]	massage	pain, ROM					no							
	TMS	pain, ROM					no							
	Corset	pain, ROM					no							
Helliwell et al. [20]	analgesics	symptoms						no						
Nwuga [20]	SWD	range						yes						
Berquist-Ullman and Larsson [22]	physiotherapy	pain					no		no					faster recovery
Postacchini et al. [23]	placebo	pain					yes			no			no	
	bed rest	pain					no			no			no	
	physiotherapy	pain					no			no			no	
	drugs	pain					no			no			no	
Cherkin et al. [30]	exercise	pain, disability								no		no		
	booklet									no		no		
Andersson et al. [31]	usual care	pain, disability									no			
Blomberg and coworkers [24–28]	physiotherapy	pain								yes		yes	yes	

SWD = short wave diathermy, ROM = range of movement, SLR = straight leg raising.

health care, disability, and quality of life measures; and the only study that showed sustained improvements in these measures.

Of the studies that compared manipulative therapy with placebo [15,18,22,23], three did not show any greater effectiveness with respect to relief of pain [15,18,22]. When reviewers have used these studies to conclude that manipulative therapy is superior to placebo [8,9], the outcomes with respect to which this conclusion applies are mean number of days to recovery [22], reduced sick-leave at 3 weeks [18], and

greater reduction in pain at 3 weeks, but not subsequently at 2 and 6 months [23].

On balance, the data show that manipulative therapy is not superior to placebo or to other treatments for the relief of pain beyond 3 weeks after treatment. The one virtue of manual therapy might be that, in the short term, it brings about a more rapid recovery in some patients [11,12,18–21]; but in the longer term, it does not provide any significantly greater reduction of pain.

The one exception to this pattern is the demonstrated superiority of medical manipulative therapy over usual care[23-27]. However, the index treatment in the studies describing this result[23,27] consisted of more than manipulative therapy. It also involved stretching exercises and injections of corticosteroids. Although the authors felt that the manipulative therapy was the cardinal ingredient of their treatment, they recognised that its efficacy could not be dissected from the possible influences of the other interventions. Perhaps what the results show is that concerted treatment by a medical practitioner using a variety of physical and pharmacological interventions is superior to conventional care for acute low back pain (see Chapter 11).

If manual therapy is the major and effective component of combined therapy, it would seem that experience or comprehensive training is required to realise that effect. Providing primary care physicians with a short course in manual therapy achieves little improvement in outcomes[32]. A study that assessed the efficacy of teaching primary care practitioners a sequence of eight manual therapy techniques found that although a slightly greater proportion of patients achieved complete recovery, patients who received manual therapy did not exhibit a greater improvement in functional status, pain, or days lost from work[32].

Key points

- Manipulative therapy is not more effective than either placebo or other interventions for the relief of pain beyond 2 weeks after treatment.
- Manipulative therapy may accelerate recovery in the short-term, but offers no greater long-term gains.
- Manipulative therapy coupled with stretching exercises and steroid injections achieves greater long-term gains in pain, disability, quality of life, and sick-leave than usual care.

References

1 Agency for Health Care Policy and Research. Acute Low Back Pain in Adults: Assessment and Treatment. US Department of Health and Human Services, Rockville, MD, 1994.

2 Royal College of General Practitioners, Chartered Society of Physiotherapy, Osteopathic Association of Great Britain, British Chiropractic Association, National Back Pain Association. Clinical Guidelines for the Management of Acute Low Back Pain. Royal College of General Practitioners, London, 1996.

3 Faas A, Chavannes AW, Koes BW, van den Hoogen JMM, Mens JMA, Smeele IJM, Romeijnders ACM, van der Laan JR. NHG-Standaard 'Lage-Rugpijn'. Huisarts Wet 1996; 39: 18–31.

4 Assendelft WJJ, Koes BW, Knipschild PG, Bouter LM. The relationship between methodological quality and conclusions in reviews of spinal manipulation. J Am Med Assoc 1995; 274: 1942–1948.

5 Koes BW, Assendelft WJJ, van der Heijden GJMG, Bouter LM et al. Spinal manipulation and mobilisation for back and neck pain: a blinded review. Br Med J 1991; 303: 1298–1303.

6 Shekelle PG, Adams AH, Chassin MR, Hurwitz EL, Brook RH. Spinal manipulation for low back pain. Ann Int Med 1992; 117: 590–598.

7 Koes BW, Assendelft WJJ, van der Heijden GJMG, Bouter LM. Spinal manipulation for low back pain: an updated systematic review of randomized clinical trials. Spine 1996; 21: 2860–2873.

8 van Tulder MW, Koes BW, Bouter LM. Conservative treatment of acute and chronic nonspecific low back pain. A systematic review of randomized controlled trials of the most common interventions. Spine 1997; 22: 2128–2156.

9 van Tulder MW, Waddell G. Conservative treatment of acute and subacute low back pain. In: Nachemson A, Jonsson E (eds) Neck and Back Pain: The Scientific Evidence of Causes, Diagnosis, and Treatment. Lippincott, Williams and Wilkins, Philadelphia, 2000: 241–269.

10 Delitto A, Cibulka MT, Erhard RE, Bowling RW, Tenhula JA. Evidence for use of an extension–mobilization category in acute low back syndrome: a prescriptive validation pilot study. Phys Ther 1993; 73: 216–228.

11 MacDonald RS, Bell CMJ. An open controlled assessment of osteopathic manipulation in non-specific low-back pain. Spine 1990; 15: 354–370.

12 Hadler NM, Curtis P, Gillings DB, Stinnett S. A benefit of spinal manipulation as adjunctive therapy for acute

low-back pain: a stratified controlled trial. Spine 1987; 12: 703–705.

13 Mathews W. Morkel M, Mathews J. Manipulation and traction for lumbago and sciatica: physiotherapeutic techniques used in two controlled trials. Physiother Pract 1988; 4: 201–206.

14 Rasmussen GG. Manipulation in treatment of low-back pain: a randomised clinical trial. Man Med 1979; 1: 8–10.

15 Glover JR, Morris JG, Khosla T. Back pain: a randomized clinical trial of rotational manipulation of the trunk. Br J Ind Med 1974; 31: 59–64.

16 Waterworth RF, Hunter IA. An open study of diflunisal, conservative and manipulative therapy in the management of acute mechanical low back pain. NZ Med J 1985; 98: 372–375.

17 Godfrey CM, Morgan PP, Schatzker J. A randomised trial of manipulation for low-back pain in a medical setting. Spine 1984; 9: 301–304.

18 Wreje U, Nordgren B, Aberg H. Treatment of pelvic joint dysfunction in primary care: a controlled study. Scand J Prim Care 1992; 10: 310–315.

19 Farrell JP, Twomey LT. Acute low back pain: comparison of two conservative treatment approaches. Med J Aust 1982; 1: 160–164.

20 Helliwel PS, Cunliffer G. Manipulation in low-back pain. Physician 1987; April: 187–188.

21 Nwuga VCB. Relative therapeutic efficacy of vertebral manipulation and conventional treatment in back pain management. Am J Phys Med 1982; 61: 273–278.

22 Bergquist-Ullman M, Larsson U. Acute low back pain in industry. Acta Orthop Scand 1977; Suppl 170.

23 Postacchini F, Facchini M, Palieri P. Efficacy of various forms of conservative treatment in low back pain. A comparative study. Neuro-Orthopedics 1988; 6: 28–35.

24 Blomberg S, Svardsudd K, Mildenberger F. A controlled, multicentre trial of manual therapy in low-back pain; initial status, sick-leave and pain score during follow-up. Scand J Prim Health Care 1992; 10: 170–178.

25 Blomberg S, Svardsudd K, Tibblin G. Manual therapy with steroid injections in low-back pain: improvement of quality of life in a controlled trial with four months' follow-up. Scand J Prim Health Care 1993; 11: 83–90.

26 Blomberg S, Tibbin G. A controlled, multicentre trial of manual therapy with steroid injections in low-back pain: functional variable, side-effects and complications during four months follow-up. Clin Rehabil 1993; 7: 49–62.

27 Blomberg S, Hallin G, Grann K, Berg E, Sennerby U. Manual therapy with steroid injections — a new approach to treatment of low back pain: a controlled multicenter trial with an evaluation by orthopedic surgeons. Spine 1994; 19: 569–577.

28 Blomberg S, Svardsudd K, Tibbin G. A randomised study of manual therapy with steroid injections in low-back pain: telephone interview follow-up of pain, disability, recovery and drug consumption. Eur Spine J 1994; 3: 246–254.

29 Pope MH, Phillips RB, Haugh LD, Hsieh CYJ, MacDonald L, Haldeman S. A prospective randomised 3-week trial of spinal manipulation, transcutaneous muscle stimulation, massage and corset in the treatment of subacute low back pain. Spine 1994; 19: 2571–2577.

30 Cherkin DC, Deyo RA, Battie M, Street J, Barlow W. A comparison of physical therapy, chiropractic manipulation, and provision of an educational booklet for the treatment of patients with low back pain. New Engl J Med 1998; 339: 1021–1029.

31 Andersson GBJ, Lucente T, Davis AM, Kappler RE, Lipton JA, Leurgans S. A comparison of osteopathic spinal manipulation with standard care for patients with low back pain. New Engl J Med 1999; 341: 1426–1431.

32 Curtis P, Carey TS, Evans P, Rowane MP, Garrett JM, Jackman A. Training primary care physicians to give limited manual therapy for low back pain. Patient outcomes. Spine 2000; 25: 2954–2961.

8. Patient education

Some authorities [1] believe that patient education, by way of pamphlets or booklets, is a desirable, but neglected, component of medical management of back pain. The objective is to empower the patient by providing them with information so that they have the appropriate insight to be able to take a greater responsibility for their own care, and thereby to rely less on passive medical therapy.

In the context of low back pain, patient education should be distinguished from back school (see Section 10). The latter is a formal, structured process of education involving classes and regular, repeated, direct contact with an instructor. In contrast, patient education is a less structured process characterised more by the issue of printed information than the use of repeated, face-to-face classes.

8.1. Efficacy

Several controlled studies have assessed the efficacy of patient education for acute low back pain. Collectively, they paint a picture of limited effectiveness, if any, of this intervention.

One study compared the outcomes of four groups of patients with acute back pain attending general practices [2]. The groups were treated with: (1) bed rest, exercises, and education consisting of a tape–slide presentation and a two-page printed summary;

(2) exercises and education; (3) bed rest only; and (4) no intervention. No differences in outcome were detected between any of the groups with respect to pain or physical activities. Indeed, the impression was that exercises and education were doing more harm than good.

A study of patients with acute or chronic back pain attending general practices explicitly evaluated the issue of a 21-page booklet compared to no issue of information [3]. It found no differences with respect to absence from work, and referrals for physiotherapy, hospital care or laminectomy; but it did report a significant reduction in the number of consultations for back pain during the ensuing 1 year. This result has been heralded as positive in favour of the use of booklets [4], but close inspection of the data is sobering. The significant reduction was derived from a X^2-squared analysis of a table listing the number of patients in each treatment group who consulted zero, one, two, three, four and more than four times in the year. The difference was indeed significant, but not uniform in direction. The intervention group showed a reduction of 10–30% in using zero, one, two, and three consultations, but an increase of 3–13% of four or more than four consultations. Thus, in addition to being not uniform, the reported 'reduction' was modest, at best. Some 84% of the patients found the booklet useful, but only 68% still had a copy at 1-year follow-up.

A study in a Health Maintenance Organization [5] compared usual care, an educational booklet, and the educational booklet coupled with a 15-min session with a clinic nurse. The nurse intervention resulted in higher patient satisfaction and higher perceived knowledge, but otherwise the groups did not differ with respect to worry, symptoms, functional status or health-care use at 1, 3, 7, and 52 weeks after intervention.

A study of the impact of an educational booklet addressing the behavioural differences between 'confronters' and 'avoiders' found significant improvements in beliefs amongst workers who did not have back pain, but not amongst workers affected by back pain [6]. However, absenteeism appeared to be significantly reduced in the intervention group during the year of intervention.

While not proving the efficacy of a patient education booklet, the study of Cherkin et al. [7] showed that provision of a booklet was no less effective for the management of acute low back pain than chiropractic manipulation or McKenzie therapy, and was considerably less expensive.

Despite the lack of positive evidence, guidelines authorities have maintained that an educational booklet is nonetheless useful in the management of acute back pain [1,8]. British authorities credit that booklets are relatively weak interventions, but claim that they are effective when they are part of an integrated package [4]. They also serve to standardise information given to patients by different physicians, and thereby reduce confusion. Booklets are perceived as a useful adjunct to the physician's message [4].

A recent study, however, challenges this belief. The study [9] compared the efficacy of providing advice to exercise, providing an information booklet, and providing both a booklet and advice to exercise. A control group received advice to stay active and analgesics. The patients who received advice to exercise and those who received the booklet each achieved slightly greater improvements in their pain than did the control group. The difference from control amounted to between 2 and 9 points on a 100-point scale. Paradoxically, the group who received *both* the booklet and advice to exercise showed no greater improvement than the control group, and ipso facto, had less improvement than either group who received only advice to exercise or only the booklet. Thus, whereas a booklet or advice to exercise, can achieve slightly better outcomes, adding a booklet to advice confers no benefit.

When education booklets were supplemented by instructional videos on back self-management and on exercises, together with four 2-hr classes conducted by a lay person, patients reported less disability and significantly less worry about back pain, at 6 and 12 months after treatment [10].

Key points

- Patient education booklets have little or no effect on the symptoms and resulting disability of acute low back pain.
- Nevertheless, patient education booklets are no less effective than some forms of passive intervention, and are considerably less expensive.
- They may achieve increased patient satisfaction, reduced use of health care, and reduced absenteeism.
- Patient education provided by a lay-person may help patients worry less about their back pain, and be slightly less disabled.

References

1   Royal College of General Practitioners, Chartered Society of Physiotherapy, Osteopathic Association of Great Britain, British Chiropractic Association, National Back Pain Association. Clinical Guidelines for the Management of Acute Low Back Pain. Royal College of General Practitioners, London, 1996.

2   Gilbert JR, Taylor DW, Hildebrand A, Evans C. Clinical trial of common treatments for low back pain in family practice. Br Med J 1985; 291: 791–794.

3   Roland M, Dixon M. Randomized controlled trial of an educational booklet for patients presenting with back pain in general practice. J Roy Coll Gen Pract 1989; 39: 244–246.

4   Burton AK, Waddell G, Burtt R, Blair S. Patient educational material in the management of low back pain in primary care. Bull Hosp Joint Dis 1996; 55: 138–141.

5   Cherkin DC, Deyo RA, Street JH, Hunt M, Barlow W. Pitfalls of patient education. Limited success of a program for back pain in primary care. Spine 1996; 21: 345–355.

6   Symonds TL, Burton AK, Tilotson KM, Main CJ. Absence resulting from low back trouble can be reduced by psychosocial intervention at the work place. Spine 1995; 20: 2738–2745.

7   Cherkin DC, Deyo RA, Battie M, Street J, Barlow W. A comparison of physical therapy, chiropractic manipulation, and provision of an educational booklet for the treatment of patients with low back pain. New Engl J Med 1998; 339: 1021–1029.

8   Agency for Health Care Policy and Research. Acute Low Back Pain in Adults: Assessment and Treatment. US Department of Health and Human Services, Rockville, 1994.

9   Little P, Roberts L, Blowers H, Garwood J, Cantrell T, Langridge J, Chapman J. Should we give detailed advice and information booklets to patients with back pain? A randomized controlled factorial trial of a self-management booklet and doctor advice to take exercise for back pain. Spine 2001; 26: 2065–2072.

10 Von Korff M, Moore JE, Lorig K, Cherkin DC, Saunders K, Gonzalez, L, Rutter C, Comite F. A randomized trial of a lay person-led self-management group intervention for back pain patients in primary care. Spine 1998; 23:2608–2615.

9. Functional Restoration

Functional Restoration is a programme of management of back pain, based on sports medicine principles, in which the complaint of pain is essentially disregarded, and management instead focuses on improving the patient's capacity for movement and for tasks specific to their occupation. A hallmark of the programme is the use of back-testing machines to monitor objectively changes in range of movement and muscle strength, with regular provision of feedback of gains to the patient.

A typical programme requires a 3-week live-in period with activities for 57 hours/week, involving specific exercises, work-simulation and work-hardening, coupled with education and cognitive–behavioural training [1].

9.1. Efficacy

There have been no trials of Functional Restoration for acute low back pain. Such data as do obtain relate only to chronic low back pain. Yet even for chronic back pain, the data are conflicting (see Chapter 17). Therefore, there is no basis in evidence for recommended formal, functional restoration programmes for acute low back pain. There is, however, some evidence to support a program that is similar in some respects to Functional Restoration.

This intervention has been popularised in Sweden for the management of *subacute* low back pain. It involves

- measurements of functional capacity, mobility, fitness and strength;
- graded exercises, prescribed and supervised by a physical therapist, in accordance with the patient's capacity and personal work demands, undertaken in an operant conditioning manner i.e. rewarding and praising progress and gains;
- a workplace visit; and
- back school.

This program differs from classical Functional Restoration in not relying on machines to measure functional capacity; in relying on a single therapist instead of a team; and not including formal psychological intervention. It is essentially a simplified functional restoration program.

Graded activity has been assessed in a single randomised, controlled study, with different aspects having been reported in different publications [2,3]. At 1 year after treatment, when compared with those treated under usual care, patients treated with graded activity exhibited greater spinal mobility, greater strength and greater fitness; they returned to work some 5 weeks sooner, and spent 8 weeks less per year on sick leave [2]. Their average pain scores and pain behaviours were not different to those of patients treated under usual care, but they were subjectively less disabled, and a smaller proportion of patients (53% vs 80%) still complained of pain [3].

These data indicate that a graded activity program may be appropriate for patients who fail to respond to early management of acute low back pain. It should be noted that any efficacy of graded activity seems to be pertinent only to subacute back pain. When similar programs have been applied to patients with acute low back pain, the results achieved were no better than those achieved by usual care [4].

Key points

- For patients with subacute back pain, a graded activity program under operant conditioning, coupled with a workplace visit, may assist patients to return to work in a fitter and less disabled state.

References

1   Mayer TG, Gatchel RJ, Kishino N, Keeley J, Capra P, Mayer H, Barnett J, Mooney V. Objective assessment of spine function following industrial injury. A prospective study with comparison group and one-year follow-up. Spine 1985; 10: 482–493.
2   Lindstrom I, Ohlund C, Eek C, Wallin L, Peterson LE, Nachemson A. Mobility, strength, and fitness after a graded activity program for patients with subacute low back pain. A randomized prospective clinical study with a behavioural therapy approach. Spine 1992; 17: 641–649.
3   Lindstrom I, Ohlund C, Nachemson A. physical performance, pain, pain behavior and subjective disability in patients with subacute low-back pain. Scand J Rehab Med 1995; 27: 153–160.
4   Sinclair SJ, Hogg-Johnson S, Mondloch MV, Shields SA. The effectiveness of an early active intervention program for workers with soft-tissue injuries. The early claimant cohort study. Spine 1997; 22: 2919–2931.

10. Back school

Back school is a course of instruction aimed at providing patients with a better understanding of their problems, and at helping patients take responsibility for their pain, while relieving their pain and functional disability [1,2]. It involves face-to-face interaction with patients in classroom-like settings.

10.1. Efficacy

The original study of back school [1] reported significant improvements over control in only one parameter — the prevalence of sick leave longer than 21 days. Why 21 days was chosen as the critical marker was not explained. No significant differences in sick leave were reported at times shorter or longer than 21 days. Nor were there any differences with respect to pain or with respect to recurrences, duration of recurrences of back pain, duration of absences, or the development of chronicity.

Despite these meagre results, back school was strongly popularised [2–4], and defended [5]. Subsequent studies yielded conflicting results and a mixture of confounding influences.

A pragmatic review [6], published in 1987, described 15 studies, of which, those with no controls reported favourable or encouraging results, but those in which some form of control or comparison was used found no advantage for back school.

A systematic review, published in 1994 [7], identified 15 controlled studies and found them to vary considerably in methodological quality. Four of these studies explicitly addressed acute low back pain. A subsequent systematic review from the same group [8] covered the same literature. One of the four stud-

ies found back school to be no more effective than advice not to strain and to use analgesics when needed [9]. Another found back school to be less effective than McKenzie exercises [10]. A third study was poorly reported; it did not indicate the nature of the control treatment or the number of patients treated [11]. The fourth study was the original study of back school, in which there was no greater improvement in pain, recurrences, duration of absences, or the development of chronicity [1]. The review concluded that "there is no evidence that a back school is effective for acute low back pain, because of contradictory results" [8].

A study not covered by these reviews provided further evidence for the lack of efficacy of back school for acute low back pain. Adding back school to standard care offered no significant advantage in terms of pain, disability, spinal function, return to work, absenteeism or recurrence [12].

Key points

- There is no evidence that back school is a worthwhile intervention for acute low back pain.
- There is evidence that back school offers no advantages in terms of pain, disability, recurrences and return to work.

References

1 Bergquist-Ullman M, Larsson U. Acute low back pain in industry. Acta Orthop Scand 1977; Suppl 170.
2 Forssell MZ. The back school. Spine 1981; 6: 104–106.
3 Hall H. Back school (an overview with reference to the Canadian Back Education Units). Clin Orthop 1983; 179: 10–17.
4 Matmiller AW. The Californian back school. Physiotherapy 1980; 66: 118–122.
5 Hall H, Hadler NM. Controversy. Low back school: education or exercise? Spine 1995; 20: 1097–1098.
6 Linton SJ, Kamwendo K. Low back schools: a critical review. Phys Ther 1987; 67: 1375–1383.
7 Koes BW, van Tulder MW, van der Windt DAWM, Bouter LM. The efficacy of back schools: a review of randomized clinical trials. J Clin Epidemiol 1994; 47: 851–862.
8 van Tulder MW, Koes BW, Bouter LM. Conservative treatment of acute and chronic nonspecific low back pain. A systematic review of randomized controlled trials of the

most common interventions. Spine 1997; 22: 2128–2156.
9 Lindequist S, Lundberg B, Wikmark R, Bergstad, Loof G, Ottermark AC. Information and regime at low back pain. Scand J Rehab Med 1984; 16: 113–116.
10 Stankovic R, Johnell O. Conservative treatment of acute low-back pain. A prospective randomised trial: McKenzie method of treatment versus patient education in mini-back school. Spine 1990; 15: 120–123.
11 Morrison GEC, Chase W, Young V, Roberts WL. Back pain. Treatment and prevention in a community hospital. Arch Phys Med Rehabil 1988; 69: 605–609.
12 LeClaire R, Esdaile JM, Suissa S, Rossignol M, Proulx R, Dupuis M. Back school in a first episode of compensated acute low back pain: a clinical trial to assess efficacy and prevent relapse. Arch Phys Med Rehabil 1996; 77: 673–679.

11. Behavioural therapy

Anxiety and depression are classical psychological symptoms that occur commonly, if not regularly, as a result of chronic pain[1]. They arise early in the evolution of back pain, being established during the acute phase; and persist at similar levels, without deterioration, into the chronic phase[2,3]. However, rather than anxiety and depression, frustration is the cardinal psychological distress reported by patients with acute low back pain[2]. This is accompanied by a variety of behavioural and cognitive responses that contribute to the patient's disability[3].

Recognition of the contribution that psychological factors make to the disability associated with back pain served as the impetus for behavioural interventions. In particular, the fear–avoidance model (Chapter 5) predicts that behavioural therapy should reduce this disability.

Two main types of behavioural therapy have been used for back pain — operant conditioning and cognitive therapy. At times, therapists have used a combination of both.

11.1. Operant conditioning

Operant conditioning addresses maladaptive behaviours. It aims to reduce or eliminate pain behaviours, and to restore well behaviours. This is achieved by changing reinforcement patterns[4]. Attention is given for health-related activity, whereas pain behaviours are met with inattention.

Part of the process is time-contingent prescription of medication, exercises and rest, as opposed to pain-contingent use. Medications are permitted at regular but set times, but not on demand. Exercise targets are set and must be met. Rest and attention are used to reinforce meeting exercise targets; but are withheld for failure to meet the quota[4]. Graphs and records are maintained to provide patients with feedback on progress. The spouse and family members are also made aware of how they reinforce pain behaviours, and are trained in how to avoid doing so, and in how to reinforce well behaviours.

11.2. Cognitive therapy

Cognitive therapy addresses how patients cope with their pain. Coping involves both what a person does and what they think and say to themselves[2]. Although there are many variants of cognitive therapy, they have in common:

- the assumption that an individual's feelings and behaviours are influenced greatly by their thoughts;
- the use of structured techniques to help patients identify, monitor, and change maladaptive thoughts, feelings, and behaviours; and
- an emphasis on teaching skills that patients can apply to a wide variety of problems[5].

Three basic phases of cognitive therapy have been identified[4].

(1) Patients are taught to reconceptualise pain by emphasising how pain can be controlled through thoughts, feelings, and beliefs. The patient is taught to modify their appraisal of their environment and to manage stress more effectively. To this end, the patient must not only know what to do but also must believe that they are capable of applying the necessary skills. A person's belief in their own effectiveness will determine whether they will try to cope, or they will avoid situations that they view as beyond their capability.

(2) Patients are taught skills such as relaxation, use of imagery, and attention diversion that they can use to cope with exacerbations of their pain, or the day-to-day pain itself.

(3) Patients are trained to practice and consolidate what is taught, with special attention to situations that could lead to relapse.

11.3. Efficacy

Despite its popularity for the management of chronic low back pain, few controlled studies have assessed behavioural therapy for acute low back pain. A systematic review[4] found that there was no evidence on the effectiveness of behavioural therapy for acute low back pain. A subsequent review[5] identified one study[6], upon which the review concluded that there is limited evidence that behavioural therapy may be effective for acute low back pain[5].

The study cited[6] has been promoted as the definitive study of operant conditioning for acute low back pain. The methods section of the report, however, reveals that it was not a study of operant conditioning in that neither of the study groups underwent changes in reinforcement. Rather, it was a study of the merits of time-contingent versus pain-contingent prescription of analgesic, exercises, and activity limits. No differences were found at 6 weeks after treatment, but differences emerged at 12 months. The patients treated by time-contingent strategies fared significantly better with respect to health care utilisation, claimed impairment, pain drawings, and being overall well, but not with respect to vocational status or activity level. The improvements, however, were modest — ranging between 22% and 35%, on average.

Although not cited in the earlier review[4], another study[7] was included in the later review[5], but not in the context of behavioural therapy, but as evidence for the efficacy of activity. That study[7], however, compared combinations of two approaches and two interventions. Patients were either allowed to "let pain be their guide" or to follow a graded, gradual reactivation programme. Each group further received either behavioural counselling limited to explanations of how the rehabilitation process was to be applied to their particular lives, or control counselling which was a non-directive discussion. There were no significant differences between groups with respect to any outcome measure at 6 months.

A more recent study[8], not yet covered by any systematic reviews, assessed the efficacy of a behavioural intervention. The intervention consisted of two 2-hr group sessions supplemented by an individualised interview. The groups were given instruction in back anatomy, 'red flags', factors contributing to fluctuations in pain, pacing of exercises and activity, basics of posture and body mechanics, cognitive restructuring, handling back pain flare-ups, and work-ing with health-care providers. These measures were reinforced by a back-care book and a videotape that emphasised resuming normal activities.

The outcomes of the intervention group were compared with those patients treated under usual care, and were assessed at 3, 6, and 12 months. In the self-care group, pain intensity was some 10% less than in the usual care group at 3 and at 6 months, but there was no difference at 12 months. The self-care group was less disabled at 3 months but not at 6 or 12 months. The self-care group reported less interference with activities at 3 and 6 months, and had fewer worries and lower scores on the fear–avoidance scale at all follow-up periods. The differences in outcome, when they did occur, were only about 20% in favour of the self-care group.

These results show that a brief cognitive–behavioural intervention can be modestly effective in reducing worries about back pain and reducing fears. Effects on other outcomes were limited in magnitude and duration.

11.4. Discussion

The study of Moore et al.[8] provides the most encouraging data, to date, for behavioural therapy for acute low back pain. In many respects, the intervention provided is consistent with the New Zealand Guidelines for acute low back pain[9]. These guidelines recommend a governing principle to the effect that:

> "What can be done to help this person experience less distress and disability?"

Specific interventions[9] require the doctor to:

- regularly review the patient's progress;
- acknowledge any difficulties the patient has in maintaining activity of daily living and in resuming work;
- be encouraging and helpful in these respects;
- maintain positive co-operation between the patient and their employer;
- explain that having more time off work will reduce the likelihood of successful return to work;

- promote self-management and self-responsibility;
- provide incentives and feedback.

To this list may be added ergonomic advice that enables the patient to undertake, or persevere with, activities in a manner that does not aggravate their pain, but for which the patient's native approach is inappropriate or counter-productive; i.e. new or better ways of doing things when the old ways seem to threaten aggravation of pain.

Others have also followed similar guidelines. Indahl et al.[10] emphasised explanation, reassurance, return to work, and self-management, and achieved major and sustained reductions in work disability. The Australian National Musculoskeletal Medicine Initiative[11] employed the same principles, and achieved major improvements in pain and disability, less chronicity, and fewer recurrences (Chapter 11). In both instances, a form of behavioural

intervention was paramount in the treatment, but it was not formal behavioural therapy, in the sense either that it was called operant conditioning or cognitive therapy, or that it was delivered by a psychologist. The intervention was provided by a physiatrist in the first study, and by primary care practitioners in the second instance. In these physician-led interventions, the behavioural intervention was incorporated seamlessly with physical interventions, in which the physician personally instructed the patient in exercises and activities, and with the physician personally encouraging return to work. In contrast, Moore et al.[8] seem to have relied on their book and videotape to cover these dimensions of the patients' rehabilitation. It may be that greater personal involvement in all aspects of the patient's rehabilitation, not just their behavioural problems, is critical to achieving greater outcomes.

Key points

- There is little evidence of effectiveness for behavioural therapy for acute low back pain.
- Behavioural therapy may be modestly more effective than usual care in reducing worries and fears.
- Without resorting to formal psychological intervention, the principles of behavioural therapy can be successfully integrated, to good effect, into a comprehensive medical rehabilitation program delivered by a single practitioner, with an emphasis on reducing fears and resuming activity.

References

1 Gamsa A. Is emotional disturbance a precipitator or a consequence of chronic pain? Pain 1990; 42: 183–195.
2 Philips HC, Grant L. Acute back pain: a psychological analysis. Behav Res Ther 1991; 29: 429–434.
3 Philips HC, Grant L. The evolution of chronic back pain problems: a longitudinal study. Behav Res Ther 1991; 29: 435–441.
4 van Tulder MW, Koes BW, Bouter LM. Conservative treatment of acute and chronic nonspecific low back pain. A systematic review of randomized controlled trials of the most common interventions. Spine 1997; 22: 2128–2156.
5 van Tulder MW, Waddell G. Conservative treatment of acute and subacute low back pain. In: Nachemson A, Jonsson E (eds) Neck and Back Pain: The Scientific Evidence of Causes, Diagnosis, and Treatment. Lippincott, Williams and Wilkins, Philadelphia, PA, 2000: 241–269.
6 Fordyce WE, Brockway JA, Bergman JA, Spengler D. Acute back pain: a control-group comparison of behavioural vs traditional management methods. J Behav Med 1986; 9: 127–140.
7 Philips HC, Grant L, Berkowitz J. The prevention of chronic pain and disability: a preliminary investigation. Behav Res Ther 1991; 29: 443–450.
8 Moore JE, Von Korff M, Cherkin D, Saunders K, Lorig K. A randomised trial of a cognitive–behavioural program for enhancing back pain self care in a primary setting. Pain 2000; 88: 145–153.
9 Kendall NAS, Linton SJ, Main CJ. Guide to Assessing Psychosocial Yellow Flags in Acute Low Back Pain: Risk Factors for Long-term Disability and Work Loss. Accident Rehabilitation and Compensation Insurance Corporation of New Zealand and the National Health Committee, Wellington, 1997.
10 Indahl A, Velund L, Reikeraas O. Good prognosis for low back pain when left untampered: a randomized clinical

trial. Spine 1995; 20: 473–477.
11 McGuirk B, King W, Govind J, Lowry J, Bogduk N. The Safety, Efficacy, and Cost-Effectiveness of Evidence-Based Guidelines for the Management of Acute Low Back Pain in Primary Care. Spine 2001; 26: 2615–2622.

12. Belts and corsets

Corsets and similar orthoses have been an arcane but traditional intervention for low back pain. Biomechanics studies have shown that wearing belts does reduce flexion–extension and lateral bending of the lumbar spine to a moderate extent, but has no effect on rotation, electromyographic activity of the back muscles, or intra-abdominal pressure [1].

Evidence of the efficacy of belts and corsets for acute low back pain is elusive. Such studies as have been conducted have addressed chronic low back pain or mixed populations of patients with acute, subacute, and chronic low back pain.

An early systematic review [2] was somewhat encouraging in its conclusions, reporting that: "the efficacy of orthoses for treating low-back pain remains controversial, although there are some promising results in the literature". Closer examination of the literature reveals that of three trials that included patients with acute low back pain, two found negative results [3,4]. The one positive study reported that patients who wore orthoses improved more than patients treated with advice alone [5].

A subsequent review [6], involving one of the authors of the earlier review [2], made no mention of belts and corsets for acute low back pain. A later review [7] cited no literature, but explicitly concluded that there is no evidence available on the use of lumbar corsets of back belts in acute low back pain.

A very large, prospective study found that neither wearing back belts nor having a policy that required belt use reduced the incidence of back injury claims or low back pain [8].

Key point
- Belts and corsets are not indicated for the management of acute low back pain.

References

1 van Poppel MNM, de Looze MP, Koes BW, Smid T, Bouter LM. Mechanism of action of lumbar supports: a systematic review. Spine 2000; 25: 2103–2113.
2 Koes BW, van den Hoogen HMM. Efficacy of bed rest and orthoses of low-back pain. A review of randomized clinical trials. Eur J Phys Med Rehabil 1994; 4: 86–93.
3 Doran DM, Newel DJ. Manipulation in treatment of low-back pain: a multicentre study. Br Med J 1975; 2: 161–164.
4 Hsieh CJ, Phillips RB, Adams AH, Pope MH. Functional outcomes of low-back pain: comparison of four treatment groups in a randomized controlled trial. J Manip Physiol Ther 1992; 15: 4–9.
5 Valle-Jones JC, Walsh H, O'Hara J, O'Hara H, Davey NB, Hopkin-Richards H. Controlled trial of a back support (Lumbotrain) in patients with non-specific low-back pain. Curr Med Res Opin 1992; 12: 604–612.
6 van Tulder MW, Koes BW, Bouter LM. Conservative treatment of acute and chronic nonspecific low back pain. A systematic review of randomized controlled trials of the most common interventions. Spine 1997; 22: 2128–2156.
7 van Tulder MW, Waddell G. Conservative treatment of acute and subacute low back pain. In: Nachemson A, Jonsson E (eds) Neck and Back Pain: The Scientific Evidence of Causes, Diagnosis, and Treatment. Lippincott, Williams and Wilkins, Philadelphia, PA, 2000: 241–269.
8 Wassell JT, Gardner LI, Landsittel DP, Johnston JJ, Johnston JM. A prospective study of back belts for prevention of back pain and injury. J Am Med Assoc 2000; 284: 2727–2732.

13. Traction

Traction is a traditional treatment for low back pain that has increasingly lost favour, as international authorities have decried passive treatments, and pressed for activation and self-rehabilitation. Furthermore, as traction has been subjected to scrutiny its rationale has proved elusive.

13.1. Rationale

There is clear evidence that spinal traction separates vertebral bodies. However, in the lumbar spine, much of the separation observed arises from flattening of the lumbar lordosis [1]. Furthermore, there is no reason to believe that any biomechanical effect of traction persists once the traction is released and the patient resumes an upright posture For example, in one small study, although traction did reduce disc herniations in two of three patients, the protrusions reappeared within 14 min after release of the force [2].

When traction is used to treat radicular pain, the implicit mechanism is decompression of the affected spinal nerve. However, since compression of spinal nerves is not a mechanism for back pain, decompression cannot be the rationale for the use of traction for back pain.

It has been proposed that perhaps spinal pain might be relieved by "increasing non-nociceptive input and recruitment of descending inhibition" [3]. While perhaps attractive as a conjecture, such a statement falls short of actually constituting evidence of how traction might relieve spinal pain. The nature and source of the 'non-nociceptive input' is not specified. Such explanations reflect a treatment looking for a rationale, and presuppose that the treatment actually does work. Another proposition is that traction serves to stretch spinal tissues [3], but in that event, it is questionable whether elaborate and passive traction offers any advantage to simple stretching exercises that patients can undertake, themselves.

Some proponents argue that traction decreases intervertebral disc pressure [4]. The data to this effect, however, are limited and conflicting. In less than a handful of cases, one study showed a decrease in disc pressure [4], but another did not [5]. Nevertheless, the proposition that traction reduces intervertebral disc pressures is confounded by the lack of a cogent theory as to how raised disc pressure causes back pain and why that pain should stay relieved once the traction is released and the patient resumes an upright posture.

13.2. Efficacy

Paradoxically, a systematic review [6] concluded, on the basis of two low-quality studies, that there is limited evidence that traction is effective for acute low back pain. Inspection of that literature, however, reveals that the patients were treated for sciatica. Moreover, one of the studies regarded as having a positive result actually found no difference with respect to relief of pain or improvement in straight-leg raising. In an earlier review [7] from the same group, that study was recorded as reporting a negative result. Most of the literature covered by the earlier review [7] addressed the use of traction for sciatica, and nearly all studies reported negative results.

The most recent review [8] found only two studies, and concluded that: "because of poor methodologic quality and small sample sizes, there is conflicting evidence on the effectiveness of traction for acute low back pain. It is not possible to make any judgment on the effectiveness of traction for acute low back pain." [8]. Assessment of the original studies reveals that this conclusion was generous.

The study [9] regarded as constituting positive evidence enrolled a mixture of patients with acute low back pain and sciatica. The index treatment was a special form of auto-traction. The control treatment was a corset. At 1 week after treatment, 15% of patients treated by traction had fully recovered, compared with none in the control group. However, by 3 weeks after treatment, there were no significant differences between the proportions of patients fully recovered, partially recovered or not recovered, in each of the groups. Nor were there any differences between the proportions of patients with persisting symptoms at 3 months. Thus, traction offered only a short-lived advantage to a small proportion of patients.

The study [10] regarded as constituting negative evidence enrolled patients with sciatica, not back pain; and included patients with acute and with chronic symptoms. It compared traction with sham traction. Immediately after treatment, both groups achieved a modest reduction in pain (20–30%) with no significant difference between the groups. Insufficient numbers of patients completed a 3-month follow-up to allow a comparison to be made at that stage. Notwithstanding the lack of efficacy, this study is not a legitimate assessment of traction for acute low back pain. It was explicitly a study of traction for sciatica.

A more recent study reported the results at 5 weeks[11] and at 3 and 6 months[12] of patients with subacute or chronic back pain treated with traction or with sham traction. On all outcomes measured, there were no significant differences between the two treatments.

Key points

- When compared with wearing a corset, traction has only a short-lived effect in a minority of patients.
- When compared with sham traction, traction has no demonstrable therapeutic effect.
- For lack of efficacy, traction is not indicated for acute low back pain.

References

1   Twomey L. Sustained lumbar traction. An experimental study of long spine segments. Spine 1985; 10: 146–149.

2   Matthews JA. Dynamic discography: a study of lumbar traction. Ann Phys Med 1968; 9: 275–279.

3   Krause M, Refshauge KM, Dessen M, Boland R. Lumbar spine traction: evaluation of effects and recommended application for treatment. Man Ther 2000; 5: 72–81.

4   Ramos G, Martin W. Effects of vertebral axial decompression on intradiscal pressure. J Neurosurg 1994; 81: 350–353.

5   Andersson GBJ, Schultz AB, Nachemson AL. Intervertebral disc pressures during traction. Scand J Rehabil Med 1983; 9: 88–91.

6   van Tulder MW, Koes BW, Bouter LM. Conservative treatment of acute and chronic nonspecific low back pain. A systematic review of randomized controlled trials of the most common interventions. Spine 1997; 22: 2128–2156.

7   van der Heijden GJMG, Beurskens AJHM, Koes BW, Assendelft WJJ, de Vet HCW, Bouter LM. The efficacy of traction for back and neck pain: a systematic, blinded review of randomized clinical trial methods. Phys Ther 1995; 75: 93–104.

8   van Tulder MW, Waddell G. Conservative treatment of acute and subacute low back pain. In: Nachemson A, Jonsson E (eds) Neck and Back Pain: The Scientific Evidence of Causes, Diagnosis, and Treatment. Lippincott, Williams and Wilkins, Philadelphia, PA, 2000: 241–269.

9   Larsson U, Choler U, Lidstrom A, Lind G, Nachemson A, Niulsson B, Roslund J. Auto-traction for treatment of lumbago–sciatica. Acta Orthop Scand 1980; 51: 791–798.

10 Matthews JA, Hickling J. Lumbar traction: a double-blind controlled study for sciatica. Rheumatol Rehabil 1975; 14: 222–225.

11 Beurskens AJ, de Vet HC, Koke AJ, Lindeman E, Regtop W, van der Heijden GJ, Knipschild PG. Efficacy of traction for non-specific low back pain: a randomised clinical trial. Lancet 1995; 346: 1596–1600.

12 Beurskens AJ, de Vet HC, Koke AJ, Regtop W, van der Heijden GJ, Lindeman E, Knipschild PG. Efficacy of traction for non-specific low back pain: 12-week and 6-month results of a randomized clinical trial. Spine 1997; 22: 2756–2762.

14. Acupuncture

The use of acupuncture in Western societies is a politically delicate issue. Not only is it promoted as a singular therapy both within medicine and by lay groups, it is a complementary medical practice identified with particular ethnic groups and philosophies. Any challenge to the purported efficacy of acupuncture, therefore, is easily misconstrued as an assault on rights of practice, philosophies, and ethnic minorities. Any desire to use or to receive acupuncture is based on ideological or cultural grounds, not on biomedical evidence.

14.1. Efficacy

Three systematic reviews have addressed the efficacy of acupuncture for acute low back pain[1-3]. One declared that there is no evidence on the use of acupuncture in acute low back pain[1]. Another found three studies that reported results immediately after treatment, with no further follow-up[2]. Even then, only marginally significant differences were reported, and the confidence intervals of the odds ratios in favour of acupuncture intersected the critical value of 1. The third review[3] explained the dissonance between these other two reviews. No study actually addressed the efficacy of acupuncture explicitly or exclusively for acute low back pain. The three available studies[4–7] enrolled a mixture of patients with acute and chronic low back pain. The third review[3] recognized that these studies showed that acupuncture achieved marginally better results than sham acupuncture, but the lack of follow-up caused the reviewers to consider the evidence in favour of acupuncture to be no better than 'neutral'.

Key point

- There is no evidence to justify the use of acupuncture as a treatment for acute low back pain.

References

1   van Tulder MW, Waddell G. Conservative treatment of acute and subacute low back pain. In: Nachemson A, Jonsson E (eds) Neck and Back Pain: The Scientific Evidence of Causes, Diagnosis, and Treatment. Lippincott, Williams and Wilkins, Philadelphia, PA, 2000: 241–269.

2   Ernst E, White AR. Acupuncture for back pain. A meta-analysis of randomized controlled trials. Arch Intern Med 1998; 158: 2235–2241.

3   van Tulder MW, Cherkin DC, Berman B, Lao L, Koes BW. The effectiveness of acupuncture in the management of acute and chronic low back pain. A systematic review within the framework of the Cochrane Collaboration Back Review Group. Spine 1999; 24: 1113–1123.

4   Duplan B, Cabanel G, Piton JL, Grauer JI, Phelip X. Acupuncture et lombosciatique a la phase aigue: Etude en double aveugle de trente cas. Sem Hop Paris 1983; 58: 3109–3114.

5   Lopacz S, Gralewski Z. Proba oceny winikow leczenia bolowych zespolow ledzwiowo-krzyzowych metoda igloterapii lub sugestii. Neur Neurochir Pol 1979; 13: 405–409.

6   Mencke VM, Wieden TE, Hoppe M, Porschke W, Hoffman O, Herget HF. Akupunktur des schulter-arm-syndrome und der lumbalgie-ischalgie: zwei prospective doppelblind-studien (teil 1). Akupunkt Theor Prax 1988; 16: 204–215.

7   Mencke VM, Wieden TE, Hoppe M, Porschle W, Hoffman O, Herget HF. Akupunktur des schulter-arm-syndrome und der lumbalgie–ischalgie: zwei prospective doppelblind-studien (teil 2). Akupunkt Theor Prax 1988; 17: 5–14.

15. Transcutaneous electrical nerve stimulation

Transcutaneous electrical nerve stimulation (TENS) is an attractive modality for the treatment of back pain. It involves the application to the back of electrodes driven by a battery-operated source that delivers a current whose pulse-width, frequency, and amplitude can be varied.

A systematic review[1] found only two trials of the effectiveness of TENS. It concluded that there is no evidence that TENS is an effective treatment for acute low back pain, because of the contradictory results.

The methodologically stronger of the two studies reviewed found that TENS offered no additional benefit to an exercise program alone[2].

Key point

- For lack of efficacy, TENS is not indicated in the management of acute low back pain.

References

1 van Tulder MW, Koes BW, Bouter LM. Conservative treatment of acute and chronic nonspecific low back pain. A systematic review of randomized controlled trials of the most common interventions. Spine 1997; 22: 2128–2156.

2 Herman E, Williams R, Stratford P, Fargas-Babjak A, Trott M. A randomized controlled trial of transcutaneous electrical nerve stimulation (CODETRON) to determine its benefits in a rehabilitation program for acute occupational low back pain. Spine 1994; 19: 561–568.

Medical Management of Acute and Chronic Low Back Pain. An Evidence-Based Approach
Pain Research and Clinical Management, Vol. 13
Nikolai Bogduk and Brian McGuirk

CHAPTER 13

Chronic low back pain

Chronic back pain is formally defined as back pain that has lasted longer than 3 months (Chapter 2). Technically, therefore, a patient will have developed chronic back pain the moment that their acute low back pain reaches 91 days in duration.

A more liberal, and pragmatic, definition would allow inclusion of patients who, during the course of their acute low back pain, show no signs of improvement. The lack of improvement suggests that these patients are likely to become chronic, whereupon it may be inefficient to wait until they satisfy the temporal criterion for chronic back pain before being managed accordingly. Given that even good treatment may take up to a month or so to show effects, this concession would apply to patients who are not showing improvement by the second month of acute back pain.

This concession, however, presupposes that the patient with acute back pain has been managed earnestly in an appropriate manner, as outlined in Chapter 11. A patient with back pain that has lasted 2 months, but who has not yet been managed well, could still respond to good management for acute back pain. Therefore, the passage of 2 months without improvement should not automatically be a basis for considering the patient to have become chronic. Similarly, even a patient who has technically passed the 3-month mark might still be eligible for management under the guidelines for acute low back pain, if their previous treatment had not been according to those principles.

Notwithstanding these considerations and exceptions, a practitioner may encounter de novo a patient with chronic low back pain. This may be a patient who has not responded to good management by other practitioners during their acute phase. They may be a patient who has not improved despite concerted and specialist assistance concerning yellow flag and occupational issues. Or they may be a new patient who presents with long-standing low back pain, about whom there is no doubt that their pain is chronic in a temporal sense, and for whom reassurance, encouragement, and simple measures are either not convincing or not indicated in the practitioner's estimation.

An approach can be adopted for these patients that is analogous in structure to that recommended for acute low back pain. The practitioner should be aware of the pre-test probabilities of diagnosis. They should assess the patient, by way of history and physical examination. They may consider undertaking investigations. Eventually they will want to implement a plan of management.

Whereas these components of management for chronic low back pain are categorically the same as those for acute low back pain, their elements and the evidence-base of each are distinctly different. Although some principles might overlap, the data are different.

The following chapters systematically outline:

- background information concerning chronic low back pain as an entity;
- an approach to the assessment of patients with chronic low back pain; and
- options for treatment.

Readers should note the differences, from those applicable to acute low back pain, concerning the causes of back pain, the utility of investigations, and the strength of evidence concerning various interventions.

Medical Management of Acute and Chronic Low Back Pain. An Evidence-Based Approach
Pain Research and Clinical Management, Vol. 13
Nikolai Bogduk and Brian McGuirk
© *2002 Elsevier Science B.V. All rights reserved*

CHAPTER 14

Causes and sources of chronic low back pain

1. Introduction

Whereas the causes of acute low back pain are largely unknown (Chapter 3), opposite data apply for chronic low back pain. Epidemiological studies have provided information on the prevalence of certain entities that are common amongst patients with uncomplicated, chronic low back pain. This information provides a working basis for planning the investigation of these patients.

It is often cited that a cause cannot be determined in 80% of patients with low back pain [1,2], or conversely, that a diagnosis is possible in only some 10–15% of cases [3]. The source of this figure is difficult to track down, but it seems to have been endorsed and enshrined by the report of the Quebec Task Force on Low Back Pain, which was published in 1987 [4]. When viewed in context, the figure is probably valid; but it reflects the opinions and practices in place in 1987 and before. Indeed, techniques of investigation, in use in 1987 and before, would not have been capable of providing a diagnosis.

History and physical examination alone are insufficient for making a valid diagnosis of low back pain. The limitations that apply for acute low back pain (Chapters 6 and 7) apply equally for chronic low back pain. There are simply no pathognomonic features on history that allow a diagnosis to be made with certainty. At best, history might reveal clues to a possible red flag condition, but that suspicion would need to be confirmed by imaging or by other investigations. No technique of physical examination has sufficient reliability and validity to allow a patho-anatomic diagnosis to be made. Plain X-rays do not provide for a diagnosis in most cases of either acute low back pain (Chapter 8) or chronic low back pain (see Chapter 15). Nor does CT scanning. MRI is able to reveal certain conditions, but it was not in common use in 1987.

It is, therefore, both understandable and not surprising that, in 1987, the cause of back pain could not be determined in 80% of cases. Indeed, it is surprising that this figure is as low as it is. It may well be that the 20% of conditions that allegedly could be diagnosed were either false-positive diagnoses, such as spondylosis, spondylolisthesis, and spondylolysis, or conditions, such as sciatica, that do not pertain to back pain.

Since 1987, new diagnostic tests have been developed, evaluated, and implemented. The use of these tests has reversed the figures. If appropriate tests are used, a diagnosis of chronic low back pain can be made in at least 50% of cases, and perhaps in as many as 70% of cases. It is no longer true that chronic back pain cannot be diagnosed.

2. Red flag conditions

Tumours and infections are rare causes of acute low back pain. They are not appreciably more common in patients with chronic low back pain.

If the prevalence of a serious condition is $P\%$ amongst patients with acute low back pain; and if $Z\%$ of these patients develop chronic back pain; and if it is assumed that all patients with a serious condition develop chronic back pain; the prevalence of a serious condition amongst patients with chronic back pain is $(P/Z)\%$. In the case of tumours, $P = 1\%$. If 30% of acute patients become chronic, the prevalence of tumours amongst chronic patients will be 3%. Even if only 15% of patients become chronic, the prevalence of tumours will be only 7%.

Although small, the prevalence of red flag conditions in patients with chronic back pain is not zero. Accordingly, practitioners have a duty of care to recognise these conditions. However, the figure is so low that practitioners should not be surprised that the vast majority of patients with chronic low back pain will not have a red flag condition.

3. Structural abnormalities

It is tempting, but incorrect, to attribute chronic low back pain to structural abnormalities seen on plain radiographs, particularly when the practitioner is not aware of other possibilities, or does not have other tests at their disposal. Such structural abnormalities include congenital abnormalities, spondylolysis, spondylolisthesis, and spondylosis.

The data concerning these conditions as a cause of back pain were reviewed in the context of acute low back pain (Chapter 8). However, those data are no less relevant in the context of chronic low back pain, and bear reiteration because of their importance in preventing wrongful diagnosis.

3.1. Congenital anomalies

Congenital anomalies such as transitional vertebrae, non-dysjunction (congenital fusion), and spina bifida occulta, occur equally commonly in symptomatic and asymptomatic individuals[5]. Consequently, they cannot be inferred to be the cause of pain.

3.2. Spondylolisthesis

Large-scale epidemiological studies have shown that in adults, spondylolisthesis is not associated with back pain[5]. Finding spondylolisthesis on a radiograph, therefore, does not constitute establishing the diagnosis. In one study[6], women with spondylolis-

thesis were found to have a greater risk of back pain, but the risk was only marginal and insufficient to render the observation diagnostic.

3.3. Spondylolysis

Pars defects occur in some 7% of asymptomatic individuals[7], and are equally common in symptomatic and asymptomatic individuals from the general population[5]. Finding a pars defect on a radiograph does not make it diagnostic of the patient's pain. Only amongst sportspeople are pars defects more common than in the general population, but even then the higher prevalence is not enough to render the finding diagnostic (Chapter 8).

For this condition to be implicated as the cause of back pain, evidence other than its radiographic presence is required. The definitive test to determine if a pars defect is symptomatic is to anaesthetise the defect[8]. Relief of pain implies that the defect is actually the source pain, and predicts surgical success[8].

3.4. Spondylosis

Spondylosis, disc degeneration, facet degeneration, or osteoarthritis, do not constitute legitimate diagnoses of the cause or source of back pain. The correlations between pain and the presence of these conditions are too weak to render the finding diagnostic (Chapter 8).

4. Instability

In some circles the term 'instability', is used as a diagnostic entity. The implication is that the patient has something biomechanically wrong in their back, and that this somehow is the cause of their pain. Furthermore, since the cause of pain is biomechanical in nature, its treatment should be mechanical. The notion of lumbar instability, however, has become very controversial, as evident in several reviews[9,10] and symposia[11-13]. Physicians have abused the term, and have applied it clinically without discipline and without due regard to available biomechanical definitions and diagnostic criteria.

The nature of instability, the various biomechanical definitions, and various clinical classifications have been reviewed in detail elsewhere [14]. To repeat that review in full here could be daunting for some readers, and distracting from the purpose at hand, which is the differential diagnosis of chronic low back pain. Instability does not qualify as such a diagnosis.

Bioengineers have tendered various definitions of instability. Some define it in terms of loss of stiffness in spinal motion segments [15,16], but this definition does not embrace the risk of sudden catastrophic failure that the term 'instability', implies [17]. Others have defined instability as an increase in the neutral zone of intervertebral movements [18]. While attractive, this definition has been applied only in experimental settings. No techniques, at present, allow its detection in patients. Another approach defines instability as an increase in the ratio between the magnitude of translation and the magnitude of rotation that a motion segment exhibits during flexion–extension of the lumbar spine [19–21]. Changes in this ratio are detectable, in vivo, but require multiple X-ray exposures, and meticulous biomechanical analysis of the images. For this reason, the techniques available have not emerged from the laboratory into conventional clinical practice.

Clinicians have classified instability according to the nature of lesions that can be demonstrated radiographically [16,22], and which ostensibly or putatively threaten the integrity of the lumbar spine (Table I). In this regard, whether or not fractures, infections, and neoplasms actually cause instability, or not, is immaterial. A diagnosis is established upon demonstrating the lesion, and does not require the formal demonstration of instability in a biomechanical sense. The nature of the lesions found is sufficient to believe that they compromise the stability of the spine.

The same cannot be said of spondylolisthesis and degenerative instability. Although spondylolisthesis looks threatening on radiographs, this condition rarely progresses in adults [23] or teenagers [24]. Furthermore, biplanar radiographic studies have shown that grade 1 and grade 2 spondylolisthesis are associated with reduced range of motion, rather than instability [25]. Some patients with spondylolisthesis may exhibit forward slipping upon standing from a lying position [26], but it is not clear whether the extent of slip is such cases is abnormal. In some patients, movement abnormalities may be revealed using special techniques that involve the patient standing loaded with a 20-kg pack, and hanging by their heads from an overhead bar [27,28]. These extreme measures, however, have been criticised as unrealistic and cumbersome [17]. Furthermore, precision studies have now shown that the motion patterns of patients with spondylolisthesis are indistinguishable from those with degenerative disc disease [29].

Several types of instability have been attributed to degeneration of the lumbar spine [16,22]. These include rotational, retrolisthetic, and translational instability; and each is supposed to be defined by an abnormal range of motion of a lumbar motion segment in the respective direction. Rotational instability was postulated as a hypothetical entity [30], and certain qualitative radiographic signs have been attributed to it [31], but neither the reliability nor the validity of these signs has been established. Retrolisthetic instability is supposed to be defined by an abnormal retrolisthesis during extension of the lumbar spine [32], but such movements also occur in asymptomatic individuals [33,34].

Translational instability is the most studied form of putative instability. It is defined by an abnormal magnitude of forward translation during flexion of the lumbar spine. The difficulty lies in setting the upper limit of normal for this translation. Posner et al. [35] prescribed a limit of 2.3 mm for L1–L4, and 1.6 mm for L5. Boden et al. [36], however, showed that many asymptomatic individuals exhibited static slips

TABLE I

Classification of lumbar segmental instabilities

I	Fractures and fracture-dislocations
II	Infections of the anterior elements
III	Neoplasms
IV	Spondylolisthesis
V	Degenerative

of such magnitude. Accordingly, they emphasised that a dynamic slip should be demonstrated before instability is considered. Moreover, they found that even dynamic slips of up to 3 mm could occur in asymptomatic individuals; only 5% of the asymptomatic population exhibit slips greater than 3 mm. Accordingly, Boden et al.[36] advocated that 3 mm be the threshold for diagnosing anterior translational instability. Hayes et al.[33], however, subsequently showed that dynamic slips of 4 mm occurred in 20% of asymptomatic individuals; and proposed that 4 mm might be a better threshold.

Despite all this effort at defining and refining the diagnostic criteria for translational instability, no-one has demonstrate that it is at all related to the cause of pain. Nor has it been shown that rectifying or preventing the slip consistently and successfully abolishes symptoms. Consequently, not even the best studied of the instabilities, has been shown to be relevant as a diagnosis.

5. Failed back surgery syndrome

Perhaps the most difficult condition to assess and to manage is back pain that persists after spinal surgery, or is worse after and despite spinal surgery. The IASP taxonomy[37] recognises this condition as 'lumbar spinal pain or radicular pain after failed spinal surgery'. More colloquially, it is known as 'failed back surgery syndrome'.

The diagnostic criteria are lumbar spinal pain, for which no other cause has been found or can be attributed, associated with an unsuccessful attempt at treating the pain in the same region by surgical means[37]. The definition and diagnostic criteria do not presuppose or require any particular mechanism or cause for the pain. They require only low back pain and a history of failed surgical therapy.

Systematically, there are three main classes of possible reasons why surgery may have failed to relieve a patient's pain:

(1) correct operation, wrong diagnosis
(2) correct diagnosis, wrong operation
(3) wrong diagnosis, wrong operation.

It may be that an operation was correctly performed but for the wrong indication, the pain stemming from a source that was not corrected by the operation. An example might be performing an arthrodesis of an L5 spondylolisthesis in a patient whose pain actually stemmed from an L4–L5 disc.

It may be that a correct patho-anatomic diagnosis was made but the operation performed was incorrect. An example might be performing a posterolateral fusion for discogenic pain, but the painful disc has been left in situ and remains painful[38,39]. Or, perhaps the correct operation was selected but poorly executed.

It may be that an incorrect diagnosis was made and an inappropriate operation was performed on structures totally unrelated to the patient's pain. An example might be performing a laminectomy and discectomy for an asymptomatic disc bulge. Another might be performing surgery on a patient with somatisation rather than an explicit anatomic source of pain. In this regard, it is perhaps sobering to recognise that of patients attending a particular pain clinic, with a history of at least two previous spinal operations, some 70% did not satisfy the criteria for their first operation, as prescribed by the American Academy of Orthopaedic Surgeons and the North American Society of Neurological Surgeons[40].

Out of these various possibilities, arise the permutations that:

- the patient may still have their original cause of pain, and it is still amenable to (correct) management, including surgical management;
- the patient may still have their original cause of pain, but it is no longer amenable to surgical management because of the anatomical changes that have been wrought by the surgery;
- the patient has a new cause of pain, such as neuroma formation, arachnoiditis, nerve injury, epidural scarring or pain somehow caused by irritation of tissues in the back by a fusion mass or by instrumentation.

In the event that a patient still has their original cause of pain, they could be managed as if their failed surgery was simply incidental. Such cases would be characterised by relatively simple previous surgery that has not seriously altered spinal anatomy. Structures that might be the original source of pain are still accessible both for investigations and for treatment.

More devastating and frustrating are situations where possible sources of pain are no longer accessible. An example would be a patient with extensive bilateral, intertransverse fusions that prevent conventional access to the intervertebral discs or zygapophysial joints for the conduct of diagnostic tests.

Although any number of possible new causes of pain might be imagined and invoked, these largely defy objective diagnosis. Invoking such explanations serves only to provide a possible explanation for the pain. It does not alter management.

One can imagine that, during extensive spinal surgery, many small nerves in the back are cut and sacrificed. These include the branches of the lumbar dorsal rami and the nerves to the intervertebral discs. When cut, these nerves might develop *neuromas*, some of which might become painful. In effect, the pain that they produce would be similar to, if not indistinguishable from the patient's original pain, for it is mediated by the same nerves as the original pain, even though the actual source of pain is different. Such neuromas, however, would be inaccessible to clinical examination, and invisible on contemporary techniques of medical imaging. Consequently they cannot be diagnosed; and they cannot be specifically treated.

One can imagine that spinal surgery might cause *adhesions* in the epidural space. Some authorities have invoked such scarring as a cause of pain, and have advocated lysis of such scarring percutaneously or under epiduroscopy as a treatment[41,42]. However, there are no techniques whereby it can be proven that this scarring is the actual cause of pain, and there are no data to this effect. Epiduroscopic lysis of adhesions is practised on the basis of a presumptive diagnosis.

One can imagine that *fusion masses* might cause pain in a variety of ways. Sharp or irregular edges

could impinge on adjacent muscles; or muscles might strain against scar tissue enveloping a fusion mass. The latter might also apply to screws, rods or other hardware implanted into the spine. Such problems might be diagnosed by anaesthetising the painful site with local anaesthetic. However, short of removing the offending material there is no established method of treating this phenomenon.

Blood or oil-based contrast media can cause chronic inflammation of the leptomeninges — referred to as *arachnoiditis*. This condition can be demonstrated by MRI or by myelography, and is attractive as an explanation for failed back surgery syndrome. However, arachnoiditis may be asymptomatic, and its relationship to pain is imperfect. There are no established diagnostic criteria; nor is there any specific therapy.

It is the futility of pursuing a patho-anatomic diagnosis in most patients with failed back surgery syndrome that has driven authorities to recognise this condition simply as a syndrome. Doing so limits treatment options but does not eliminate them entirely (see Chapter 16).

However, encouraging new work is appearing. Failed back surgery syndrome may not be as undiagnosable and as untreatable as previously believed. If investigated with appropriate techniques, such as discography, many of these patients prove to have internal disc disruption. This constitutes a condition that was originally present but not diagnosed, and for which the surgery undertaken was inappropriate.

6. Internal disc disruption

Internal disc disruption (IDD) is a condition that befalls lumbar intervertebral discs. Anatomically it is characterised by biochemical degradation of the matrix of the nucleus pulposus and the development of radial fissures that extend into the anulus fibrosus. Those fissures can be graded according to the extent to which they penetrate the anulus and what they do in the anulus (Fig. 1). Fissures of grade I, II,

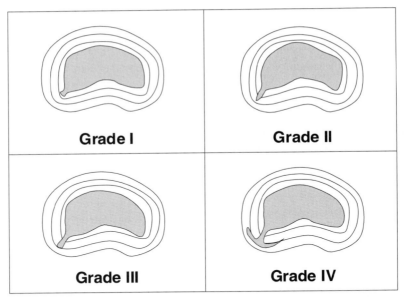

Fig. 1. The appearance and grading of fissures in the anulus fibrosus of lumbar intervertebral discs.

and III, extend into the inner, middle, and outer third of the anulus fibrosus [43]. A grade IV fissure is a grade III fissure that, from its tip, also extends circumferentially around the anulus, assuming the shape of a ship's anchor [44]. All of these changes occur in a disc that externally is intact. Its contour is normal, or essential so. This external integrity of the disc distinguishes IDD from disc protrusions and disc herniations.

Biophysically, internal disc disruption is characterised by severe disturbances in the stress distribution within the disc. In a normal lumbar disc, stress is distributed fairly uniformly across the nucleus pulposus and the inner anulus fibrosus [45] (Fig. 2). Some normal discs may have a slightly greater stress in the posterior anulus. Discs with IDD do not conform to this pattern. Across the nucleus pulposus, stress is absent or chaotically irregular; the uniform stress profile is not evident. Within the anulus, the stress is greater than normal, particularly in the posterior anulus (Fig. 3).

Radiographically, IDD can be demonstrated by CT-discography: a procedure in which contrast medium is injected into the nucleus of the disc and an axial view of its dispersal is obtained by comput-

erised axial tomography. The contrast medium fills the nucleus and any radial fissures, which renders the characteristic features of IDD visible on CT scans of the disc [43].

These various features are strongly correlated with one another. There is a strong correlation (Table II) between the radiologic features of IDD

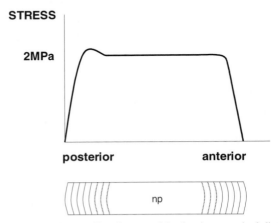

Fig. 2. The stress profile of a normal lumbar intervertebral disc. The curve shows the magnitude of stress across a section of the intervertebral disc as illustrated in the lower inset. np, nucleus pulposus. Based on Adams et al. [45].

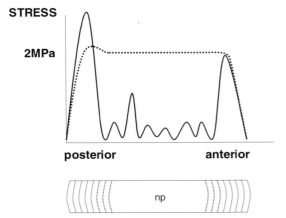

STRESS

2MPa

posterior   **anterior**

np

Fig. 3. The stress profiles of an internally disrupted lumbar intervertebral disc. The curve shows the magnitude of stresses across a section of the disc, as illustrated in the inset. Stresses are irregular and reduced across the nucleus pulposus (np), and increased in the posterior anulus fibrosus. Based on McNally et al.[48].

TABLE III

The correlation between abnormal stress profiles and pain from a lumbar intervertebral disc

Stress	Disc	
	Painful	Not painful
Nuclear stress		
Depressurised	11	0
Normal	7	13
	Fisher's exact test; $P = 0.017$	
Anular stress		
Stressed	17	2
Normal	1	11
	Fisher's exact test; $P = 0.001$	

Based on McNally et al.[48].

and whether the disc is painful or not [46,47], as determined by disc stimulation (see Chapter 19). There is a strong correlation between abnormal stress profiles and whether or not the disc is painful [48] (Table III). Furthermore, IDD is not synonymous with disc degeneration or age changes. It is a distinct and separate condition. Degenerative changes correlate with age, but radial fissures are unrelated to age, and are independently related to pain, irrespective of age [46].

The aetiology of IDD is still being explored, but the best available evidence suggests that it is caused by fatigue failure. Repeated, but submaximal, loading of the disc in compression eventually causes a small fracture in the superior vertebral endplate of the disc. Biophysically, this fracture compromises the load-bearing behaviour of the disc, and abnormal stress profiles develop immediately [45]. Biochemically, the fracture precipitates a degradation of the nuclear matrix, either by lowering the pH of the nucleus, which favours degradation in favour of synthesis of normal matrix; or by permitting an active immune reaction to the proteins of the nucleus [49,50].

How IDD becomes painful remains controversial. The putative mechanisms cannot be tested because no-one has yet devised a precision technique to study the neurophysiology of intervertebral discs in vivo. Nevertheless, a combination of two theories obtains [50], and a third has emerged.

While so long as a degraded nucleus remains contained within the anulus fibrosus, there is no anatomical means for it to become painful, for there are no nerve endings in the nucleus or in the deeper layers of the anulus. However, if a radial fissure develops, degraded matrix components and inflammatory chemicals can reach the nerve endings in the outer third of the anulus. This establishes a basis for *chemical* nociception. Effectively, the disc feels like a sterile abscess.

Meanwhile, a radial fissure compromises the function of the anulus fibrosus. Normally, the loads

TABLE II

The correlation between the grade of anular disruption and reproduction of pain by disc stimulation

Pain reproduction	Anular disruption			
	Grade III	Grade II	Grade I	Grade 0
Exact	43	29	6	4
Similar	32	36	21	8
Dissimilar	9	11	6	2
None	16	24	67	86

The numbers refer to the number of patients exhibiting the features tabulated. Based on Moneta et al.[46]. $\chi^2 = 148$; $P < 0.001$.

applied to any sector of the anulus are shared across all the lamellae of the anulus. A radial fissure involves disruption of the inner lamellae, leaving only the outer lamellae still intact. The affected sector of the anulus, however, is still subject to normal loads. Those loads have to be shared by a decreased number of lamellae. This establishes a basis for *mechanical* nociception. Essentially, the remaining lamellae are strained by normal loads.

These two mechanisms can combine. The biochemical changes not only produce chemical nociception, they also sensitise the nerve endings of the anulus, rendering them more susceptible to mechanical stimulation.

The emerging theory of pain from IDD places the source not in the anulus fibrosus but in the vertebral endplate[51]. The theory maintains that the fractured endplate is less able than normal to withstand the pressures exerted on the disc during activities of daily living. In essence, the weakened endplate bows under compression, and the pain arises from the bending bone of endplate. This theory and the anulus mechanism are not mutually exclusive. A patient with a disrupted disc and a painful anulus could well have pain also from a weakened endplate.

The clinical features of IDD are protean. They consist of pain at rest (stemming from chemical nociception), aggravated by movements (as a result of mechanical nociception from the anulus and/or the endplate). There would be no neurological signs (because the disc is intact externally, and does not irritate nerve roots). There are no radiological abnormalities (because X-rays do not show discs, and CT does not reveal the internal architecture of the disc).

Because no other clinical features distinguish painful IDD, it cannot be diagnosed clinically. It looks, feels, and behaves like any other back pain. X-rays and CT look normal. For these reasons, IDD cannot be diagnosed using physical examination or conventional medical imaging. For these reasons, it would not have been diagnosed back in 1987, when the Quebec Task Force felt that 80% of back pain could not be diagnosed. However, IDD can be identified using MRI and CT-discography (see Chapters 15 and 19).

The diagnostic criteria for IDD are that the affected disc must be painful when stimulated in the course of discography, and that it exhibits a grade III or greater fissure[52]. A formal study, using these criteria stringently, found that the prevalence of IDD was 39% ($\pm 10\%$) amongst patients with chronic low back pain attending centres specialising in the investigation of spinal pain[53]. This promotes IDD as the most common cause of chronic low back pain.

7. Zygapophysial joint pain

Studies in normal volunteers have shown that noxious stimulation of the zygapophysial joints of the lumbar spine can cause back pain and referred pain into the lower limb[54−56]. These studies provide prima facie evidence that these joints might be a source of chronic low back pain. Complementary studies have shown that some patients can have their chronic low back pain relieved by anaesthetisation of one or other of their lumbar zygapophysial joints, under controlled conditions[57−59].

In older patients attending a rheumatology practice[58], and in heterogeneous patients attending a pain clinic[59], the prevalence of zygapophysial joint pain is about 40% ($\pm 13\%$). Amongst younger patients with a history of injury, the prevalence is lower — about 15% ($\pm 5\%$)[57]. Depending on the age group and history of the patient, zygapophysial joint pain is either as common or somewhat less common than IDD as a basis for chronic back pain.

There are no clinical features that distinguish lumbar zygapophysial joint pain from other causes of back pain. It cannot be diagnosed by clinical examination[57,59,60]. It cannot be diagnosed by CT scanning[61]. It can only diagnosed by controlled diagnostic blocks[57−59]. These blocks were not in common use when the Quebec Task Force reported that back pain could not be diagnosed.

8. Sacroiliac joint pain

Belief in the sacroiliac joint as a source of low back pain waxed and waned throughout the 20th century. Arguments for and against this belief, however, were based solely on assertion and opposition. Objective evidence became available in the 1990s.

Studies in normal volunteers showed that noxious stimulation of the sacroiliac joint could produce low back pain [62]. Complementary studies, using diagnostic blocks of this joint, showed that in patients with chronic back pain, the prevalence of sacroiliac joint pain was of the order of 13% (±7%) [63] or 19% (±10%) [64], i.e. about 15%. Sacroiliac joint blocks were not in common use in 1987 when the Quebec Task Force found that back pain could not be diagnosed.

9. Summary

Contrary to prevailing, and nihilistic, opinion, back pain can be diagnosed. Later chapters outline how this can be done. It is not true that 80% of back pain cannot be diagnosed. That figure obtains only if one relies on techniques that are unable to provide a diagnosis. On the contrary, if appropriate techniques are used, a diagnosis is possible in some 75% of cases.

The pre-test chances of IDD being the cause are 40%. The pre-test chances of it being zygapophysial joint pain are 15% in injured workers, and 40% in older individuals. The pre-test chances of the source of pain being the sacroiliac joint are about 20%. It has also been shown that only rarely do patients have a combination of these disorders. They have one or the other but not both [65]. Consequently, one can sum their individual prevalences. Using the mean figures yields a sum of 70% (40 + 15 + 15%). Even using the worst-case figures, based on the 95% confidence intervals of the prevalences, yields 46% (29 + 10 + 7%).

Whatever the correct figure, back pain does not defy diagnosis. There are certain conditions that the practitioner can expect that their patient could have. The management of chronic back pain is predicated both by an awareness of this epidemiology, and a decision as to whether the practitioner wishes or chooses to pursue a diagnosis or not.

Key points

- Red flag conditions, such as tumours and infections are uncommon, if not rare, causes of chronic low back pain.
- The presence on radiographs of congenital abnormalities, spondylolisthesis, spondylolysis, or spondylosis is not diagnostic of the cause of chronic back pain.
- In the absence of operational criteria, instability does not constitute a valid diagnosis.
- Some authorities recognise persistent pain after back surgery as a syndrome in its own right, without regard to the mechanisms or causes of pain.
- Causes such as arachnoiditis, neuroma formation, and fusion impingement, lack operational diagnostic criteria.
- The most common, detectable causes of chronic low back pain are internal disc disruption, zygapophysial joint pain, and sacroiliac joint pain.
- Respectively, the prevalence of these conditions in patients with chronic low back pain are:

internal disc disruption	39% (29–49%)
zygapophysial joint pain	15% (10–20%)
sacroiliac joint pain	15% (7–23%)

References

1 Kirwan EO. Back pain. In: Wall PD, Melzack R (eds) Text Book of Pain, 2nd edn. Churchill Livingstone, Edinburgh, 1989, pp 335–340.

2 White AA. The 1980 symposium and beyond. In: Frymoyer JW, Gordon SL (eds) New Perspectives on Low Back Pain. American Academy of Orthopaedic Surgeons, Park Ridge, 1989: 3–17.

3 Frymoyer W. Epidemiology. In: Frymoyer JW, Gordon SL (eds) New Perspectives on Low Back Pain. American Academy of Orthopaedic Surgeons, Park Ridge, 1989: 19–33.

4 Quebec Task Force on Spinal Disorders. Scientific approach to the assessment and management of activity-related spinal disorders: a monograph for clinicians. Spine 1987; 12: S1–S59.

5 van Tulder MW, Assendelft WJJ, Koes BW, Bouter LM. Spinal radiographic findings and nonspecific low back pain. A systematic review of observational studies. Spine 1997; 22: 427–434.

6 Virta L, Ronnemaa T. The association of mild–moderate isthmic lumbar spondylolisthesis and low back pain in middle-aged patients is weak and it only occurs in women. Spine 1993; 18: 1496–1503.

7 Moreton RD. Spondylolysis. J Am Med Assoc 1966; 195: 671–674.

8 Suh PB, Esses SI, Kostuik JP. Repair of a pars interarticularis defect — the prognostic value of pars infiltration. Spine 1991; 16 (Suppl 8): S445–S448.

9 Nachemson AL. Instability of the lumbar spine: pathology, treatment, and clinical evaluation. Neurosurg Clin North Am 1991; 2: 785–790.

10 Pope MH, Frymoyer JW, Krag MH. Diagnosing instability. Clin Orthop 1992; 279: 60–67.

11 Kirkaldy-Willis WH. Presidential symposium on instability of the lumbar spine: introduction. Spine 1985; 10: 254.

12 Nachemson A. Lumbar spine instability: a critical update and symposium summary. Spine 1985; 10: 290–291.

13 Wiesel S. Editor's corner. Semin Spine Surg 1991; 3: 91.

14 Bogduk N. Clinical Anatomy of the Lumbar Spine and Sacrum, 3rd edn. Churchill-Livingstone, Edinburgh, 1997, pp 215–225.

15 Frymoyer JW, Pope MH. Segmental instability. Semin Spine Surg 1991; 3: 109–118.

16 Panjabi MM. The stabilizing system of the spine. Part II. Neutral zone and instability hypothesis. J Spinal Disord 1992; 5: 390–397.

17 Ashton-Miller JA, Schultz AB. Spine instability and segmental hypermobility biomechanics: a call for the definition and standard use of terms. Semin Spine Surg 1991; 3: 136–148.

18 Pope MH, Panjabi M. Biomechanical definitions of spinal instability. Spine 1985; 10: 255–256.

19 Gertzbein SD, Seligman J, Holtby R, Chan KW, Ogston N, Kapasouri A, Tile M. Centrode characteristics of the lumbar spine as a function of segmental instability. Clin Orthop 1986; 208: 48–51.

20 Gertzbein SD, Seligman J, Holtby R, Chan KH, Kapasouri A, Tile M, Cruickshank B. Centrode patterns and segmental instability in degenerative disc disease. Spine 1985; 10: 257–261.

21 Weiler PJ, King GJ, Gertzbein SD. Analysis of sagittal plane instability of the lumbar spine in vivo. Spine 1990; 15: 1300–1306.

22 Hazlett JW, Kinnard P. Lumbar apophyseal process excision and spinal instability. Spine 1982; 7: 171–176.

23 Fredrickson BE, Baker D, McHolick WJ, Yuan HA, Lubicky JP. The natural history of spondylosis and spondylolisthesis. J Bone Joint Surg 1984; 66A: 699–707.

24 Danielson BI, Frennered AK, Irstam LKH. Radiologic progression of isthmic lumbar spondylolisthesis in young patients. Spine 1991; 16: 422–425.

25 Pearcy M, Shepherd J. Is there instability in spondylolisthesis? Spine 1985; 10: 175–177.

26 Lowe RW, Hayes TD, Kaye J, Bag RJ, Luekens A. Standing roentgenograms in spondylolisthesis. Clin Orthop 1976; 117: 80–84.

27 Friberg O. Lumbar instability: a dynamic approach by traction–compression radiography. Spine 1987; 12: 119–129.

28 Kalebo P, Kadziolka R, Sward L. Compression–traction radiography of lumbar segmental instability. Spine 1990; 15: 351–355.

29 Axelsson P, Johnsson R, Stromqvist B. Is there increased intervertebral mobility in isthmic adult spondylolisthesis? A matched comparative study using roentgen stereophotogrammetry. Spine 2000; 25: 1701–1703.

30 Farfan HF, Gracovetsky S. The nature of instability. Spine 1984; 9: 714–719.

31 Kirkaldy-Willis WH, Farfan HF. Instability of the lumbar spine. Clin Orthop 1982; 165: 110–123.

32 Knutsson F. The instability associated with disk degeneration in the lumbar spine. Acta Radiol 1994; 25: 593–609.

33 Hayes MA, Howard TC, Gruel CR, Kopta JA. Roentgenographic evaluation of lumbar spine flexion–extension in asymptomatic individuals. Spine 1989; 14: 327–331.

34 La Rocca H, MacNab I. Value of pre-employment radiographic assessment of the lumbar spine. Ind Med Surg 1970; 39: 31–36.

35 Posner I, White AA, Edwards WT, Hayes WC. A biomechanical analysis of the clinical stability of the lumbar and lumbosacral spine. Spine 1982; 7: 374–389.

36 Boden SD, Davis DO, Dina TS, Patronas NJ, Wiesel SW. Abnormal magnetic-resonance scans of the lumbar spine in asymptomatic subjects. J Bone Joint Surg 1990; 72A: 403–408.

37 Merskey H, Bogduk N (eds). Classification of Chronic Pain. Descriptions of Chronic Pain Syndromes and Definitions of Pain Terms, 2nd edn. IASP Press, Seattle, WA, 1994, p 179.

38 Weatherly CR, Prickett CR, O'Brien JP. Discogenic pain

persisting despite solid posterior fusion. J Bone Joint Surg 1986; 68B: 142–143.

39 Barrick WT, Schofferman JA, Reynolds JB, Godlthwaite ND, McKeehen M, Keaney D, White AH. Anterior lumbar fusion improves discogenic pain at levels of prior postero-lateral fusion. Spine 2000; 25: 853–857.

40 Long DM, Filtzer DL, BenDebba M, Hendler NH. Clinical features of the failed-back syndrome. J Neurosurg 1988; 69: 61–71.

41 Manchikanti L, Bakhit CE. Percutaneous lysis of epidural adhesions. Pain Phys 2000; 3: 46–64.

42 Manchikanti L, Singh V, Kloth D, Slipman CW, Jasper JF, Trescot AM, Varley KG, Atluri SL, Giron C, Curran MJ, Rivera J, Baha G, Bakhit CE, Reuter MW. Interventional techniques in the management of chronic pain: part 2.0. Pain Phys 2001; 4: 24–96.

43 Sachs BL, Vanharanta H, Spivey MA, Guyer RD, Videman T, Rashbaum RF, Johnson RG, Hochschuler SH, Mooney V. Dallas discogram description: a new classification of CT/discography in low-back disorders. Spine 1987; 12: 287–294.

44 Aprill C, Bogduk N. High intensity zone: a diagnostic sign of painful lumbar disc on magnetic resonance imaging. Br J Radiol 1992; 65: 361–369.

45 Adams MA, McNally DS, Wagstaff J, Goodship AE. Abnormal stress concentrations in lumbar intervertebral discs following damage to the vertebral bodies: cause of disc failure? Eur Spine J 1993; 1: 214–221.

46 Moneta GB, Videman T, Kaivanto K, Aprill C, Spivey M, Vanharanta H, Sachs BL, Guyer RD, Hochschuler SH, Raschbaum RF, Mooney V. Reported pain during lumbar discography as a function of anular ruptures and disc degeneration. A re-analysis of 833 discograms. Spine 1994; 17: 1968–1974.

47 Vanharanta H, Sachs BL, Spivey MA, Guyer RD, Hochschuler SH, Rashbaum RF, Johnson RG, Ohnmeiss D, Mooney V. The relationship of pain provocation to lumbar disc deterioration as seen by CT/discography. Spine 1987; 12: 295–298.

48 McNally DS, Shackleford IM, Goodship AE, Mulholland RC. In vivo stress measurement can predict pain on discography. Spine 1996; 21: 2500–2587.

49 Bogduk N. The lumbar disc and low back pain. Neurosurg Clin North Am 1991; 2: 791–806.

50 Bogduk N. Clinical Anatomy of the Lumbar Spine and Sacrum, 3rd edn. Churchill Livingstone, Edinburgh, 1997, pp 205–212.

51 Heggenness MH, Doherty BJ. Discography causes end plate deflection. Spine 1993; 18: 1050–1053.

52 Merskey H, Bogduk N (eds). Classification of Chronic Pain. Descriptions of Chronic Pain Syndromes and Definitions of Pain Terms, 2nd edn. IASP Press, Seattle, WA, 1994, pp 180–181.

53 Schwarzer AC, Aprill CN, Derby R, Fortin J, Kine G, Bogduk N. The prevalence and clinical features of internal disc disruption in patients with chronic low back pain. Spine 1995; 20: 1878–1883.

54 Mooney V, Robertson J. The facet syndrome. Clin Orthop 1976; 115: 149–156.

55 McCall IW, Park WM, O'Brien JP. Induced pain referred from posterior lumbar elements in normal subjects. Spine 1979; 4: 441–446.

56 Fukui S, Ohseto K, Shiotani M, Ohno K, Karasawa H, Nagaauma Y. Distribution of referred pain from the lumbar zygapophyseal joints and dorsal rami. Clin J Pain 1997; 13: 303–307.

57 Schwarzer AC, Aprill CN, Derby R, Fortin J, Kine G, Bogduk N. Clinical features of patients with pain stemming from the lumbar zygapophyseal joints. Is the lumbar facet syndrome a clinical entity? Spine 1994; 19: 1132–1137.

58 Schwarzer AC, Wang S, Bogduk N, McNaught PJ, Laurent R. Prevalence and clinical features of lumbar zygapophyseal joint pain: a study in an Australian population with chronic low back pain. Ann Rheum Dis 1995; 54: 100–106.

59 Manchikanti L, Pampati V, Fellows B, Bakhit CE. Prevalence of lumbar facet joint pain in chronic low back pain. Pain Phys 1999; 2: 59–64.

60 Schwarzer AC, Derby R, Aprill CN, Fortin J, Kine G, Bogduk N. Pain from the lumbar zygapophyseal joints: a test of two models. J Spinal Disord 1994; 7: 331–336.

61 Schwarzer AC, Wang S, O'Driscoll D, Harrington T, Bogduk N, Laurent T. The ability of computed tomography to identify a painful zygapophyseal joint in patients with chronic low back pain. Spine 1995; 20: 907–912.

62 Fortin JD, Dwyer AP, West S, Pier J. Sacroiliac joint: pain referral maps upon applying a new injection/arthrography technique: Part I: asymptomatic volunteers. Spine 1994; 19: 1475–1482.

63 Schwarzer AC, Aprill CN, Bogduk N. The sacroiliac joint in chronic low back pain. Spine 1995; 20: 31–37.

64 Maigne JY, Aivaliklis A, Pfefer F. Results of sacroiliac joint double block and value of sacroiliac pain provocation tests in 54 patients with low-back pain. Spine 1996; 21: 1889–1892.

65 Schwarzer AC, Aprill CN, Derby R, Fortin J, Kine G, Bogduk N. The relative contributions of the disc and zygapophyseal joint in chronic low back pain. Spine 1994; 19: 801–806.

Medical Management of Acute and Chronic Low Back Pain. An Evidence-Based Approach
Pain Research and Clinical Management, Vol. 13
Nikolai Bogduk and Brian McGuirk

CHAPTER 15

Assessment

1. Introduction

The assessment of a patient with chronic low back pain shares the same principles as pertain to the assessment of acute low back pain, although with certain modifications. Taking a history remains important. Physical examination remains unproductive. Imaging assumes a relatively greater importance. Psychological assessment becomes more significant. Certain investigations, not indicated for acute low back pain, become relevant for chronic back pain.

2. History

The protocol for taking a history of chronic low back pain can be the same as the protocol for acute low back pain (Chapter 6). Understandably, the history will be longer, and the patient will probably have undergone a large number of treatments (which, by definition, will have failed to provide relief). Nevertheless, following a systematic protocol ensures that no, possibly significant, aspect of the patient's history is overlooked.

Taking a history, in terms of the site of pain, its spread, quality, frequency, duration, aggravating factors, and relieving factors (Chapter 6), serves to describe the patient's complaint. However, neither alone, nor in combination, are these various features likely to provide a patho-anatomic diagnosis. No pattern of pain, no pattern of aggravating or relieving factors, points to any particular condition. Indeed, the most common causes of chronic back pain (Chapter 14) are indistinguishable from one another clinically. Certain negative caveats, however, apply.

Widespread pain, extending out of the lumbar region into the thoracic region and beyond, does not constitute low back pain. Something else is going on. Patients with such pain may well have started with a focal low back pain; they may still have a lumbar source of pain; but their symptoms reflect more than a focal source. They may have developed spreading, central hyperalgesia, driven by their original source of pain. They may have a somatization disorder[1]. These conditions, their diagnosis, and their management are not covered by the evidence-base for low back pain, and are beyond the province of this text.

Some may consider them important differential diagnoses of back pain, but they are characterized by widespread pain in a single, confluent area. The pain may encompass the lumbar region but it extends caudad into the lower limbs, and cephalad into the thoracic region and even beyond. This distribution distinguishes it from low back pain. To a purist, widespread pain is not a differential diagnosis of low back pain which, by definition, is pain confined to the lumbosacral region, with or without referral to the lower limbs (Chapter 2). Widespread pain is a different entity.

However, widespread pain should not be confused with somatic referred pain, which starts in the lumbosacral region and spreads into one or both lower limbs. Somatic referred pain, however, does not extend cephalad to encompass the thoracic or other regions.

Nor does widespread pain pertain to patients with multiple sources of musculoskeletal pain. A patient with neck pain or shoulder pain is quite entitled also to develop back pain as a separate, but additional, problem; just as a patient with osteoarthritis of the

Name:					Low Back Pain		
D.O.B.			M.R.N.				
Presence of			*Cardiovascular*			*Endocrine*		
Trauma	Y	N	Risk factors?	Y	N	Corticosteroids?	Y	N
Night Sweats	Y	N	*Respiratory*			*Musculoskeletal*		
Recent Surgery	Y	N	Cough?	Y	N	Pain elsewhere?	Y	N
Catheterisation	Y	N	*Urinary*			*Neurological*		
Venipuncture	Y	N	Haematuria?	Y	N	Symptoms/signs	Y	N
Occupational exposure	Y	N	Retention?	Y	N	*Skin*		
Hobby exposure	Y	N	Stream problems?	Y	N	Infections?	Y	N
Sporting exposure	Y	N	*Reproductive*			Rashes?	Y	N
(Overseas) travel	Y	N	Menstrual problems?	Y	N	*G.I.T.*		
Illicit drug use	Y	N	*Haemopoietic*			Diarrhoea?	Y	N
Weight loss	Y	N	Problems?	Y	N			
History of Cancer	Y	N						
Comments					*Signature:*		
					Date:		

Fig. 1. A checklist for red flag clinical indicators, suitable for inclusion in medical records used in general practice, developed by the author for the National Musculoskeletal Medicine Initiative.

hip is entitled to get back pain. Multiple, concurrent musculoskeletal complaints do not necessarily imply a single, unifying cause; nor should the practitioner be driven to find such a single cause. Patients with multiple complaints do not have a single, confluent region of pain. Each concurrent complaint is circumscribed, rendering it discrete topographically; each has a different history, and different aggravating factors. The cardinal distinction is that each regional pain problem would make perfect sense if it occurred in isolation, as the patient's only complaint. The presentation is rendered complicated only by the simultaneity of more than one concurrent complaint. The apparent complexity is simplified by reducing the presentation to each of its regional components. Each component can then be assessed and managed separately. Whereupon, the patient's back pain is but one of several problems that the patient has.

As with acute low back pain, *associated features are paramount* in detecting red flag conditions. The red flag checklist (Fig. 1) serves just as well for chronic low back pain as it does for acute low back pain. Encountering a positive response to any item on this checklist does not make a diagnosis of a red flag condition, but it does prompt further consideration, and possibly investigation, for a serious medical condition. On the other hand, nil responses to all items on the checklist allow the practitioner and the patient to be reassured that a serious condition is extremely unlikely to be the cause of pain.

In patients with chronic low back pain, neurological signs or symptoms can have various implications. Most critically, their onset may indicate that the lesion responsible for the back pain has progressed or extended to involve the nervous system. On the other hand, the patient may have developed neurological complications, such as arachnoiditis, as a result of previous investigations or treatment. Whatever the possible causes, neurological features constitute a complication. The patient is suffering more than just back pain, and assessing the cause of their neurological impairment becomes more critical than finding the cause of their back pain. Consequently, the investigation of such patients is driven by the neurological features, not by their pain.

Quite deliberately, the investigation and management of neurological disorders is not addressed in this text. The investigation and management of intraspinal and extraspinal tumours, and of myelopathy should follow conventional lines. For radicular pain and radiculopathy, their assessment and management according to evidence-based principles has been addressed elsewhere[2]. For present purposes, however, the important principle is that the investigation of neurological disorders should not be confused with, or misportrayed as appropriate for, the investigation of uncomplicated chronic low back pain. Thus, for example, whereas CT scanning may be appropriate for the investigation of numbness and weakness, it is not indicated when pain is the only presenting feature.

References

1   DSM-IV. Diagnostic and Statistical Manual of Mental Disorders, 4th edn. American Psychiatric Association, Washington, DC, 1994, pp 446–452.
2   Bogduk N, Govind J. Medical Management of Acute Lumbar Radicular Pain. An Evidence-Based Approach. Newcastle Bone and Joint Institute, Newcastle, 1999.

3. Physical examination

The fact that a patient has chronic low back pain instead of acute low back pain does not change the evidence-base concerning physical examination (Chapter 7). Although a practitioner may 'look', 'feel', and 'move', no clinical test that he or she might perform has sufficient reliability and validity to allow the formulation of a patho-anatomic diagnosis. Nevertheless, physical examination may be relevant and appropriate to provide a description of disability, and to serve as a baseline against which improvements might be measured, but this is not tantamount to establishing a diagnosis.

Nor will a neurological examination provide a diagnosis. If a patient has neurological signs, they no longer simply have back pain. They have a neurological disorder that invites investigation and management in its own right, as if the back pain was irrelevant.

With respect to the three most common causes of chronic low back pain — internal disc disruption, zygapophysial joint pain, and sacroiliac joint pain (Chapter 14), there is mixed evidence concerning the utility of physical examination as a means of providing a diagnosis.

A positive response for centralization under the McKenzie system of assessment correlates with the presence of internal disc disruption[1]. The correlation is insufficiently strong to be diagnostic, but the positive likelihood ratio of 2.4, that has been found for this assessment, increases the chances of internal disc disruption being the cause of pain from a pre-test likelihood of 40% to a post-test likelihood of 60%[2].

There are no tests that are diagnostic of zygapophysial joint pain[3–5], but certain features increase the likelihood that zygapophysial joints are the source of pain. An idiosyncrasy of these features is that some involve a combination of positive and negative features. It is the absence, rather than the presence, of certain features that implicates the zygapophysial joints. The features are age greater than 65 years, pain relieved by recumbency, and *absence* of aggravation of pain by coughing, forward flexion, rising from flexion, hyperextension, and extension–rotation[6]. If five or more of these features are evident, the likelihood ratio for zygapophysial joints being the source of pain is 3.0[7]. Nevertheless, because the prevalence of zygapophysial joint pain is low, even with this likelihood ratio, the diagnostic confidence that the zygapophysial joints are the source of pain remains low. For a prevalence of 15%, the diagnostic confidence is barely 35%. For a prevalence of 40%, the diagnostic confidence is only 67%.

Some investigators have found certain physical tests of sacroiliac joint pain to be reliable[8]. Others have denied this[9]. However, both agree that no test has been shown to be valid for sacroiliac joint pain[8,10]. Accordingly, sacroiliac joint pain cannot be diagnosed by physical examination.

A certain set of physical tests has achieved an application and notoriety that is dissonant with the purpose for which it was originally introduced. These are the so-called Waddell's inorganic tests[11]. They involve: assessing the patient's response to simulated axial loading and simulated rotation; the response to straight-leg raising in the sitting position; and noting overreaction to physical examination, and any inappropriate distribution of numbness and weakness. These tests were introduced to help practitioners recognize patients whose problems encompassed more than just a physical impairment, and for whom a more detailed psychological assessment might be warranted. In essence, they were no more than screening tests that served as a bridge between physical assessment and psychological assessment.

These tests, however, rapidly became misused. Instead of being used as a means of progressing to psychological assessment in an unobtrusive and compassionate manner, they were applied to define ingenuine patients, particularly in medicolegal assessments. The tests were originally named 'nonorganic physical signs', and this probably facilitated their abuse. Patients with nonorganic signs could be diagnosed as not having an organic cause for their pain.

The misuse became so rampant that the original author had occasion to redress the issue[12]. With a colleague, he emphasized that the tests constituted only a psychological screen, and were not a substitute for complete psychological assessment; nor were they a test of credibility or veracity. Furthermore, they were not a basis for denying proper treatment, be that physical, psychological or a combination of both.

Nor are the tests prognostic of outcome. Several studies have determined the extent to which return to work correlates with positive responses to one or

more of the tests[13–16]. The results of those studies were conveniently summarized in the most recent study[16]. Of interest is the negative likelihood ratio of the tests, viz. their ability to predict failure to return to work. For various combinations of responses to the tests, the negative likelihood ratios are barely less than 1.0, most being between 0.60 and 0.90, the least being 0.48[16]. Such ratios indicate only about a 10% greater risk of not returning to work.

The nonorganic signs are not diagnostic, nor are they predictive. They serve explicitly and only to alert practitioners to consider that something more than an organic lesion is affecting the patient.

References

1   Donelson R, Aprill C, Medcalf R, Grant W. A prospective study of centralization of lumbar and referred pain. Spine 1997; 33: 1115–1122.
2   Bogduk N, Lord SM. Commentary on: A prospective study of centralization of lumbar and referred pain: a predictor of symptomatic discs and anular competence. Pain Med J Club J 1997; 3: 246–248.
3   Schwarzer AC, Aprill CN, Derby R, Fortin J, Kine G, Bogduk N. Clinical features of patients with pain stemming from the lumbar zygapophysial joints. Is the lumbar facet syndrome a clinical entity? Spine 1994; 19: 1132–1137.
4   Schwarzer AC, Wang S, Bogduk N, McNaught PJ, Laurent R. Prevalence and clinical features of lumbar zygapophyseal joint pain: a study in an Australian population with chronic low back pain. Ann Rheum Dis 1995; 54: 100–106.
5   Schwarzer AC, Derby R, Aprill CN, Fortin J, Kine G, Bogduk N. Pain from the lumbar zygapophyseal joints: a test of two models. J Spinal Disord 1994; 7: 331–336.
6   Revel M, Poiraudeau S, Auleley GR, Payan C, Denke A, Nguyen M, Chevrot A, Fermanian J. Capacity of the clinical picture to characterize low back pain relieved by facet joint anesthesia. Proposed criteria to identify patients with painful facet joints. Spine 1998; 23: 1972–1977.
7   Bogduk N. Commentary on the capacity of the clinical picture to characterize low back pain relieved by facet joint anesthesia. Pain Med J Club J 1998; 4: 221–222.
8   Dreyfuss P, Michaelsen M, Pauza K, McLarty J, Bogduk N. The value of history and physical examination in diagnosing sacroiliac joint pain. Spine 1996; 21: 2594–2602.
9   van der Wurff P, Hagmeijer RHM, Meyne W. Clinical tests of the sacroiliac joint. A systematic methodological review. Part I: reliability. Man Ther 2000; 5: 30–36.
10   van der Wurff P, Meyne W, Hagmeijer RHM. Clinical tests

of the sacroiliac joint. A systematic methodological review. Part 2: validity. Man Ther 2000; 5: 89–96.

11 Waddell G, McCulloch JA, Kummel E, Venner RM. Nonorganic physical signs in low-back pain. Spine 1980; 5: 117–125.

12 Main CJ, Waddell G. Spine Update. Behavioral responses to examination. A reappraisal of the interpretation of 'nonorganic signs'. Spine 1998; 23: 2367–2371.

13 Bradish CF, Lloyd GJ, Aldam CH, Albert J, Dyson P, Doxey NCS, Mitson GL. Do nonorganic signs help to predict the return to activity of patients with low-back pain? Spine 1988; 13: 557–560.

14 Wernecke MW, Harris DE, Lichter RL. Clinical effectiveness of behavioral signs for screening chronic low-back pain patients in a work-oriented physical rehabilitation program. Spine 1993; 18: 2412–2418.

15 Kummel BM. Nonorganic signs of significance in low back pain. Spine 1996; 21: 1077–1081.

16 Fritz JM, Wainner RS, Hicks GE. The use of nonorganic signs and symptoms as a screening tool for return-to-work in patients with acute low back pain. Spine 2000; 25: 1925–1931.

4. Psychological assessment

The impetus for psychological assessment stems from the recognition of chronic back pain as an illness that involves more than just a complaint of pain [1,2]. It involves reactions and responses to that pain and its persistence. These reactions produce distress and suffering, and result in pain behaviours. Recognizing these responses becomes as much part of the assessment as recognizing the physical symptoms and signs. Failure to recognize psychological dimensions of a patient's problem can compromise the effectiveness of medical management [1,2]. Meanwhile, psychologists contend that certain psychological features can and should be targeted for treatment in their own right [2].

Psychological assessment does not equate to the pursuit of a pejorative diagnosis, such as malingering. A review of the literature [3] found that malingering is a rare phenomenon amongst patients with chronic pain; and its diagnosis is fraught with difficulties; yet pain behaviours are often mistaken for, or misrepresented as evidence of, malingering. As a medical diagnosis, malingering has no valid operational criteria [4]; it is no more than a suspicion or

an opinion that the patient is complaining of pain falsely, but deliberately, motivated by an external incentive such as to avoid responsibilities or obtain financial gain. Like several other purely psychological diagnoses, the diagnosis of malingering requires that there be no physical basis for the patient's complaint; but physical examination (see above) and conventional medical imaging (see below) can neither detect nor refute a cause of chronic back pain, in the majority of cases. Therefore, this requirement cannot be satisfied using conventional investigations. For such reasons, experts have warned that physicians should desist from believing that malingering can be conclusively identified in some way; that referrals to professionals for such a determination should be discouraged; and claims that such a determination has some validity should be viewed with caution [3].

Nor is psychological assessment acquitted by attributing the patient's complaints to 'secondary gain'. Although popular, this concept has a fragile foundation in the scientific literature [5]. A thorough review of this topic has found that research on this phenomenon is weak and constrained by many methodological flaws [5]. Nevertheless, certain pertinent conclusions can be drawn. Foremost, the presence of alleged secondary gain does not add to the validity of identifying patients with psychiatric disorders versus organic disorders [5]. Nor does the receipt of financial benefits change behaviour [5]; and the secondary losses that patients suffer often outweigh the benefits perceived by others of alleged secondary gains [5].

There is no universally accepted protocol for psychological assessment of the patient with chronic low back pain. Various experts and individuals have developed their own particular approach. Furthermore, options apply, as to whether the assessment should be undertaken by interview or by the application of questionnaires; and as to whether the assessment is the responsibility of the patient's attending practitioner or should be delegated to specialist professionals.

Many practitioners may feel uncomfortable conducting a psychological assessment. For lack of training or experience, they may feel that they do not know what to do; they may feel it is not their responsibility; or they may feel that they do not have the time to undertake an assessment. Accordingly, they may prefer to engage specialist professionals in order to avoid engaging in psychological assessment themselves.

However, if a practitioner is to remain involved in the management of a patient, and even if they do not undertake the psychological assessment themselves, they should be aware of what psychologists can and might do. Without resorting to formal questionnaires and similar devices, a practitioner can undertake a psychological assessment at least to identify potential problems relevant to the patient and to their management. What to look for can be distilled from what the various questionnaires are designed to detect.

Fear–avoidance behaviour applies as much to chronic low back pain as it does to acute low back pain (Chapter 5). If a patient's fears and beliefs were not recognized and successfully addressed during the acute phase of their illness, they will constitute an important component of the chronic phase. Mistaken beliefs and unconstructive behaviours compound the patient's disability and may interfere with recovery. Enquiring about physical, domestic, social, and vocational issues (Chapter 10) reveals how patients have reacted and responded to their pain, and what impact the pain has had on them. In that regard, it should constitute a standard part of the medical assessment. Obtaining that information constitutes a first step towards a psychological assessment.

The Fear–Avoidance Behaviour Questionnaire (FABQ)[6] scores responses to questions about what the patient believes about the relationship between their pain and physical activity and work. It asks if the patient believes that physical activity makes the pain worse, or harms the back. It asks if the patient believes that work is responsible for the pain, and will make it worse; and if the patient cannot or should not return to work. These same issues can be addressed in the course of a normal interview without necessarily administering a formal questionnaire (Chapter 10).

Patients with chronic low back pain may be involved in compensation claims. These patients may have fears, beliefs, and expectations that pertain to what they must go through and what they will achieve by pursuing their claim. Not to imply that the claim is unjustified, but some of these beliefs and expectations may be unrealistic, and counterproductive to recovery; and for that reason should be explored, and resolved, if necessary.

A particular focus of psychologists has been how patients cope with, and adjust to, chronic pain. To measure these features quantitatively, they have developed and implemented a variety of instruments to assess these processes, such as the Vanderbilt Pain Management Inventory (VPMI), the Coping Strategies Questionnaire (CSQ), Ways of Coping Checklist (WCCL), and the Multidimensional Health Locus of Control (MHLC) scale. Experts have commented on the utility of these instruments and how they have been applied in research studies[2,7].

What research studies have shown of significance in this regard is that a substantial proportion of patients with chronic pain believe that their problems are not under their own control, but are attributed to chance, luck, or to the actions of other people[2,7–10], or believe that pain is enduring and mysterious[11]. These patients tend to have greater psychological distress, feel helpless, and use praying and hoping to cope with pain[7,8]. Furthermore, they tend to catastrophize[2,8–11], i.e. over-rate and overstate the negative aspects of their problems and their effects. Indeed, catastrophizing, in itself, has been shown to be related to reports of higher levels of pain, disability, and distress[12].

Such beliefs and behaviours are regarded by some as maladaptive[8,9]. Instead of taking responsibility for their own rehabilitation, these patients may pursue and become dependent on passive treatments despite the fact that they do not work. If for no other reason, these beliefs and behaviours should be recognized so as to prevent the futile pursuit of passive therapies. As well, psychologists contend that these beliefs should be targeted as part of any treatment, with the prospect that the beliefs can be changed and that the patient might develop successful pain management skills[7–9,11,13].

Depression is a specific symptom exhibited by many patients with chronic pain. Indeed, it is so prevalent that it can be expected to be expressed, to some degree or other, by any patient with chronic low back pain. Specialist units can identify and quantify depression through the administration of instruments such as the Beck Depression Inventory (BDI) [14] or the Zung Depression Index [15]. For screening purposes in less specialist settings, other approaches are possible, in which depression is assessed as an important, but only one of several, factors that constitute general psychological distress.

The Symptom Checklist-90 Revised (SCLR-90R) is an instrument that can be easily and rapidly administered in conventional practice. It screens for abnormalities in nine specific categories — somatization, obsessive–compulsive traits, interpersonal sensitivity, depression, anxiety, hostility, phobic anxiety, paranoid ideation, and psychoticism. When applied to patients with chronic low back pain, it shows elevations particularly in the scales for somatization, depression, obsessive–compulsive, and psychoticism [16,17]. Respectively, these scales reflect attentional focus on physical sensations, depression, pain-related rumination and frustration, and feelings of isolation as well as loss of control [17]. These features do not indicate a primary psychological disorder, nor do they indicate general psychological distress. Rather, they reflect a characteristic cluster of psychological symptoms that are the consequence of experiencing chronic pain. In less formal and more colloquial terms, the SCL-90R shows that patients with chronic back pain feel their pain, are pre-occupied with it, are depressed, and feel unable to do anything about it. Practitioners not wishing to administer instruments such as the SCL-90R, can, nevertheless, explore these issues by conventional interview, in order to determine the extent to which patients are distressed by their chronic low back pain.

Another instrument for assessing psychological distress is the Distress and Risk Assessment Method (DRAM) [18]. This is a simple and straightforward method of assessment, whose results correlate significantly with other psychometric instruments such as the CSQ, MHLC, BDI, and the Minnesota Multiphasic Personality Inventory [18]. The principal components of the DRAM enquire about somatic fea-

TABLE I

Elements assessed by the Distress and Risk Assessment Method [17]

Somatic perception	Depression
Heart rate increase	Feels downhearted
Feeling hot all over	Feels best in morning
Sweating all over	Has crying spells or feels like it
Sweating in a particular part of the body	Has trouble getting to sleep at night
Pulse in neck	Feels that nobody cares
Pounding in head	Eats as much as used they to
Dizziness	Still enjoys sex
Blurring of vision	Losing weight
Feeling faint	Has trouble with constipation
Everything appearing unreal	Heart beats faster than usual
Nausea	Gets tired for no reason
Butterflies in stomach	Mind is as clear as it used to be
Pain or ache in stomach	Tends to wake up too early
Stomach churning	Finds it easy to do the things they used to
Desire to pass water	Is restless and cannot keep still
Mouth becoming dry	Is hopeful about the future
Difficulty swallowing	Is more irritable than usual
Muscles in neck aching	Finds it easy to make a decision
Legs feeling weak	Feels quite guilty
Muscles twitching or jumping	Feels useful and needed
Tense feeling across forehead	Life is pretty full
Tense feeling in jaw muscles	Feels that they would be better of if dead
	Still able to enjoy the things they used to

tures and features of depression (Table I). Using a questionnaire format [18], responses to these items can be scored to determine levels of distress. High scores correlate with higher reported levels of pain, and with poorer outcome from treatment. Practitioners not wishing to administer the questionnaire format can, nevertheless, screen patients for significant distress by enquiring about the items listed in Table I. By referring to the table, or the original instrument [18], they can ensure that they do not omit particular symptoms of distress.

4.1. Synopsis

It is difficult to recommend exactly to what extent an individual practitioner should become engaged in the psychological domain of a patient with chronic low back pain. This depends on whether the practitioner feels capable of pursuing psychological matters; whether they are prepared to afford the effort to pursue them fully; and whether they believe there is merit in doing so.

The merit of defining psychological problems is two-fold. First and foremost, patients with a high degree of psychological distress respond more poorly to conventional treatment. Recognizing psychological distress, therefore, serves to prevent prescribing routine treatment that is destined to fail, which in turn will compound the patient's distress. Secondly, psychologists contend that various elements of psychological distress can be formally treated, and that these problems, rather than the patient's physical complaints, should be the priority of treatment. The efficacy of such treatment is addressed in Chapter 17.

For these reasons, psychological assessment cannot be ignored. The question that remains is whether the practitioner is responsible for the assessment or whether they should refer the patient for assessment by a specialist. An appropriate answer is that both apply.

For patients with high levels of psychological distress, or with particular maladaptive beliefs, the time necessary to explore the problems in detail, and the techniques for their management, will be beyond the province of 'physically oriented' practitioners. Such patients will require specialist intervention. However, that should not excuse the practitioner from becoming aware of the psychological problems and understanding them. Referrals should not be dismissive: summarily sending the patient 'off to the psychologist'. They should be undertaken with insight. That requires at least a prima facie assessment of the problems at hand, and with which the practitioner is seeking assistance. To that end, the precepts outlined in this section, should enable the practitioner to formulate a preliminary assessment that can be explained to the patient, and which becomes the basis for a cogent referral to a specialist.

References

1 Waddell G. A new clinical model for the treatment of low-back pain. Spine 1987; 12: 632–644.
2 Keefe, FJ, Bradley LA, Main CJ. Psychological Assessment of the pain patient for the general clinician. In: Pain 1999 — An Updated Review. Refresher Course Syllabus. IASP Press, Seattle, WA, 1999: 219–230.
3 Fishbain DA, Cutler R, Rosomoff HL, Rosomoff RS. Chronic pain disability exaggeration/malingering and submaximal effort research. Clin J Pain 1999; 15: 244–274.
4 DSM-IV. Diagnostic and Statistical Manual of Mental Disorders, 4th edn. American Psychiatric Association, Washington, DC, 1994, p 683.
5 Fishbain DA, Rosomoff HL, Cutler RB, Rosomoff RS. Secondary gain concept: a review of the scientific evidence. Clin J Pain 1995; 11: 6–21.
6 Waddell G, Newton M, Henderson I, Somerville D, Main CJ. A fear–avoidance beliefs questionnaire (FABQ) and the role of fear–avoidance beliefs in chronic low back pain and disability. Pain 1993; 52: 157–168.
7 Jensen MP, Turner JA, Romano JM, Karoly P. Coping with chronic pain: a critical review of the literature. Pain 1991; 47: 249–283.
8 Crisson JE, Keefe FJ. The relationship of locus of control to pain coping strategies and psychological distress in chronic pain patients. Pain 1988; 35: 147–154.
9 Rosenstiel AK, Keefe FJ. The use of coping strategies in chronic low back pain patients: relationship to patient characteristics and current adjustment. Pain 1983; 17: 33–44.
10 Strong J, Ashton R, Stewart A. Chronic low back pain: toward an integrated psychosocial assessment model. J Consult Clin Psychol 1994; 62: 1058–1063.
11 Williams DA, Keefe FJ. Pain beliefs and the use of cognitive–behavioral coping strategies. Pain 1991; 46: 185–190.
12 Severeijns R, Vlaeyen JWS, van der Hout MA, Weber WEJ. Pain catastrophizing predicts pain intensity, disability, and psychological distress independent of the level of physical impairment. Clin J Pain 2001; 17: 165–172.
13 Jensen MP, Turner JA, Romano JM, Lawler BK. Relationship of pain-specific beliefs to chronic pain adjustment. Pain 1994; 57: 301–309.
14 Zung WWK. A self-rating depression scale. Arch Gen Psychiatry 1965; 32: 63–70.
15 Beck AT, Ward CH, Mendelson M, Mock J, Erbaugh J. An inventory for measuring depression. Arch Gen Psychiatry 1961; 4: 561–571.
16 Kinney RK, Gatchel RJ, Mayer TG. The SCL-90R evaluated as an alternative to the MMPI for psychological screening of chronic low-back pain patients. Spine 1991; 16: 940–942.
17 Peebles JE, McWilliams LA, MacLennan R. A comparison of symptom checklist 90 — revised from patients chronic pain from whiplash and patients with other musculoskeletal injuries. Spine 2001; 26: 766–770.

18 Main CJ, Wood PLR, Hollis S, Spanswick CC, Waddell G. The distress and risk assessment method. A simple patient classification to identify distress and evaluate the risk of poor outcome. Spine 1992; 17: 42–52.

5. Medical imaging

With respect to reliability and validity, the evidence concerning medical imaging is the same for chronic low back pain is it was for acute low back pain (Chapter 8). What differs is its utility.

Given that history and physical examination are not diagnostic, and given that the patient's pain has persisted, the possibility of a serious but occult lesion obtains. The probability of a red flag condition is low (Chapter 6), and even less so if the patient has no red flag indicators. Nevertheless, failure to improve constitutes a criterion for checking and ensuring that the patient does not have a demonstrable lesion that has not yet progressed to produce neurological or systemic features. Medical imaging is the paramount means of doing so, but the critical issue is what constitutes the appropriate screening test.

Plain radiographs can show bone, but bone lesions are rare causes of back pain, be it acute or chronic. Plain radiographs may detect myeloma or osseous metastases, if these are advanced; but plain radiographs may fail to detect these and other conditions of bone. Plain radiographs will not detect lesions in soft tissues. Thus, one cannot be certain that a normal radiograph has effectively excluded serious causes of pain. Conversely, plain radiographs will detect structural abnormalities that are not related to pain (Chapter 8) but which might be misrepresented as the cause of pain. This constitutes a possible distraction from pursuing the real cause. Plain radiography, therefore, is not an appropriate screening test for chronic low back pain. Its false-negative rate and its false-positive rate provide a false sense of security that either an occult lesion has been excluded, or that the cause of pain has been found.

Resorting to CT scanning does not improve the situation. CT may be appropriate for the pursuit of neurological signs, but that is not a surrogate for pursuing back pain. CT is not indicated for low back pain.

As a screening test for low back pain, magnetic resonance imaging (MRI) has the virtues of having high sensitivity and high specificity. It demonstrates the surrounding soft tissues of the lumbar spine as well as the internal architecture of the vertebral bodies and intervertebral discs. It is able to demonstrate bone lesions and haemopoietic lesions. It is able to demonstrate intradural and extradural lesions. For these reasons, it is the best available screening test for patients with persistent back pain. Its disadvantages are cost and relative inaccessibility in some places in the world. However, both seem to be improving. As MRI becomes more accessible its costs come down. Furthermore, if practitioners have been disciplined in their use of medical imaging for patients with acute back pain, they will have used plain films rarely and CT scans not at all. Those savings could offset the cost to society of the use of MRI for patients with chronic pain.

Accordingly, if a practitioner is concerned about occult lesions, MRI constitutes the investigation of choice. It reveals and excludes more lesions more thoroughly than either plain films or CT. If MRI is not available, plain films and CT are not substitutes; they are inferior options.

Yet, upon obtaining MRI, a practitioner should be cognisant that the likely yield of red flag conditions is low. Most scans will be normal or reveal only age-related changes. Degenerative changes and disc bulges are no more a diagnosis of chronic back pain than they are a diagnosis of acute back pain (Chapter 8). However, there are certain features that MRI can reveal that are pertinent to chronic low back pain.

5.1. High-intensity zone

The high-intensity zone (HIZ) is a feature that can occur in the posterior anulus of a lumbar intervertebral disc. It is seen on T2-weighted images, and consists of a bright signal surrounded by the dark signal of fibres of the anulus fibrosus anterior and posterior to it (Fig. 2). It constitutes the appearance in sagittal section of the circumferential portion of

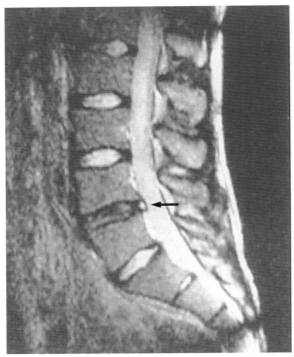

Fig. 2. The appearance of a high-intensity zone in an anulus fibrosus (arrow).

TABLE II

The prevalence and validity of the high intensity zone as a sign of painful internal disc disruption, as reported by various studies

Source	Prevalence	Sensitivity	Specificity	LR
1	28%	0.71	0.89	6.5
2	45%	na	na	na
3	na	0.27	0.95	5.4
4	na	0.52	0.90	5.2
5	na	0.78	0.74	3.0
6	na	0.31	0.90	3.1
7	na	0.09	0.93	1.3

LR, positive likelihood ratio; na, data not provided.

a grade IV anular fissure. A particular feature of the HIZ, as originally described, is that it is an ultra-bright signal: one that rivals and exceeds the brightness of the cerebrospinal fluid [11]. This feature distinguishes it from other types of fissures that can occur in the anulus fibrosus, and which may or may not be symptomatic.

When originally described, the HIZ was found to have a prevalence of 28% in 500 patients with chronic low back pain, and a strong correlation with the affected disc having a painful, grade III or grade IV fissure [1]. In that respect, it had a positive-predictive value of 89%, and a positive likelihood ratio of 6.0. Accordingly, it was heralded as a sign that occurred in a minority of patients but one that was diagnostic of internal disc disruption [1]. This gave MRI an unprecedented utility. Not only did MRI have a role as a screening test for red flag conditions, it had the ability to indicate the source of pain, at least in a proportion of patients.

Subsequent studies have provided a mixture of corroborating and dissenting results (Table II). Only one other study has measured the prevalence of high-intensity zones in patients with chronic low back pain [2]. An HIZ was detected in 45% of 156 patients. Other studies have investigated selected samples of patients to determine the correlation between the HIZ and discogenic pain. Although various studies have disputed the sensitivity of this sign, all have agreed on a high specificity (Table II). Furthermore, all but one study found reasonable or high positive likelihood ratios. These consistencies indicate that although the HIZ will not necessarily detect all cases of internal disc disruption, when present, it is very unlikely to be false-positive.

Underlying the variation in the data are several technical and conceptual issues. Not all studies that have looked for the HIZ have used the same settings to obtain heavily T2-weighted images. The study with the lowest sensitivity used images in which the signal from the cerebrospinal fluid was not starkly white, and disregarded the criterion of an extremely bright signal. An HIZ is not just any white spot in the anulus.

Reservations have been raised concerning the validity of the HIZ on the grounds that it commonly occurs in asymptomatic patients [8,9]. In this regard, the HIZ was never promoted as an unqualified sign of back pain. This sign does not discriminate between patients with and without back pain, but its validity applies in patients who do have back pain. In such patients, the HIZ strongly indicates that the affected disc is the source of the patient's pain, and predicts that the disc will have internal disc disruption with a grade III or grade IV fissure.

5.2. Endplate changes

Between 20% and 50% of patients with chronic back pain exhibit abnormalities evident in one or more vertebral endplates [10–12]. Typically, these consist of high-intensity signals that are associated with fissuring of the cartilage and increased vascularity in the subchondral bone. Although endplate changes can occur concurrently with high-intensity zones, they can also occur independently [12]. e

When present, these endplate changes are strongly associated with the affected disc being painful. One study [12] found the sensitivity of endplate changes to be low (0.23), but the specificity was high (0.97), yielding a likelihood ratio of 7.7. Another [4] found similar sensitivity (0.22) and specificity (0.95), but a smaller likelihood ratio (4.4). Nevertheless, these ratios provide a diagnostic confidence of internal disc disruption being the cause of pain of 83% and 75%, respectively.

Key points

- History is not diagnostic in the assessment of patients with chronic back pain, but it is an important tool in screening for red flag indicators.
- Physical examination is not diagnostic but certain tests can increase the likelihood of internal disc disruption, or zygapophysial joint pain, being the basis of the patient's complaint.
- The importance of psychological assessment lies in identifying patients who are distressed by their pain and have difficulty coping. Doing so avoids misdirecting these patients to inappropriate passive therapy, and they may benefit from more behaviourally orientated interventions.
- Plain radiography and CT are not indicated in the investigation of back pain.
- MRI constitutes an optimal screening test for occult lesions.
- High-intensity zone lesions and vertebral endplate changes are strongly indicative that the affected disc is the source of the patient's pain.

References

1 Aprill C, Bogduk N. High-intensity zone: a diagnostic sign of painful lumbar disc on magnetic resonance imaging. Br J Radiol 1992; 65: 361–369.

2 Rankine JJ, Gill P, Hutchinson CE, Ross ERS, Williamson JB. The clinical significance of the high-intensity zone on lumbar spine magnetic resonance imaging. Spine 1999; 24: 1913–1920.

3 Saifuddin A, Braithwaite I, White J, Taylor BA, Renton P. The value of lumbar spine magnetic resonance imaging in the demonstration of anular tears. Spine 1998; 23: 453–457.

4 Ito M, Incorvaia KM, Yu SF, Fredrickson BE, Yuan HA, Rosenbaum AE. Predictive signs of discogenic lumbar pain on magnetic resonance imaging with discography correlation. Spine 1998; 23: 1252–1260.

5 Schellhas KP, Pollei SR, Gundry CR, Heithoff KB. Lumbar disc high-intensity zone; correlation of magnetic resonance imaging and discography. Spine 1996; 21: 79–86.

6 Smith BMT, Hurwitz EL, Solsberg D, Rubinstein D, Corenman DS, Dwyer AP, Kleiner J. Interobserver reliability of detecting lumbar intervertebral disc high-intensity zone on magnetic resonance imaging and association of high-intensity zone with pain and anular disruption. Spine 1998; 23: 2074–2080.

7 Ricketson R, Simmons JW, Hauser BO. The prolapsed intervertebral disc. The high-intensity zone with discography correlation. Spine 1996; 21: 2758–2762.

8 Stadnik TW, Lee RR, Coen HL, Neirynck EC, Buissert TS, Osteaux MJ. Annular tears and disk herniation: prevalence and contrast enhancement on MR images in the absence of low back pain or sciatica. Radiology 1998; 206: 49–55.

9 Buirski G, Silberstein M. The symptomatic lumbar disc in patients with low-back pain: magnetic resonance imaging appearances in both a symptomatic and control population. Spine 1993; 18: 1808–1811.

10 de Roos A, Kressel K, Spritzer C, Dalinka M. MR imaging of marrow changes adjacent to end plates in degenerative lumbar disc disease. Am J Roentgenol 1987; 149: 531–534.

11 Modic MT, Steindberger PM, Ross JS, Masaryk TJ, Carter JR. Degenerative disc disease: assessment of changes in vertebral body marrow with MR imaging. Radiology 1988; 166: 193–199.

12 Braithwaite I, White J, Saifuddin A, Renton P, Taylor BA. Vertebral end-plate (Modic) changes on lumbar spine MRI: correlation with pain reproduction at lumbar discography. Eur Spine J 1998; 7: 363–368.

Medical Management of Acute and Chronic Low Back Pain. An Evidence-Based Approach
Pain Research and Clinical Management, Vol. 13
Nikolai Bogduk and Brian McGuirk

CHAPTER 16

Treatment strategies

No single approach to the treatment of chronic low back pain has been validated. Guidelines for the management of acute low back pain are abundant [1-4]. Evidence-based guidelines for chronic low back pain are scarce. It would seem that chronic low back pain and its management is an issue too complex to be reduced to simple guidelines that are universally palatable and acceptable.

If one were to take an overview of what is available for chronic back pain and what currently happens, one would find a diverse field characterized by tensions. These tensions are caused by differences in history, competing concepts, and how practitioners react to the impact of innovations, including the advent of evidence-based medicine (Fig. 1).

From a historical perspective, the oldest strategies for chronic low back pain are conservative monotherapies and surgery. Prior to about 1980, patients with chronic low back pain would seek, receive, or be referred for conservative therapy. Typically, this would be of a single form, e.g. drugs, traction, ultrasound, exercises, or loosely defined 'physical therapy'. If one of these treatments did not work, another would be tried. If none of them worked, surgery was the next step. Being the oldest strategy, this approach is steeped in tradition and is still used in many circles.

Around 1980, this strategy was challenged. The failure of conservative monotherapies and the failure of surgery to eliminate chronic back pain prompted the advent of a behavioural approach. It was argued that conservative therapy and surgery were not working because the patients had impairments and disabilities that were not being addressed by passive, conservative therapies and not being corrected by surgery. Paramount amongst these impairments were psychological and behavioural problems, such as depression, fear, and inappropriate beliefs and attitudes. The correct approach to chronic low back pain required that these behavioural dimensions of the patient's problem be addressed together with their functional capacity. Since it was well known (at the time) that back pain could not be diagnosed and could not be treated medically or surgically, it was pointless making pain the target of therapy. Nevertheless, the patient would be helped by reducing their psychological distress and improving their physical behaviour. Indeed, this has become the prevailing strategy at present [5].

As greater attention came to be paid to the management of chronic low back pain, some individuals recognized that conservative therapies and surgery did not work, and even behavioural approaches did not work for some patients. This prompted innovations in the form of 'high-tech' treatments. Archetypical of these interventions are spinal cord stimulation and intraspinal delivery of drugs.

Conceptually, 'high-tech' interventions shared with conservative therapies and surgery the feature of being monotherapies. Application of the therapy was what the patient required. The therapy would stop, or substantially relieve, their pain. With behavioural therapy, 'high-tech' interventions shared the feature that a patho-anatomic diagnosis could not be made and was not required. Treatment was symptomatic and could be applied without a diagnosis.

The latest strategy to join this system is what

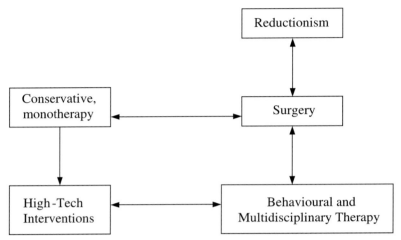

Fig. 1. A schematic representation of the tensions that apply between various strategies for the management of chronic low back pain.

can be referred to as reductionism. This strategy assumed that patients with chronic back pain did have a lesion, but it was not being diagnosed. As a result, conservative therapies and even surgery were being applied empirically and without attention to a valid diagnosis. For that reason, they were not working. Nor was it appropriate to relegate patients to palliative, symptomatic or behavioural therapy when a cause of pain might be found. The objective of the reductionist strategy became to pin-point the source of pain and to stop the pain.

In essence, contemporary tensions can be reduced to a tri-polar system (Fig. 2). One pole is persistence with monotherapies — being single types of treatment delivered by essentially a single individual, and which include conservative therapies, traditional surgery, and high-tech interventions. The second pole is multidisciplinary behavioural therapy — being multiple interventions, delivered by a team of professionals, but focusing on psychological distress, beliefs, attitudes and physical performance, rather than on pain. The third pole is the reductionist strategy, which involves finding the source of pain with the view to stopping it.

The cardinal tension between monotherapy and both the reductionist and multidisciplinary strategy is the belief that monotherapy does not work; that either reductionism or multidisciplinary therapy should be the preferred approach. Between reduc-

tionism and multidisciplinary therapy is the mutual belief that the other does not work. Compounding this latter tension is the belief, held by some[6], that the reductionist approach is futile and misguided. Reductionism imposes a further tension in that pursuing a precision diagnosis requires specialized skills and facilities, which are not widely available, and cannot be implemented by conventional practitioners.

Pervading these tensions is yet another factor — cost. Conservative therapies become costly when perpetuated to no avail. High-tech interventions are costly, as are multidisciplinary programs. Reductionist interventions can become costly if used in an undisciplined manner, and can be very costly if surgery becomes the method of treatment.

In the past, practitioners would have been drawn to one or other of these three poles by training, by familiarity, or out of convenience. Some practitioners may have found themselves, and their patients, victims of the tensions: torn between one or other strategy, or bouncing from one to the other. Choices were made for pragmatic, practical, or ideological reasons. The advent of evidence-based medicine, provides some degree of salvation. Instead of hearsay, anecdote, and public relations, practitioners can evaluate how well the various options work, according to the evidence. This is explored in the succeeding chapters.

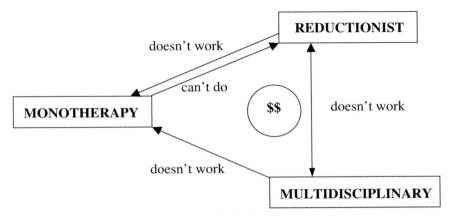

Fig. 2. The tri-polar tensions between strategies for the management of chronic low back pain.

References

1 Agency for Health Care Policy and Research. Acute Low Back Pain in Adults: Assessment and Treatment. US Department of Health and Human Services, Rockville, MD, 1994.

2 Royal College of General Practitioners, Chartered Society of Physiotherapy, Osteopathic Association of Great Britain, British Chiropractic Association, National Back Pain Association. Clinical Guidelines for the Management of Acute Low Back Pain. Royal College of General Practitioners, London, 1996.

3 Faas A, Chavannes AW, Koes BW, van den Hoogen JMM, Mens JMA, Smeele IJM, Romeijenders ACM, van der Laan JR. NHG-Standaard 'Lage-Rugpijn'. Huisarts Wet 1996; 39: 18–31.

4 National Advisory Committee on Core health and Disability Services, Accident Rehabilitation and Compensation Insurance Corporation. Clinical Practice Guidelines. Acute Low Back Problems in Adults: Assessment and Treatment. Core Services Committee, Ministry of Health (New Zealand), Wellington, 1995.

5 Waddell G, Main CJ. A new clinical model of low back pain and disability. In: Waddell G (ed) The Back Pain Revolution. Churchill Livingstone, Edinburgh, 1998: 223–240.

6 Loeser JD. Mitigating the dangers of pursuing care. In: Pain Treatment Centres at a Crossroads: A Practical ad Conceptual Reappraisal, Progress in Pain Management, Vol 7. IASP Press, Seattle, WA, 1996, pp 101–108.

Medical Management of Acute and Chronic Low Back Pain. An Evidence-Based Approach
Pain Research and Clinical Management, Vol. 13
Nikolai Bogduk and Brian McGuirk

CHAPTER 17

Monotherapy

1. Introduction

A monotherapy is an intervention that consists of delivering to the patient a treatment of a single kind, by a single individual (assistants notwithstanding). In particular, monotherapies are passive, in that the treatment is supposed to achieve its effect without any active participation by the patient. The patient takes a drug, or submits to the application of manual forces or devices. The role of the patient is no more than to receive the treatment, for it is the treatment that provides the therapeutic effect.

In recent years, various monotherapies have come under scrutiny. They have been subjected to systematic reviews of the literature. The available evidence from these reviews is not flattering. No monotherapy has been found to be curative of chronic low back pain, and few have been shown even to be helpful.

One of the reasons for this lack of efficacy is a fundamental problem faced by nearly all monotherapies — lack of diagnosis. While so long as practitioners rely on history and physical examination to make a diagnosis, they are thwarted in their objective. Physical examination lacks reliability, validity or both, and for that reason cannot be used to make a diagnosis (Chapter 15). Nor does conventional medical imaging help (Chapter 15). For most patients with chronic low back pain, medical imaging demonstrates a totally normal lumbar spine or changes normal for age. Consequently, monotherapies cannot be based on a patho-anatomic diagnosis or expected to rectify a structural or physiological abnormality, for the latter cannot be reliably and validly detected.

The reputation of efficacy of monotherapies rests on anecdote and assertion, but turns on the available evidence.

2. Drug therapy

2.1. Analgesics

Systematic reviews have concluded that there is limited evidence that analgesics provide short-term, symptomatic relief of chronic low back pain[1,2]. This conclusion is based on just one small study, that showed that paracetamol is equally effective as diflunisal[3]. That study, however, showed only that 7 out of 13 patients treated with paracetamol reported mild or no back pain at 4 weeks after commencing treatment, compared to 13 out 16 patients treated with diflunisal. There are no long-term data on the efficacy of analgesics for chronic low back pain.

2.2. NSAIDs

There is limited evidence that non-steroidal anti-inflammatory drugs (NSAIDs) are more effective than placebo[1,2], and there is strong evidence that various NSAIDs are equally effective[1,2]. However, NSAIDs do not eliminate pain. The literature attests to an average reduction in pain of only 10%[4] or less[5]; and NSAIDs are not superior to manipulation, physiotherapy, back school or application of an anti-oedema gel[6]. Furthermore, the efficacy of NSAIDs has typically been studied for periods of only 2–4 weeks, and 6 weeks at the most. There are no long-term data on the efficacy of NSAIDs for chronic low back pain [1,2].

2.3. Antidepressants

Although antidepressants are often used as a co-analgesic, the evidence fails to show any superiority over placebo [1,2,7].

2.4. Muscle relaxants

One study [8] has demonstrated that tetrazepam is significantly more effective than placebo in reducing pain. This efficacy, however, was assessed only at 10 days after commencing treatment. At that time, patients taking tetrazepam had an average reduction of pain of 50%; patients taking placebo had a 30% reduction. There are no long-term data on the effi-cacy of tetrazepam, and no data on any other muscle relaxants for chronic low back pain [1,2].

2.5. Opioids

The use of opioids for chronic back pain has been subjected to two controlled trials. One compared the efficacy of naproxen, oxycodone, and oxycodone combined with sustained release morphine [9]. The other compared sustained-release morphine with benztropine as a placebo-control [10]. Each study showed similar outcomes.

Opioids are more effective than naproxen or placebo for relieving pain, but the average effect is little more than a reduction by 10 points on a 100-point visual analogue scale. Opioids, however, do not improve the psychological or functional status of patients treated. Accordingly, opioids offer a modest to trivial palliative effect for pain, but no other therapeutic benefits.

Key points

- There is very little evidence of the efficacy of drug treatment for chronic low back pain.
- Analgesics and NSAIDs offer only limited relief of pain. Their efficacy beyond 6 weeks is unknown.
- Antidepressants provide no greater relief of pain than placebo.
- Only one study has addressed muscle relaxants, and showed only that tetrazepam was superior to placebo in relieving pain over a 10-day period.
- Even opioids are only palliative; they do not eliminate chronic low back pain, and they do not improve psychological or physical function.

References

1 van Tulder MW, Koes BW, Bouter LM. Conservative treatment of acute and chronic nonspecific low back pain. A systematic review of randomized controlled trials of the most common interventions. Spine 1997; 22: 2128–2156.

2 van Tulder MV, Goossens M, Waddell G, Nachemson A. Conservative treatment of chronic low back pain. In: Nachemson A, Jonsson E (eds) Neck and Back Pain: The Scientific Evidence of Causes, Diagnosis, and Treatment. Lippincott, Williams and Wilkins, Philadelphia, PA, 2000: 271–304.

3 Hickey RF. Chronic low back pain: a comparison of diflunisal with paracetamol. NZ Med J 1982; 95: 312–314.

4 Videman T, Osterman K. Double-blind parallel study of piroxicam versus indomethacin in the treatment of low back pain. Ann Clin Res 1984; 16: 156–160.

5 Berry H, Bloom B, Hamilton EBD, Sinson DR. Naproxen sodium, diflunisal, and placebo in the treatment of chronic back pain. Ann Rheum Dis 1982; 41: 129–132.

6 Postacchini F, Facchini M, Palieri P. Efficacy of various forms of conservative treatment in low back pain: a comparative study. Neuro-Orthop 1988; 6: 28–35.

7 Turner JA, Denny MC. Do antidepressant medications relieve chronic low back pain? J Fam Pract 1993; 37: 545–553.

8 Arbus L, Fajadet B, Aubert D, Morre M, Goldberger E. Activity of tetrazepam (myolastan) in low back pain: a double-blind trial vs placebo. Clin Trials J 1990; 27: 258–

267.

9 Jamison RN, Raymond SA, Slawsby EA, Nedeljkovic SS, Katz NP. Opioid therapy for chronic noncancer back pain. A randomized prospective study. Spine 1998; 23: 2591–2600.

10 Moulin DE, Iezzi A, Amireh R, Sharpe WKJ, Boyd D, Merskey H. Randomised trial of oral morphine for chronic non-cancer pain. Lancet 1996; 347: 143–147.

3. Traction

Systematic reviews of traction for chronic low back pain [1–3] have been confounded by a lack of appropriate studies. The older literature essentially assessed the efficacy of traction for sciatica rather than for back pain. Even so, that literature showed little or no attributable benefit for traction when compared to other interventions or to sham traction [1,3]. The one study that has explicitly addressed the treatment for low back pain found it to be no more effective than sham traction [4,5].

Key point

- Traction is no more effective than sham treatment for chronic low back pain.

References

1 van der Heijden GJMG, Beurskens AJHM, Koes BW, Assendelft WJJ, de Vet HCW, Bouter L. The efficacy of traction for back and neck pain: a systematic, blinded review of randomized clinical trial methods. Phys Ther 1995; 75: 93–104.

2 van Tulder MW, Koes BW, Bouter LM. Conservative treatment of acute and chronic nonspecific low back pain. A systematic review of randomized controlled trials of the most common interventions. Spine 1997; 22: 2128–2156.

3 van Tulder MV, Goossens M, Waddell G, Nachemson A. Conservative treatment of chronic low back pain. In: Nachemson A, Jonsson E (eds) Neck and Back Pain: The Scientific Evidence of Causes, Diagnosis, and Treatment. Lippincott, Williams and Wilkins, Philadelphia, PA, 2000: 271–304.

4 Beurskens AJ, de Vet HC, Koke A, Lindeman E, Regtop W, van der Heijden GJ, Knipschild PG. Efficacy of traction for non-specific low back pain: a randomised clinical trial. Lancet 1995; 346: 1596–1600.

5 Beurskens AJ, de Vet HC, Koke AJ, Regtop W, van der Heijden GJ, Lindeman E, Knipschild PG. Efficacy of traction for nonspecific low back pain. 12-week and 60 month results of a randomized clinical trial. Spine 1997; 22: 2756–2762.

4. Manipulative therapy

For the treatment of chronic low back pain, systematic reviews [1,2] have concluded that: "there is strong evidence that manipulative therapy provides more effective short-term pain relief than a placebo treatment; and that there is moderate evidence that manual therapy is more effective than usual care by a general practitioner, bed rest, analgesics and massage, for short-term pain relief. There is limited and conflicting evidence of any long-term effects" [2]. However, if the original data are consulted, from the studies covered by these reviews, it can be shown that the conclusions drawn are not as strong as they first seem (Table I).

One study [12] was used by the systematic reviews [1,2] as providing evidence that manipulation was effective. That study, however, used manipulation as a co-intervention. The main thrust of the study was to demonstrate the efficacy of prolotherapy (see below). It is in that context that the authors portrayed their intervention; and it is in that context that their study is reviewed in the present text.

Two studies [8,9], rated by the reviews [1,2] as methodologically weak, showed manipulative therapy to be superior to analgesics and massage at 2 and 3 weeks after treatment, with respect to reducing pain. In contrast, two studies [5,6], rated as methodologically stronger, found no greater benefit than from sham treatment at 2 and 4 weeks. None of these studies provided longer-term follow-up.

The weakest study [11] found no greater benefit from manipulative therapy, compared to a variety of other interventions, at 3 weeks and 2 months; and no benefit at 6 months. On the other hand, one weak study [10], found manipulation to be superior to drugs and massage at 6 months. In that study, the patients treated by manipulation improved their pain scores from 1.8, on a 3-point scale, to 0.7, whereas the con-

TABLE I

The studies of manual therapy for acute low back pain, indicating the control used, the outcome measure used, and whether or not manual therapy was shown to be better than control at the follow-up time indicated

Study	Control used	Outcome measure	Follow-up Weeks				Months				Comments
			2	3	4	6	2	3	6	12	
Koes et al. [3,4]	physical therapy	pain, function		no		no	no	no		yes	difference small
	usual care by GP	pain, function		no		no	no				
	placebo SWD, US	pain function		no		no	no				
	physical therapy	global perceived effect		no		no	no	no	no		difference small
	usual care by GP	global perceived effect		yes		yes	yes				difference small
	placebo SWD, US	global perceived effect		no		no	no				
Triano et al. [5]	back education	pain, disability	no								
	sham manipulation	pain, disability	no								
Gibson et al. [6]	SWD, sham SWD	pain			no						
Herzog et al. [7]	back school	pain, disability									No differences immediately after treatment
Evans et al. [8]	analgesics	patient satisfaction		yes							
Waagen et al. [9]	massage	pain	yes								
Arkuszewski [10]	drugs, massage	pain							yes		30% no pain vs 12%
Postacchini et al. [11]	physical therapy	pain, disability		no			no	no			
	NSAID			no			no	no			
	back school			no			no	no			
	placebo gel			no			no	no			

GP, general practitioner; SWD, shortwave diathermy; US, ultrasound.

trol group improved from 1.8 to 1.0; 32% of patients treated by manipulation were free of pain, compared to 12% in the control group.

The data from the strongest study[3] are difficult to relate, because of the intricate way that they were presented and analysed. On an intention-to-treat analysis, manipulation was not better than physical therapy, usual care by a general practitioner, or placebo therapy with shortwave diathermy and ultrasound, with respect to pain and function at 3, 6, or 12 weeks after treatment. A difference in favour of manipulative therapy occurred only in comparison with usual care by a general practitioner, and only with respect to an outcome measure called 'global perceived effect'. This measure was not explicitly defined, but seems to have been the patient's assessment of the degree of 'benefit' that they obtained from their assigned treatment. Significant differences, when they occurred, however, did not lie in greater numbers of

patients being fully relieved of their symptoms. They amounted to greater proportions of patients feeling between 10% and 60% better, and fewer patients feeling worse. There were no differences in 'global perceived effect' between manipulation, physiotherapy, and placebo treatment.

When an alternative analysis was used[3], which censored patients who dropped out or changed treatments, manipulation was found to be superior to placebo, with respect to improvement in pain and 'global perceived effect', at 6 weeks. Again the difference was due only to a greater proportion of patients feeling partially better. A difference at 12 weeks was not demonstrated.

A report of the long-term results of this study[4] provided comparisons only between manipulative therapy and physiotherapy. It found no difference in 'global perceived effect' but a difference in favour of manipulation, with respect to reduction in pain.

The difference, however, was small, amounting to an improvement of 4.5 on a 10-point scale, compared with 3.8.

Overall, the data on manipulative therapy for chronic low back pain, show limited and inconsistent effectiveness. The weaker studies showed conflicting short-term results, and conflicting long-term results[5-11]. When compared to sham manipulation or to placebo treatment, most studies have not found manipulation to be superior[5,6,11]. Even the strongest study[3] found no superiority to placebo, on an intention-to-treat analysis. A difference emerged only on an alternative analysis, and was due to a larger proportion of patients achieving partial improvement.

Thus, contrary to the conclusions of the systematic reviews[1,2], the evidence is not 'strong' that manipulation is superior placebo treatment for chronic low back pain. The reviews are nevertheless correct in reporting that any efficacy is limited to short-term

effects. Yet, even so, those effects are limited to partial improvements in pain, function, and patient satisfaction.

The only consistent and lasting effect that emerged from the strongest study[3], was that manipulative therapy was superior to care by a general practitioner, with respect to 'global perceived effect'. Given that manipulative therapy was not overtly superior to placebo treatment in this study, the apparent superiority of manipulation over GP care is not so much evidence of efficacy of manipulative therapy as it is evidence of the inferiority of usual care for chronic back pain.

Accordingly, it might be conceded that manipulative therapy is a more satisfying option for patients with chronic low back pain than care by a GP, but even so, its effectiveness is limited. Patients achieve improvements in their pain, and do feel that they benefit somewhat, but few are completely or even greatly relieved.

Key points

- For the treatment of chronic low back pain, manipulative therapy has not been consistently shown to be superior to placebo.
- Manipulative therapy is perceived by patients as better than care by a GP, but is not consistently better than other, competitive treatments.
- Any long-term benefits are limited to partial improvements in pain, function, and perceived benefit.

References

1. van Tulder MW, Koes BW, Bouter LM. Conservative treatment of acute and chronic nonspecific low back pain. A systematic review of randomized controlled trials of the most common interventions. Spine 1997; 22: 2128–2156.
2. van Tulder MV, Goossens M, Waddell G, Nachemson A. Conservative treatment of chronic low back pain. In: Nachemson A, Jonsson E (eds) Neck and Back Pain: The Scientific Evidence of Causes, Diagnosis, and Treatment. Lippincott, Williams and Wilkins, Philadelphia, PA, 2000: 271–304.
3. Koes BW, Bouter LM, van Mameren H, Essers AHM, Verstegen GMJR, Hofhuizen DM, Houben JP, Knipschild PG. The effectiveness of manual therapy, physiotherapy and treatment by the general practitioner for non-specific back and neck complaints: a randomized clinical trial. Spine 1992; 17: 28–35.
4. Koes BW, Bouter LM, van Mameren H, Essers AHM, Verstegen GMJR, Hofhuizen DM, Houben JP, Knipschild PG. Randomised clinical trial of manual therapy and physiotherapy for persistent back and neck complaints: results of one year follow-up. Br Med J 1992; 304: 601–605.
5. Triano JJ, McGregor M, Hondras MA, Brennan PC. Manipulative therapy versus education programs in chronic low-back pain. Spine 1995; 20: 948–955.
6. Gibson T, Grahame R, Harkness J, Woo P, Balgrave P, Hills R. Controlled comparison of short-wave diathermy treatment with osteopathic treatment in non-specific low-back pain. Lancet 1985; 1: 1258–1261.
7. Herzog W, Conway PJW, Willcox BJ. Effects of different treatment modalities on gait symmetry and clinical measures for sacroiliac joint patients. J Manip Physiol Ther 1991; 14: 104–109.

8   Evans DP, Burke MS, Lloyd KN, Roberts EE, Roberts GM. Lumbar spinal manipulation on trial. Part 1: clinical assessment. Rheumatol Rehabil 1978; 17: 46–53.

9   Waagen GN, Haldeman S, Cool G, Lopez D, DeBoer KF. Short term trial of chiropractic adjustments for the relief of chronic low back pain. Man Med 1986; 2: 63–67.

10 Arkuszewski Z. The efficacy of manual treatment in low back pain: a clinical trial. Man Med 1986; 2: 68–71.

11 Postacchini F, Facchini M, Palieri P. Efficacy of various forms of conservative treatment in low back pain: a comparative study. Neuro-Orthop 1988; 6: 28–35.

12 Ongley MJ, Klein RG, Dorman TA, Eek BC, Hubert LJ. A new approach to the treatment of chronic low back pain. Lancet 1987; 2: 143–146.

5. Acupuncture

Reviewers have repeatedly struggled with drawing conclusions from the literature on acupuncture for chronic low back pain, largely because of the poor quality of the literature and the absence of short-term, let alone long-term, follow-up in many studies. van Tulder et al.[1] concluded that "because of contradictory results, there is no evidence that acupuncture is an effective treatment for chronic low back pain". Another team, led by van Tulder[2], and having added one extra study to their review, concluded that "because of inconsistent findings and poor quality of the studies, it is not possible to judge the effectiveness of acupuncture for chronic low back pain".

Ezzo et al.[3] addressed acupuncture for all types of chronic pain, not just back pain, and concluded that there was "limited evidence that acupuncture is better than no treatment" but that it was "premature at this time to draw conclusions about how effective acupuncture is compared to placebo, sham acupuncture or standard care for the treatment of chronic pain".

In their review, Ernst and White[4] specifically targeted chronic low back pain and concluded that acupuncture was superior to various control interventions, although there is insufficient evidence to state whether it is superior to placebo. Inspection of the original literature reveals what these conclusions mean in detail, particularly with respect to 'control interventions'.

Acupuncture has been shown to be superior to no treatment[5,6], superior to physiotherapy[7,8], superior to transcutaneous electrical nerve stimulation (TENS)[9], and comparable in effect to trigger point therapy[10]. Conspicuously, however, it has repeatedly been found to be no more effective than sham treatment[7,11–14]. The apparent superiority of acupuncture, therefore, seems to be based on the failure of the control treatments against which it has been compared, and not on any specific, greater benefit afforded by acupuncture.

Accordingly, another, and most recent, systematic review[15] found no convincing evidence to show that acupuncture is effective in the management of chronic low back pain.

Key point

- Multiple studies have failed to show that acupuncture is effective for chronic low back pain.

References

1   van Tulder MW, Koes BW, Bouter LM. Conservative treatment of acute and chronic nonspecific low back pain. A systematic review of randomized controlled trials of the most common interventions. Spine 1997; 22: 2128–2156.

2   van Tulder MV, Goossens M, Waddell G, Nachemson A. Conservative treatment of chronic low back pain. In: Nachemson A, Jonsson E (eds) Neck and Back Pain: The Scientific Evidence of Causes, Diagnosis, and Treatment. Lippincott, Williams and Wilkins, Philadelphia, PA, 2000: 271–304.

3   Ezzo J, Berman B, Hadhazy VA, Jadad AR, Lao L, Singh BB. Is acupuncture effective for the treatment of chronic pain? A systematic review. Pain 2000; 86: 217–225.

4   Ernst E, White AR. Acupuncture for back pain. A meta-analysis of randomized controlled trials. Arch Int Med 1998; 158: 2235–2241.

5   Coan RM, Wong G, Ku SL, Chan YC, Wang L, Ozer FT, Coan PL. The acupuncture treatment of low back pain: randomized controlled study. Am J Chin Med 1980; 8: 181–189.

6   Thomas M, Lundberg T. Importance of modes of acupuncture in the treatment of chronic nociceptive low back pain. Acta Anaesthesiol Scand 1994; 38: 63–69.

7   Yue SJ. Acupuncture for chronic back and neck pain. Acupunct Electrother Res 1978; 3: 323–324.

8   Gunn CC, Milbrandt WE, Little AS, Mason KE. Dry needling of muscle points for chronic low-back pain. Spine 1980; 5: 279–291.

9   Lehmann TR, Russell DW, Spratt KF. The impact of patients with nonorganic physical findings on a controlled trial of transcutaneous electrical nerve stimulation and electroacupuncture. Spine 1983; 8: 625–634.

10 Garvey TA, Marks MR, Wiesel SW. A prospective, randomized, double-blind evaluation of trigger-point injection therapy for low-back pain. Spine 1989; 14: 962–964.

11 Edelist G, Gross AE, Langer F. Treatment of low back pain with acupuncture. Can Anaesth Soc J 1976; 23: 303–306.

12 Gallachi G, Muller W. Akupunktur: bringt sie etwas? Schweiz Rundsch Med Prax 1983; 72: 779–782.

13 Macdonald AJR, Macrae KD, Master BR, Rubin A. Superficial acupuncture in the relief of chronic low back pain. Ann R Coll Surg Engl 1983; 65: 44–46.

14 Mendelson G, Selwood TS, Kranz H, Loh ST, Kidson MA, Scott DS. Acupuncture treatment of chronic back pain. Am J Med 1983; 74: 49–55.

15 van Tulder MW, Cherkin DC, Berman B, Lao L, Koes BW. The effectiveness of acupuncture in the management of acute and chronic low back pain. A systematic review within the framework of the Cochrane Collaboration Back Review Group. Spine 1999; 24: 1113–1123.

6. Injection therapies

A variety of injection therapies have been used for chronic low back pain. They involve the injection of various agents, such as local anaesthetic, local anaesthetic and corticosteroids, or sclerosants, into various sites, such as the epidural space, tender points in muscles, or ligaments.

6.1. Epidural steroids

Although epidural steroids have been included in systematic reviews of treatment for low back pain[1–3], they do not have a legitimate role in the treatment of back pain. They are expressly a treatment for radicular pain, alias sciatica[4], which is not back pain. Indeed, there have been no controlled studies of the efficacy of epidural steroids for low back pain, per se. All controlled trials have addressed the treatment of radicular pain.

The inclusion of epidural steroids in systematic reviews concerning back pain is, therefore, an indication either that reviewers misunderstand the difference between back pain and radicular pain and their treatment, or that reviews reflect the reality of clinical practice at large, in which epidural steroids are misused to treat back pain.

> **Key points**
> - Epidural steroids may be indicated for radicular pain, but they are not indicated for back pain.
> - Nor is there any evidence that they are effective for chronic low back pain.

References

1   van Tulder MW, Koes BW, Bouter LM. Conservative treatment of acute and chronic nonspecific low back pain. A systematic review of randomized controlled trials of the most common interventions. Spine 1997; 22: 2128–2156.

2   van Tulder MV, Goossens M, Waddell G, Nachemson A. Conservative treatment of chronic low back pain. In: Nachemson A, Jonsson E (eds) Neck and Back Pain: The Scientific Evidence of Causes, Diagnosis, and Treatment. Lippincott, Williams and Wilkins, Philadelphia, PA, 2000: 271–304.

3   Nelemans PJ, de Bie RA, deVet HCW, Sturmans F. Injection therapy for subacute and chronic benign low back pain. Spine 2001; 26: 501–515.

4   Bogduk N. Spine update: epidural steroids. Spine 1995; 20: 845–848.

6.2. Tender point injections

In some patients with chronic back pain, injecting local anaesthetic, with or without a corticosteroid, into tender points in the back muscles seems to relieve their pain. The available data indicate that, when compared with placebo injections, the efficacy of such injections is modest at best, and fleeting in duration.

Injections of lignocaine are more effective than injections of normal saline, but only in the hands of rheumatologists, not in the hands of general practitioners [1]. When assessed at 2 weeks after injection, lignocaine provides an average of 40% reduction in pain. Bupivacaine is more effective than normal saline, but offers a modest 10% reduction in pain, when assessed at 7 days [2]. Methylprednisolone mixed with lignocaine is more effective than normal saline in securing 'improvement' in pain, when assessed at 2 weeks [3].

Collectively, these studies favour an effect of injection therapy, but the small sample sizes used prevent the pooled outcome data from achieving statistical significance. The 95% confidence intervals of the pooled relative risk cross the critical value of 1.0 [4].

One old study reported that a greater proportion of patients achieve complete relief of pain (odds ratio: 7.7) when corticosteroids are used rather than lignocaine alone [5]. This encouraging report, however, has not been replicated.

Key point

- The injection of tender points is not an effective means of treating chronic low back pain.

References

1   Collee G, Dijkmans BAC, Vanderbroucke JP, Cats A. Iliac crest pain syndrome in low back pain: a double-blind, randomized study of local injection therapy. J Rheumatol 1991; 18: 1060–1063.
2   Hameroff SR, Crago BR, Blitt CD, Womble J, Kanel J. Comparison of bupivacaine, etidocaine, and saline for trigger-point therapy. Anaesth Analg 1981; 60: 752–755.
3   Sonne M, Christensen K, Hansen SE, Jensen EN. Injection of steroids and local anaesthetics as therapy for low back pain. Scand J Rheum 1985; 14: 343–345.
4   Nelemans PJ, de Bie RA, deVet HCW, Sturmans F. Injection therapy for subacute and chronic benign low back pain. Spine 2001; 26: 501–515.
5   Bourne IH. Treatment of chronic back pain. Comparing corticosteroid–lignocaine injections with lignocaine alone. Practitioner 1984; 228: 333–338.

6.3. Prolotherapy

A variety of agents have been used to sclerose tender muscles and ligaments. These include phenol, dextrose, and glycerine, alone or in various combinations, mixed with lignocaine. Collectively, injection of these agents has become known as prolotherapy. The professed objective of prolotherapy is to strengthen weak or injured ligaments by inducing a fibroblastic reaction to the injection [1]. Two studies have claimed success in controlled trials of prolotherapy for chronic back pain.

One study reported significantly greater improvements in pain and disability, sustained at 6 months, in patients treated with prolotherapy compared with those who had control treatment [2]. Of the 40 patients treated with prolotherapy, 35 obtained 50% or greater relief of their pain, and reduced their disability; 15 of the patients had complete relief. In the control group of 41 patients, the corresponding figures were 16 and 4 patients. Such large degrees of relief in such proportions of patients, sustained at 6 months, have not been reported for any other monotherapy for chronic low back pain. However, these patients also had preliminary injections of lignocaine, injections of trimacinolone, and a forceful manipulation, which the control group did not receive. Indeed, because manipulation was used, some reviewers have ranked this study as one that provided positive results for manipulation [3,4]. It is difficult, therefore, to disentangle the effects specifically attributable to the prolotherapy in this study.

The second study [5] compared the efficacy of prolotherapy with that of saline mixed with lignocaine. The authors reported a significantly greater proportion of patients in the prolotherapy group obtaining 50% improvement in pain or disability immediately after treatment, but at 6 months, this difference was no longer statistically significant. The group data showed no statistically significant differences between mean scores of each group for pain, disability, range of motion, or strength, at 6 months.

These studies do not offer convincing evidence of efficacy for prolotherapy. The second study did not corroborate the outstanding success reported by the first. In part, this may be due to the absence of co-interventions in the second study. The putative benefit of prolotherapy needs to be revealed in a trial less confounded by other interventions.

> **Key points**
>
> - The data on prolotherapy for chronic low back pain are limited and conflicting.
> - The efficacy seen in one study has not been corroborated by another, and has not been disentangled from the effects of co-interventions.

References

1   Liu YK, Tipton CM, Matthes DD, Bedford TG, Maynard JA, Walmer HC. An in situ study of the influence of a sclerosing solution in rabbit medial collateral ligaments and its junction strength. Conn Tiss Res 1983; 11: 95–102.

2   Ongley MJ, Klein RG, Dorman TA, Eek BC, Hubert LJ. A new approach to the treatment of chronic low back pain. Lancet 1987; 2: 143–146.

3   van Tulder MW, Koes BW, Bouter LM. Conservative treatment of acute and chronic nonspecific low back pain. A systematic review of randomized controlled trials of the most common interventions. Spine 1997; 22: 2128–2156.

4   van Tulder MV, Goossens M, Waddell G, Nachemson A. Conservative treatment of chronic low back pain. In: Nachemson A, Jonsson E (eds) Neck and Back Pain: The Scientific Evidence of Causes, Diagnosis, and Treatment. Lippincott, Williams and Wilkins, Philadelphia, PA, 2000: 271–304.

5   Klein RG, Eek BC, DeLong WB, Mooney V. A randomized double-blind trial of dextrose–glycerine–phenol injections for chronic, low back pain. J Spinal Dis 1993; 6: 23–33.

6.4. Botulinum toxin

A modern innovation in the treatment of spinal pain has been the use of injections of botulinum toxin, ostensibly to relieve pain due to muscle spasm. However, an explicit diagnosis of muscle spasm has not been a prerequisite for this treatment. Rather, it has been applied only empirically to patients with non-specific low back pain.

One study has reported the results of a randomized, controlled trial [1]. In that trial, 15 patients were treated with botulinum toxin, and 16 with injections

TABLE II

The results of treatment of low back pain with botulinum toxin or saline

Treatment	n	Three weeks Pain relief		Eight weeks Pain relief	
		>50%	<50%	>50%	<50%
Botulinum toxin	15	11	4	9	6
Saline	16	4	12	1	14
P		0.012		0.009	
Power		79%		81%	

Based on Foster et al. [1].

of saline. The results showed that botulinum toxin was significantly superior to normal saline in producing at least 50% relief of pain; and despite the relatively small sample sizes, the study had sufficient statistical power to demonstrate this difference (Table II).

Quite clearly, botulinum toxin exerts an effect than cannot be attributed to that of a placebo. However, at best, the effects of botulinum toxin are partial and limited in duration. Although a large proportion of patients achieves a worthwhile degree of relief, none have been reported to achieve complete relief of pain. Furthermore, the results attenuate over time, and there are no data as to its lasting efficacy beyond 2 months. At best, the data attest to a possible, temporary and palliative treatment for chronic low back pain.

> **Key points**
>
> For the treatment of chronic low back pain:
>
> - botulinum toxin has an effect greater than that of a placebo, but
> - it provides only partial relief of limited duration.

References

1   Foster L, Clapp L, Erickson M, Jabbari B. Botulinum toxin A and chronic low back pain. A randomized, double-blind study. Neurology 2001; 56: 1290–1293.

7. Massage

A systematic review [1], published in 1999, lamented the paucity of studies of massage therapy for low back pain. It found four studies that tested massage as a monotherapy for either acute or chronic low back pain, but usually as a control therapy. One study that explicitly involved patients with chronic low back pain [2], found massage to be superior to no treatment, with respect to improvement in pain and reduction in analgesic consumption. The review concluded that too few trials of massage therapy exist for a reliable evaluation of its efficacy [1].

Since that review [1], a randomized controlled trial has appeared, in which patients were allocated to comprehensive massage therapy, soft-tissue manipulation only, remedial exercise with posture education,

or placebo in the form of sham laser therapy [3]. Massage achieved greater improvements in function and in pain than the other treatments. At 1 month follow-up, 63% of the massage group reported no pain, compared to 27%, 14% and 0% in the other three groups, respectively.

The large proportion of patients rendered pain-free might seem surprising, but it may be due to the relatively short duration of illness in the patients treated. The author considered their patients to have subacute back pain, rather than chronic pain, but the data show that the patients had a mean duration of 12–15 weeks [3]. This indicates that half of the patients had chronic back pain and half did not. Nevertheless, the results are sufficiently encouraging that massage should be a treatment worthy of more concerted evaluation in the future.

Key points

- Although massage therapy appears to be more effective than no treatment,
- the efficacy of massage therapy for chronic low back pain, has not been properly tested and determined.

References

1 Ernst E. Massage therapy for low back pain: a systematic review. J Pain Symptom Manage 1999; 17: 65–69.
2 Konrad K, Tatrai T, Hunka A, Verecker E, Korondi I. Controlled trial of balneotherapy in treatment of low back pain. Ann Rheum Dis 1992; 51: 820–822.
3 Preyde M. Effectiveness of massage therapy for subacute low-back pain: a randomized controlled trial. Can Med Ass J 2000; 162: 1815–1820.

8. Miscellaneous

On balance, the limited evidence available indicates that *electromyographic biofeedback* is not effective

for chronic low back pain [1,2]. Nor is there any evidence that orthoses or transcutaneous electrical nerve stimulation (*TENS*) are effective [1,2]. When used to treat back pain, *magnets* are no more effective than sham magnets [3].

The one controlled study of *hydrotherapy* found that, compared to being put on a waiting list, hydrotherapy achieved no significant gains in pain but did achieve greater improvements in disability, when assessed immediately after 4 weeks of treatment [4].

Key point

- Biofeedback, orthoses, TENS, magnets, and hydrotherapy are not effective for chronic low back pain.

References

1   van Tulder MW, Koes BW, Bouter LM. Conservative treatment of acute and chronic nonspecific low back pain. A systematic review of randomized controlled trials of the most common interventions. Spine 1997; 22: 2128–2156.
2   van Tulder MV, Goossens M, Waddell G, Nachemson A. Conservative treatment of chronic low back pain. In: Nachemson A, Jonsson E (eds) Neck and Back Pain: The Scientific Evidence of Causes, Diagnosis, and Treatment. Lippincott, Williams and Wilkins, Philadelphia, PA, 2000: 271–304.
3   Collacott EA, Zimmerman JT, White DW, Rindone JP. Bipolar permanent magnets for the treatment of chronic low back pain: a pilot study. J Am Med Assoc 2000; 283: 1322–1325.
4   McIlveen B, Robertson V. A randomized controlled study of the outcome of hydrotherapy for subjects with low back or back and leg pain. Physiotherapy 1998; 84: 17–26.

9. Surgery

In the past, surgery was used to treat back pain on symptomatic grounds, and without a valid surgical diagnosis. The indications for fusion of the lumbar spine amounted to no more than persistent pain, degenerative disc disease, or assumed instability. Yet, neither degenerative disc disease nor instability is a valid diagnosis of the cause of back pain (Chapter 14). In essence, fusion was undertaken to stop movement with the expectation that doing so would stop pain. The rationale seemed to be no more that: the patient has pain; the pain is aggravated by movement; eliminating movement should stop the pain. No explicit lesion was diagnosed in order to be corrected by the surgery.

It is not surprising, therefore, that the results of surgery undertaken in this manner are less than impressive. A systematic review [1], undertaken in 1992, found no controlled trials of surgery for chronic low back pain, but collated the observational studies published available at the time. It found that whereas a satisfactory outcome was achieved in an average of 69% of patients, the success rate ranged greatly, from 95% to 16%. More recent reviewers were not persuaded by observational studies, and concluded that there is no acceptable evidence of the efficacy of any form of fusion for degenerative lumbar spondylosis, back pain or 'instability' [2,3], and no evidence on whether any form of surgery for degenerative lumbar disc disease is effective in returning patients to work [2].

These data and these conclusions pertain to surgery in general, and to surgery undertaken without a valid patho-anatomic diagnosis being made. Other data are available for surgery undertaken for specific conditions. Those are considered in Chapter 21.

Key point

- There is no evidence that surgery undertaken without a valid diagnosis is effective for chronic low back pain.

References

1   Turner JA, Ersek M, Herron L, Haselkorn J, Kent D, Ciol MA, Deyo R. Patient outcomes after lumbar spinal fusions. J Am Med Assoc 1992; 268: 907–911.
2   Gibson JNA, Grant IC, Waddell G. The Cochrane review of surgery for lumbar disc prolapse and degenerative lumbar spondylosis. Spine 1999; 24: 1820–1832.
3   Waddell G, Gibson A, Grant. IC, Surgical treatment of lumbar disc prolapse and degenerative lumbar disc disease. In: Nachemson A, Jonsson E (eds) Neck and Back Pain: The Scientific Evidence of Causes, Diagnosis, and Treatment. Lippincott, Williams and Wilkins, Philadelphia, PA, 2000: 305–325.

10. Spinal cord stimulation

Spinal cord stimulation is a method for controlling pain mediated by the spinal cord, irrespective of origin. It involves the introduction of electrodes into the epidural space. These are used to deliver a current from an implanted stimulator that inhibits the perception of pain by inducing a tingling sensation in the region in which pain is felt. With respect to back pain, its foremost application has been in the treatment of failed back surgery syndrome.

There have been no controlled studies of this intervention, but a systematic review has compiled the observational data[1]. In general, it seems that an average of 59% of patients treated achieve at least 50% relief of their pain, with leg pain being relieved more often than back pain. This relief is sustained, on the average, for up to 5 years, but attenuates by

10 years. Although 58% of patients improve their ability to undertake activities of daily living, only 30% of patients previously working remain at work, and only 13% of those previously not working return to work.

These data do not portray spinal cord stimulation as a cure for chronic back pain. Indeed, it is not particularly effective for back pain. It is effective largely for leg pain. Nevertheless, for patients with failed back surgery syndrome, for whom no other intervention appears indicated or effective, spinal cord stimulation can be regarded as an option for palliative care.

Key points

- There are no controlled data on the efficacy of spinal cord stimulation for chronic low back pain.
- The role of spinal cord stimulation would seem best to be limited to the palliation of leg pain in patients with failed back surgery syndrome.

References

1   Turner JA, Loeser JD, Bell KG. Spinal cord stimulation for chronic low back pain: a systematic literature synthesis. Neurosurgery 1995; 37: 1088–1096.

11. Intraspinal opioids

Some patients with cancer pain require increasing doses of oral opioids in order to maintain pain relief, or are unable to tolerate oral opioids. When treated with epidural or intrathecal opioids, these patients can achieve or regain pain relief with remarkably low, total daily doses of opioid. Prompted by such experience with cancer patients, physicians have used intraspinal opioids to treat patients with noncancer pain, including chronic low back, usually in the form of failed back surgery syndrome. The literature on the efficacy of intraspinal opioids, however, is limited in quantity and poor in quality.

Early studies reported various degrees of success. Two studies each described four patients with back pain amongst others with cancer pain and various forms of other, noncancer pain[1,2]. Of these studies, one reported good responses[1], the other described only fair to poor responses[2]. A larger study[3] described 43 patients with noncancer pain, 35 of whom had failed back surgery syndrome. It reported that 66% of 32 patients obtained good relief.

A relatively recent review[4] summarised the results of the two largest studies of the use of intraspinal opioids for noncancer pain[5,6]. In the first study[5], 42% of patients had failed back surgery syndrome; the rest had other forms of noncancer pain that did not involve the back. That study reported an average of 61% reduction in pain across all patients, but did not provide separate data on the patients with back pain. Furthermore, the results were derived from a survey of physicians in the USA, who were asked to undertake retrospective chart reviews of their patients. The response rate was only 50%.

The other study[6] was a retrospective review of

162 patients, 42 of whom were lost to follow-up. Of the remaining 120 patients who commenced treatment, 73 had failed back surgery syndrome; the remainder had a variety of other conditions not related to the back. Of the 73 patients, only 49 continued treatment until follow-up. In these patients, the average pain scores were 93 on a 100-point scale at inception, and reduced to 33 at 6 months, but rose to 41 at follow-up an average 3 years later. Although this reduction in pain would seem attractive, the large proportions of patients lost to follow-up or who discontinued treatment, suggests that only a minority of patients initially treated achieve lasting, worthwhile benefit. This inference is reinforced by a recent study[7] and review[8] which commented that

intrathecal treatment was often ineffective (69%) in patients with spinal pain.

Chapters in a recent textbook on the surgical management of spinal pain describe and promote intraspinal opioids for the treatment of both cancer pain and noncancer pain[9-12], but do not provide data on their efficacy for low back pain, beyond the literature cited above. It would seem that intraspinal opioids might constitute an option for the palliation of otherwise intractable, chronic low back pain, but its efficacy and cost-effectiveness remain to be validated. Indeed, in the context of noncancer pain, one commentator has lamented the lack of controlled trials, and has described intraspinal opioids as "an elegant treatment in search of an indication"[13].

Key points

- Intraspinal opioids may be an option for palliative care for patients with chronic low back pain resistant to other interventions, but
- data are lacking as to their efficacy in this regard.

References

1   Penn RD, Paice JA. Chronic intrathecal morphine for intractable pain. J Neurosurg 1987; 67: 182–186.

2   Arner S, Rawal N, Gustafson LL. Clinical experience of long-term treatment with epidural and intrathecal opioids — a nationwide survey. Acta Anaesthesiol Scand 1988; 32: 253–259.

3   Auld AW, Maki-Jokela A, Murdoch DM. Intraspinal narcotic analgesia in the treatment of chronic pain. Spine 1985; 10: 777–781.

4   Paice JA, Winkelmuller W, Burchiel K, Racz GB, Prager JP. Clinical realities and economic considerations: efficacy of intrathecal pain therapy. J Pain Symptom Manage 1997; 14: S14–S26.

5   Paice JA, Penn RD, Shott S. Intraspinal morphine for chronic pain: a retrospective, multicenter study. J Pain Symptom Manage 1996; 11: 71–80.

6   Winkelmuller M, Winkelmuller W. Long-term effects of continuous intrathecal opioid treatment in chronic pain of nonmalignant aetiology. J Neurosurg 1996; 85: 458–467.

7   Nitescu P, Dahm P, Appelgren L, Curelaru I. Continuous infusion of opioid and bupivacaine by externalised intrathecal catheters in long-term treatment of 'refractory' non-malignant pain. Clin J Pain 1998; 14: 17–28.

8   Dahm P, Nitescu P, Appelgren L, Curelaru I. Efficacy

and technical complications of long-term continuous intraspinal infusions of opioid and/or bupivacaine in refractory non-malignant pain: a comparison between the epidural and the intrathecal approach with externalised or implanted catheters and infusion pumps. Clin J Pain 1998; 14: 4–16.

9   Levy RM. Intrathecal opioids: patient selection. In: Burchiel K (ed) Surgical Management of Pain. Thieme, New York, 2002: 592–602.

10 Slavin KV, Hsu FPK, Fessler RG. Intrathecal opioids: intrathecal drug-delivery systems. In: Burchiel K (ed) Surgical Management of Pain. Thieme, New York, 2002: 603–613.

11 Follett KA. Intrathecal opioids: technique and outcomes. In: Burchiel K (ed) Surgical Management of Pain. Thieme, New York, 2002: 614–624.

12 Lazorthes Y, Sallerin B, Verdie JC, Sol JC. Intrathecal and intracerebroventricular opioids: past uses and current indications. In: Burchiel K (ed) Surgical Management of Pain. Thieme, New York, 2002: 625–632.

13 Fields H. Commentary. In: Burchiel K (ed) Surgical Management of Pain. Thieme, New York, 2002: 632.

12. Epidurolysis

Some practitioners believe that back pain can be caused by epidural adhesions, particularly in failed back surgery syndrome. However, there are no data to show that adhesions cause back pain; nor are there any techniques whereby the diagnosis can be made. Nevertheless, in accordance with their beliefs, these practitioners have developed or implemented various techniques for interrupting these adhesions. The procedures are variously known as lysis of epidural adhesions or epidurolysis.

The original procedures involved the injection, through an epidural catheter, of agents such as bupivacaine, hyaluronidase, triamcinolone, and hypertonic saline [1-4]. The most recent variant involves direct visualisation of the adhesions using an endoscope [1,5,6].

The use of the injection procedure was supported by uncontrolled trials that reported that some 25–50% of patients obtained at least 50% reduction of their pain for 3 months [1-4]. Greater proportions of patients have been reported to obtain relief, for the same period, when the endoscopic variant has been used [1,4].

The one controlled study of epidurolysis [6] showed that there was no significant difference in outcome between patients treated with hypertonic saline and hyaluronidase, hypertonic saline alone, normal saline with hyaluronidase, or normal saline alone. Despite this, the authors concluded that the results of their study confirm the benefits of percutaneous epidural neuroplasty as part of an overall pain management strategy. There have been no controlled trials of endoscopic epidurolysis.

Key point

- The available data show that epidurolysis is no more effective than placebo treatment for chronic low back pain.

References

1   Manchikanti L, Pampati V, Bakhit CE, Pakanati RR. Non-endoscopic and endoscopic adhesiolysis in post lumbar laminectomy syndrome: a one-year outcome study and cost-effectiveness analysis. Pain Physician 1999; 2: 52–58.

2   Manchikanti L, Bakhit CE. Percutaneous lysis of epidural adhesions. Pain Physician 2000; 3: 46–64.

3   Anderson SR, Racz GB, Heavner J. Evolution of epidural lysis of adhesions. Pain Physician 2000; 3: 262–270.

4   Manchikanti L, Singh V, Kloth D, Slipman CW, Jasper JF, Trescot AM, Varley KG, Atluri SL, Giron C, Curran MJ, Rivera J, Baha G, Bakhit CE, Reuter MW. Interventional techniques in the management of chronic pain: part 2.0. Pain Physician 2001; 4: 24–96.

5   Saberski LR. A retrospective analysis of spinal canal endoscopy and laminectomy outcomes data. A pilot study. Pain Physician 2000; 3: 193–196.

6   Heavner JE, Racz GB, Raj P. Percutaneous epidural neuroplasty: prospective evaluation of 0.9% NaCl versus 10% NaCl with or without hyaluronidase. Reg Anaest Pain Med 1999; 24: 202–207.

13. Behavioural therapy

Behavioural therapy is an intervention that concentrates not on the patient's back pain and its cause, but on the disability that results from the patient's attitudes, beliefs, psychological distress, and illness behaviour. In general, three behavioural treatment approaches can be distinguished: operant, cognitive, and respondent [1,2]. *Operant* treatment involves positive reinforcement of healthy behaviour, withdrawal of attention toward pain behaviour, and time-contingent prescription of medication. *Cognitive* treatment addresses what their pain means to patients, and what they expect. It seeks to modify the patient's thoughts, beliefs, and feelings about these matters. *Respondent* treatment seeks to modify the patient's physiological responses to pain, largely by reducing muscle tension by means of relaxation techniques of various sorts. *Cognitive–behavioural* therapy is a comprehensive treatment approach that includes a combination of education; identification and modification of thoughts and feelings about pain, and maladaptive beliefs and pain behaviours; the provision of coping strategies; and the use of relaxation.

The data on the efficacy of behavioural therapy for back pain are difficult to distil in their entirety. Whereas some studies focused on behavioural therapy as an isolated intervention (i.e. a monotherapy), others incorporated it into a multidisciplinary program. The use of behavioural therapy in a multidisciplinary context is addressed in Chapter 18. Its efficacy as a monotherapy for back pain is considered below.

One systematic review[3] considered the efficacy of behavioural therapy for a variety of pain problems, including rheumatoid arthritis, osteoarthritis, fibromyalgia, and temporomandibular joint pain, as well as low back pain. It concluded that: "published randomized controlled trials provide good evidence for the effectiveness of cognitive behavioural therapy and behavioural therapy for chronic pain in adults"[3]. The review found that behavioural therapy was more effective than a waiting list control condition, with respect to improving pain, and improving mood, and cognitive and behavioural function. When compared to active control treatments, behavioural therapy was modestly more effective with respect to pain experience, cognitive coping, and pain behaviour, but not with respect to other domains. However, the review[3] also commented that: "data were notably sparse on health service use, drug, intake, uptake of additional treatment, and change in work and occupational status as a consequence of treatment"[3].

A subsequent review[4], that exclusively considered the literature on behavioural therapy for chronic low back pain, offered more explicit conclusions. It found that[4]:

- there was no difference in efficacy between the various forms of behavioural therapy;
- there was strong evidence that behavioural treatment had a moderate positive effect on pain, and a small positive effect on functional status and behaviour, when compared with no treatment, placebo treatment, or being put on a waiting list;
- adding a behavioural component to a usual treatment program has no short-term or long-term effect on pain, functional status, or behaviour.

The review[4] found only one study that compared behavioural therapy directly with a competitive, active control treatment for chronic low back pain. That study found no superiority of behavioural therapy over exercise treatment[5].

In essence, a systematic review of the best, available literature has shown that behavioural therapy, as a monotherapy for chronic low back pain, is *better than no therapy*, and better than a placebo, but it is *not better than exercise* therapy, and provides *no additional benefit* when added to other interventions. What the systematic review did not reveal, however, is that the demonstrable benefits of behavioural therapy, when evident, amount to only a partial reduction in pain and only an improvement in behavioural features. Behavioural therapy does not eliminate chronic low back pain and its associated features.

Key points

- Behavioural therapy is better than no treatment and better than placebo therapy for chronic low back pain, but
- the efficacy of behavioural therapy is limited, and
- behavioural therapy is not more effective than other active interventions.
- Behavioural therapy might be suitable as a form of palliative therapy for intractable low back pain, but
- behavioural therapy is insufficiently effective to constitute a primary, or exclusive intervention.

References

1 Vlaeyen JW, Haazen IW, Schuerman JA, Kole-Snijders AMJ, van Eek H. Behavioural rehabilitation of chronic low back pain: comparison of an operant treatment, an operant-cognitive treatment and an operant-respondent treatment. Br J Clin Psychol 1995; 34: 95–118.

2 Turk DC, Flor H. Etiological theories and treatments for chronic back pain: its psychological models and interventions. Pain 1984; 19: 209–233.

3 Morley S, Eccleston C, Williams A. Systematic review and meta-analysis of randomized controlled trials of cognitive behaviour therapy and behaviour therapy for chronic pain in adults, excluding headache. Pain 1999; 80: 1013.

4 van Tulder MW, Ostelo R, Vlaeyen JWS, Linton SJ, Morley SJ, Assendelft WJJ. Behavioral treatment for chronic back pain. A systematic review within the framework of the Cochrane Back Review Group. Spine 2000; 25: 2688–2699.

5 Turner JA, Clancy S, McQuade KJ, Cardenas DD. Effectiveness of behavioral therapy for chronic low back pain: a component analysis. J Consult Clin Psychol 1990; 58: 573–579.

14. Back school

Systematic reviews, involving the same authors[1–3], and addressing essentially the same literature, have offered slightly different conclusions about the efficacy of back school in the treatment of chronic low back pain. Of the more recent reviews, one published in 1997 concluded that: "There is strong evidence that an intensive back school program in an occupational setting is more effective than no actual treatment for chronic low back pain. There is limited evidence that a back school is more effective than other conservative treatment for chronic low back pain"[1]. By the year 2000, this conclusion had changed to: "There is limited evidence that an intensive back school program in an occupational setting in Scandinavia is more effective than no actual treatment. There is conflicting evidence on the effectiveness of back schools in nonoccupational settings and outside Scandinavia"[2].

Part of the reason for this difference is that certain studies in the 1997 were reclassified in the 2000 review from studies of back school to studies of multidisciplinary treatment. The roots for this distinction can be found in a 1994 review of the same literature.

The 1994 review[3] was the longest and most detailed, and covered more literature than the subsequent reviews. It found that: "The best studies indicated that back schools may be effective in occupational settings in acute, recurrent or chronic conditions."[3]. The reviewers also found that the results were more likely to be favourable in studies of higher quality. In that respect, however, a confounder arises. The higher quality studies did not use back school as an isolated therapy. Back school was part of a multidisciplinary program.

When back school has been used as a sole therapy for chronic low back pain it has been found to be no better than a program of calisthenics[4], no better than a pamphlet[5], or detuned ultrasound[6], or being on a waiting list[7]. Adding back school to a training program confers no advantage[8], but adding back school to exercises achieves slightly better results than exercises alone[9]. One study[10] found back school to be better than either placebo or physiotherapy. This study, however, was graded as low quality by all three systematic reviews[1–3]. A high quality study[11] found back school to be more effective than no systematic treatment. The magnitude of effect, however, was small, amounting to a decrease from 90 to only 70 on a 100-point composite visual analogue scale; a decrease from 18 to 16 on a 20-point back pain index; and an improvement from 20 to 19 on the Oswestry Disability Questionnaire.

When back school has been reported and interpreted as being effective, it has been used as a part of a multidisciplinary program[12–15]. It is that literature which earlier systematic reviews regarded as good quality and providing evidence in favour of back school[1,3], but which the latest review[2] reclassified as evidence of multidisciplinary management.

In essence, the literature shows that back school is not effective, or at best marginally better than usual care, when used as a sole therapy for chronic low back pain. Any greater benefit that it offers arises from its incorporation into a multidisciplinary program. This is considered in Chapter 18.

Key point

- When used as a sole therapy, back school is not effective for chronic low back pain.

References

1   van Tulder MW, Koes BW, Bouter LM. Conservative treatment of acute and chronic nonspecific low back pain. A systematic review of randomized controlled trials of the most common interventions. Spine 1997; 22: 2128–2156.

2   van Tulder MV, Goossens M, Waddell G, Nachemson A. Conservative treatment of chronic low back pain. In: Nachemson A, Jonsson E (eds) Neck and Back Pain: The Scientific Evidence of Causes, Diagnosis, and Treatment. Lippincott, Williams and Wilkins, Philadelphia, PA, 2000: 271–304.

3   Koes BW, van Tulder MW, van der Windt DAWM, Bouter LM. The efficacy of back schools: a review of randomized clinical trials. J Clin Epidemiol 1994; 47: 851–862.

4   Donchin M, Woolf O, Kaplan L, Floman Y. Secondary prevention of low-back pain. A clinical trial. Spine 1990; 15: 1317–1320.

5   Berwick DM, Budman S, Feldstein M. No clinical effect of back schools in an HMO. A randomized prospective trial. Spine 1989; 14: 339–344.

6   Lankhorst GJ, van der Stadt RJ, Vogelaar TW, van der Korst JK, Prevo AJH. The effect of the Swedish back school in chronic idiopathic low-back pain. Scand J Rehab Med 1983; 15: 141–145.

7   Keijsers JFME, Streenbakkers WHL, Meertens RM, Bouter LM, Kok GJ. The efficacy of the back school: a randomized trial. Arthr Care Res 1990; 3: 204–209.

8   Lindequist SL, Lundberg B, Wikmark R, Bergstad B, Loof G, Ottermark AC. Information and regime at low-back pain. Scand J Rehab Med 1984; 16: 113–116.

9   Klaber Moffett JA, Chase SM, Portek I, Ennis JR. A controlled prospective study to evaluate the effectiveness of a back school in the relief of chronic low-back pain. Spine 1986; 11: 120–122.

10 Postacchini F, Facchini M, Palieri P. Efficacy of various forms of conservative treatment in low back pain: a comparative study. Neuro Orthopedics 1988; 6: 28–35.

11 Hurri H. The Swedish back school in chronic low-back pain. Part I. Benefits. Scand J Rehab Med 1989; 21: 33–40.

12 Harkapaa K, Jarvikoski A, Mellin G, Hurri H. A controlled study on the outcome of inpatient and outpatient treatment of low-back pain. Part I. Pain, disability, compliance, and reported treatment benefits three months after treatment. Scand J Rehab Med 1989; 21: 81–89.

13 Mellin G, Hurri H, Harkapaa K, Jarvikoski A. A controlled study on the outcome of inpatient and outpatient treatment of low-back pain. Part II. Effects on physical measurements three months after treatment. Scand J Rehab Med 1989; 21: 91–95.

14 Harkapaa K, Mellin G, Jarvikoski A, Hurri H. A controlled study on the outcome of inpatient and outpatient treatment of low-back pain. Part III. Long-term follow-up of pain, disability, and compliance. Scand J Rehab Med 1990; 22: 181–188.

15 Mellin G, Harkapaa K, Hurri H, Jarvikoski A. A controlled study on the outcome of inpatient and outpatient treatment of low-back pain. Part IV. Long-term effects on physical measurements. Scand J Rehab Med 1990; 22: 189–194.

15. Exercises

Similar problems apply to the literature on exercises as they do to the literature on back school. It is difficult to dissociate the benefits of exercise therapy from the benefits of co-interventions when these have been used. Furthermore, much of the literature has been devoted to comparing one type of exercise against another, rather than testing exercise against some other form of competitive therapy.

An earlier review[1] held that: "There is strong evidence that exercise therapy is effective for chronic low back pain." This conclusion was subsequently amended and elaborated in a more recent, and more extensive review[2].

For chronic low back pain, the latter review[2] found that:

- there is strong evidence that exercise therapy is more effective than usual care by a general practitioner;
- there is limited evidence that exercises provide better outcomes than back school;
- there is conflicting evidence on whether or not exercise is more effective than an inactive, sham treatment;
- there is no evidence concerning the effectiveness of either flexion exercises or extension exercises;

- there is conflicting evidence concerning the relative effectiveness of flexion versus extension exercises;
- there is strong evidence that strengthening exercises are not more effective than other types of exercises;
- there is conflicting evidence that strengthening exercises are more effective than inactive treatment.

These conclusions, and the data that support them, portray a limited efficacy for exercise therapy. Exercise is better than nothing, and better than usual care by general practitioners, but it is not consistently been shown to be better than sham therapies or passive therapies. Moreover, the effect-size of exercise therapy is not great. When compared to placebo treatments, exercise therapy offers improvements in pain scores ranging from 0% [3] to little more than 10% [4,5] or 15%, [6,7]. Exceptional in this regard is an average of 57% reduction in pain attributed to special exercises focused on coactivation of the abdominal and multifidus muscles [8]. According to the best available data, therefore, if exercises are to be used for chronic low back pain, they should be these special exercises.

Few studies on exercise have reported on return to work and continued use of health care. Success in these outcomes has been reported by and attributed to multidisciplinary programs of which exercise therapy is only one part (Chapter 18).

Key points

- Conventional exercises are better than no treatment for chronic low back pain, and better than usual care by a general practitioner.
- Exercises are not necessarily more effective than an inactive sham treatment.
- When compared to placebo treatments, exercise therapy offers improvements in pain scores ranging from 0% to little more than 15%.
- The only exercise therapy that has been shown to be achieve substantial and lasting reductions in pain are special exercises directed at coactivation of the abdominal and multifidus muscles.

References

1   van Tulder MW, Koes BW, Bouter LM. Conservative treatment of acute and chronic nonspecific low back pain. A systematic review of randomized controlled trials of the most common interventions. Spine 1997; 22: 2128–2156.

2   van Tulder M, Malmivaara A, Esmail R, Koes B. Exercise therapy for low back pain. A systematic review within the framework of the Cochrane Collaboration Back Review Group. Spine 2000; 21: 2784–2796.

3   Hansen FR, Bendix T, Skov P, Jensen CV, Kristensen JH, Krohn L, Schioeler H. Intensive, dynamic back-muscle exercises, conventional physiotherapy, or placebo-control treatment of low-back pain: a randomized, observer-blind trial. Spine 1993; 18: 98–107.

4   Frost H, Klaber Moffet JA, Moser JS, Fairbank JC. Randomised controlled trial for evaluation of fitness programme for patients with chronic low back pain. Br Med J 1995; 310: 151–154.

5   Frost H, Lamb SE, Klaber Moffet JA, Fairbank JC, Moser JS. A fitness programme for patients with chronic low back pain: 2-year follow-up of a randomized controlled trial. Pain 1998; 75: 273–279.

6   Risch SV, Norvell NK, Pollock ML, Risch ED, Langer H, Fulton M, Graves JE, Leggett SH. Lumbar strengthening in chronic low back pain patients: physiologic and psychologic benefits. Spine 1993; 18: 232–238.

7   Torstensen TA, Ljunggren AE, Meen HD, Odland E, Mowinckel P, Geijerstam S. Efficiency and costs of medical exercise therapy, conventional physiotherapy, and self-exercise in patients with chronic low back pain: a pragmatic, randomized, single-blinded, controlled trial with 1-year follow-up. Spine 1998; 23: 2616–2624.

8   O'Sullivan PB, Twomey LT, Allison GT. Evaluation of specific stabilizing exercise in the treatment of chronic low back pain with radiologic diagnosis of spondylolysis or spondylolisthesis. Spine 1997; 22: 2959–2967.

16. Summary

The results of controlled trials and of systematic reviews paint a disappointing picture of the efficacy of monotherapies for chronic low back pain.

- There are no data from controlled trials to support any efficacy for surgery, spinal cord stimulation, epidural steroids, and intraspinal opioids.
- The best quality studies have denied or failed to show any efficacy greater than that of placebo for acupuncture, injection of tender points, traction, epidurolysis, and back school.
- The data on prolotherapy are conflicting and not yet compelling.
- The only treatment shown in a controlled trial to have produced substantial and lasting reductions in pain are special exercises designed to coactivate the abdominal and multifidus muscles.
- Other monotherapies for chronic back pain achieve only limited reductions in pain, some for only short periods. These include analgesics, NSAIDs, and opioids, manipulative therapy, massage, behavioural therapy, and conventional exercises.

Individually, none of these latter treatments is curative of chronic low back pain. Nor do they achieve major and sustained reductions in pain and disability. For that reason, they cannot be countenanced as primary interventions for chronic low back pain. However, and nonetheless, the fact that some of these interventions can confer some benefit offers them a possible role, either individually or in combination, as palliative therapy for intractable low back pain. That role is perhaps, at odds with how these interventions are sometimes portrayed and publicized in practice, but the data on their efficacy really does not justify a greater therapeutic status.

For the practitioner wanting to know what to do with this information, the messages are several.

Do not expect monotherapies to 'work' for chronic low back pain. Therefore, do not prescribe them, or portray them, as 'cures'.

At best, monotherapies may be palliative and if used, should be portrayed as such. Their objective is to provide perhaps some degree of relief, but not to effect a cure. The evidence simply does not support a greater role.

Of all the monotherapies, only special exercises designed to coactivate the abdominal muscles and multifidus hold the promise of substantial and sustained reductions in back pain.

There is no evidence that submitting patients to multiple monotherapies, simultaneously or serially, achieves better outcomes. Doing so may seem expedient but it protracts the problem, and potentially compounds the patient's distress because of repeated failures of treatment.

More appropriate, and potentially more effective, is the use of other interventions, as described in Chapters 19, 20, and 21.

Medical Management of Acute and Chronic Low Back Pain. An Evidence-Based Approach
Pain Research and Clinical Management, Vol. 13
Nikolai Bogduk and Brian McGuirk

CHAPTER 18

Multidisciplinary treatment

1. Introduction

It is difficult to define accurately, and perhaps to everyone's satisfaction, exactly what constitutes multidisciplinary treatment. One approach might be to accept as multidisciplinary treatment what authors have described in papers that bear the term in their title. Another might be to accept what has been interpreted by reviewers as constituting multidisciplinary treatment. Or multidisciplinary treatment might be whatever is said to be multidisciplinary treatment by those who provide it, even though that treatment may bear only a remote relationship to the literature.

Whatever the particular definition, the essence of multidisciplinary treatment is the simultaneous application of different interventions each provided by a different professional (discipline). However, the actual components of the program, or its emphasis, differ and can be traced or related to one of three origins (Fig. 1).

Functional restoration is a system of treatment developed in Texas as the PRIDE programme, by Mayer and colleagues[1]. Conceptually, functional restoration is based on sports medicine principles, in which the complaint of pain is essentially disregarded, and management instead focuses on improving the patient's capacity for movement, using testing machines to monitor objectively changes in range of movement and muscle strength, with regular provision of feedback of gains to the patient. The cardinal interventions are specific exercises, work-simulation and work-hardening (i.e. increasing the

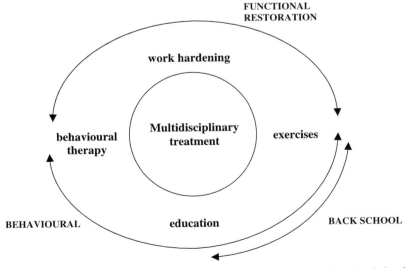

Fig. 1. The combinations, emphases, and foci of various multidisciplinary programs for chronic low back pain.

TABLE I

How authors and reviewers have classified various studies involving multidisciplinary treatment for chronic low back pain

Study	Classification				
	Multidisciplinary treatment	Functional restoration	Back school	Not specified	Not mentioned
Harkapaa and colleagues [12-15]	R2, R3, R4		R1	AU	
Bendix and colleagues [16-19]	R2, R3, AU	AU			R1
Alaranta et al. [20]	R1, R3			AU	R1
Mitchell and Carmen [21]	R2, R3	AU			R1
Peters and colleagues [6,7]	AU				R1, R2, R3
Haldorsen et al. [10]	AU				R1, R2, R3
Deardorff et al. [11]	AU				R1, R2, R3

AU, author of study; R1, van Tulder et al., 1997 [22]; R2, van Tulder et al., 2000 [23]; R3, Guzman et al. [24]; R4, Flor et al. [25].

patient's endurance for their own particular occupational demands). These interventions, however, are complemented with education (cf. back school) and cognitive–behavioural therapy. A typical programme requires a 3-week live-in period with activities for 57 hours per week [1].

The original study of functional restoration [1] reported an 86% return to work, and a reduction in surgery rates and consumption of health-care. A 2-year follow-up confirmed that 86% of patients had remained at work [2]. These results were subsequently replicated by independent investigators [3,4], and functional restoration attracted considerable endorsement, at least in the United States [5].

Other programs appear to have their origin in behavioural therapy. They emphasise psychological interventions, in the form of operant and cognitive therapy, but couple that with education and exercises [6-11]. In contrast to classical functional restoration, work-hardening, as such, is not specifically mentioned, or emphasised, in some of these studies [6-9]. The emphasis of intervention seems to have been more on the patient's psychological function and personal physical function.

A third approach consists largely of the educational aspects of back school, complemented by exercises [12-15]. Formal, cognitive–behavioural intervention has not been a component, nor has occupational intervention.

Table I indicates the problems inherent in interpreting the literature in this field. Some studies have been regarded as studies of multidisciplinary treatment by some reviewers, but not by others. Some authors did not portray their interventions as multidisciplinary treatment. Others considered they were using functional restoration, but reviewers have not recognised this classification. The authors of some studies considered that their treatment was multidisciplinary or multimodal, but these studies have not been included in reviews.

2. Efficacy

For some time, the reputation of multidisciplinary treatment was sustained by a systematic review that compiled all the literature prior to 1992 [25]. That review addressed the management of chronic pain in general, but did include many studies that dealt with low back pain. The authors concluded that multidisciplinary treatment was superior to no treatment, waiting list controls, or single-discipline treatments, but cautioned that the quality of designs and study descriptions were marginal. Subsequent reviews have been more decisive.

One systematic review [23] reported finding four high-quality randomised, controlled trials of multidisciplinary treatment for chronic back pain but of these, one concerned subacute back pain (see Chapter 12), leaving three pertinent trials [12–15,20,21]. Of the six low-quality trials identified by this review, two pertained to subacute low back pain (Chapter 12), and two pertained to the evaluation of cognitive therapy as an addition to a rehabilitation program (Chapter 18). The two remaining trials were by the same authors and were variously considered to be studies of either multidisciplinary treatment or functional restoration [16–21]. The review found that: "There is strong evidence that a multidisciplinary treatment program aimed at functional restoration is useful for patients with long-lasting, severe chronic low back pain." [23].

A more recent review [24] included the pertinent studies from the above-mentioned review, but also several additional studies. It classified the studies according to the intensity of the intervention (based on frequency and duration of the treatment), and looked carefully at the pooled results for particular outcomes. It found that:

there is strong evidence that intensive multidisciplinary biopsychosocial rehabilitation with functional restoration improves function when compared with inpatient or outpatient non-multidisciplinary rehabilitation [16,17,20];

there is moderate evidence that intensive multidisciplinary biopsychosocial rehabilitation with functional restoration reduces pain when compared with outpatient non-multidisciplinary rehabilitation or usual care [16,17,20];

there is contradictory evidence regarding vocational outcomes of intensive multidisciplinary biopsychosocial rehabilitation; whereas Bendix et al. [16] reported improvements in 'work-readiness', Alaranta et al. [20] and Mitchell and Carmen [21] showed no benefit on sickness leave. . . ;

regarding less intensive multidisciplinary biopsychosocial rehabilitation, five trials could not show improvements in pain, function, or vocational outcomes when compared with non-multidisciplinary outpatient rehabilitation or usual care [12,16,26–28].

With respect to the two major of these conclusions, an inspection of the published data provides an insight into the effect-size. In the first study of Bendix et al. [16], the intensive functional restoration program reduced disability from 15.5 on a 30-point scale to 8.5, at 4 months; and reduced back pain from 5.3, on a scale of 0–10, to 2.7. These would seem to be reasonable improvements, although few patients were rendered pain-free or fully rehabilitated.

The second study of Bendix et al. [17] reported more modest gains. Function improved from 16.9 to only 12.1, and pain from 6.1 to 5.7. Alaranta et al. [20] achieved an average reduction in pain of only 17 points on a 100-point scale. With respect to functional capacity, the significant gain reported by Alaranta et al. [20] was that a smaller proportion of their index patients suffered back problems during light activities or at rest; but there were no differences from control patients with respect to the proportion of patients being pain-free, or having problems only during moderate activities.

Bendix et al. [16,17] achieved significantly greater reductions in sick-leave and contacts with the health-care system. However, this was not the experience of Alaranta et al. [20] or of Mitchell and Carmen [21].

Of the studies not covered by systematic reviews, one [11] showed that multidisciplinary management achieved no greater reduction in pain than an untreated control group; the major gains were reduction in use of medication and a 48% return to work rate. Another [10] found no consistent advantages of multidisciplinary treatment over usual care with respect to pain, but the index patients were slightly more satisfied with their job, and were slightly less distressed psychologically. However, return-to-work rates were not better.

The third study [6,7] achieved appreciable, but modest, gains in patients treated in a multidisciplinary programme compared with patients having usual care. In general, a greater proportion of index patients were using medications appropriately, were active and had no increase in pain. These results portray multidisciplinary treatment as being palliative, but not a means of ridding patients of their pain and the difficulties it causes.

3. Synopsis

Systematic reviews [22–24] of the literature paint a picture of limited, and perhaps selective, efficacy of multidisciplinary management of chronic low back pain. When subjected to meta-analysis [24], the data do not show that multidisciplinary treatment is able to eliminate problems or achieve greater return to work. The data do show differences in efficacy between psychologically based programs and ones based on intensive exercises.

Psychologically based programs achieve palliative effects in that they may reduce distress and prevent deterioration, but there is no evidence that they restore patients to normal activities including work. In this regard, they may be appropriate when complete restoration and return to work is not a goal, or is considered unachievable.

Intensive programs focussed on exercises, are more effective than less intensive programs or programs that focus on behaviour. Yet even so, the improvements achieved are limited. Patients can expect to have less pain and be able to function somewhat better, but their problems are not eliminated. In essence, multidisciplinary treatment is tantamount to palliative care. Nevertheless, intensive programs do provide greater benefits than do usual care or less intensive, and passive interventions.

For this reason, multidisciplinary treatment has been championed as the preferred method of managing chronic low back pain [29]. Moreover, it is a form of intervention that is relatively easy to develop and provide. Professionals in the disciplines required are abundant, and the facilities required are relatively standard.

However, multidisciplinary treatment falls short of constituting a solution to the problem of chronic low back pain. Although the magnitude of each patient's problem might be reduced, the problem still persists. Disability may be reduced, but the burden of illness remains.

Key points

- Multidisciplinary therapy for chronic low back pain exists in various forms.
- Intensive physical programs achieve some improvements in functional capacity, and modest reductions in pain, but not a greater return to work.
- Less intensive physical programs are not demonstrably more effective than other interventions.
- More psychologically based programs may serve as palliative care, to reduce distress and maintain some degree of activity, but they do not eliminate pain.

References

1 Mayer TG, Gatchel RJ, Kishino N, Keeley J, Capra P, Mayer H, Barnett J, Mooney V. Objective assessment of spine function following industrial injury. A prospective study with comparison group and one-year follow-up. Spine 1985; 10: 482–493.
2 Mayer TG, Gatchel RJ, Mayer H, Kishino N, Keeley J, Mooney V. A prospective two-year study of functional restoration in industrial low back injury. J Am Med Assoc 1987; 258: 1763–1767.
3 Hazard RG, Fenwick JW, Kalisch SM, Redmond J, Reeves V, Reid S, Frymoyer JW. Functional restoration with behavioural support. A one-year prospective study of patients with chronic low-back pain. Spine 1989; 14: 157–161.
4 Burke SA, Harms-Constas CK, Aden PS. Return to work/work retention outcomes of a functional restoration program: a multi-center, prospective study with a comparison group. Spine 1994; 19: 1880–1886.
5 Hazard RG. Spine update. Functional restoration. Spine 1995; 20: 2345–2348.
6 Peters JL, Large RG. A randomised control trial evaluation in- and outpatient pain management programmes. Pain 1990; 41: 283–293.
7 Peters J, Large RG, Elkind G. Follow-up results from a randomised controlled trial evaluating in- and outpatient pain management programmes. Pain 1992; 50: 41–50.
8 Roberts AH, Sternbach RA, Polich J. Behavioral management of chronic pain and excess disability: long-term

follow-up of an outpatient program. Clin J Pain 1993; 9: 41–48.

9   Guck TP, Skultety FM, Meilman PW, Dowd ET. Multi-disciplinary pain centre follow-up study: evaluation with a no-treatment control group. Pain 1985; 21: 295–306.

10 Haldorsen EMH, Kronholm K, Skouen JS, Ursin H. Multimodal cognitive behavioural treatment of patients sick-listed for musculoskeletal pain: a randomised controlled study. Scand J Rheumatol 1998; 27: 16–25.

11 Deardorff WW, Rubin HS, Scott DW. Comprehensive multidisciplinary treatment of chronic pain: a follow-up study of treated and non-treated groups. Pain 1991; 45: 35–43.

12 Harkapaa K, Jarvikoski A, Mellin G, Hurri H. A controlled study on the outcome of inpatient and outpatient treatment of low-back pain. Part I. Pain, disability, compliance, and reported treatment benefits three months after treatment. Scand J Rehab Med 1989; 21: 81–89.

13 Mellin G, Hurri H, Harkapaa K, Jarvikoski A. A controlled study on the outcome of inpatient and outpatient treatment of low-back pain. Part II. Effects on physical measurements three months after treatment. Scand J Rehab Med 1989; 21: 91–95.

14 Harkapaa K, Mellin G, Jarvikoski A, Hurri H. A controlled study on the outcome of inpatient and outpatient treatment of low-back pain. Part III. Long-term follow-up of pain, disability, and compliance. Scand J Rehab Med 1990; 22: 181–188.

15 Mellin G, Harkapaa K, Hurri H, Jarvikoski A. A controlled study on the outcome of inpatient and outpatient treatment of low-back pain. Part IV. Long-term effects on physical measurements. Scand J Rehab Med 1990; 22: 189–194.

16 Bendix AF, Bendix T, Ostenfeld S, Bush E, Andersen A. Active treatment programs for patients with chronic low back pain: a prospective, randomized, observer-blinded study. Eur Spine J 1995; 4: 148–152.

17 Bendix AF, Bendix T, Vaegter K, Lund C, Frolund L, Holm L. Multidisciplinary intensive treatment for chronic low back pain: a randomized, prospective study. Clevel Clin J Med 1996; 63: 62–69.

18 Bendix AF, Bendix T, Lund C, Kirkbak S, Ostenfeld S. Comparison of three intensive programs for chronic low back pain patients: a prospective, randomized, observer-blinded study with one-year follow-up. Scand J Rehab Med 1997; 29: 81–89.

19 Bendix AF, Bendix T, Labriola M, Boekgaard P. Functional restoration for chronic low back pain: two-year follow-up of two randomized clinical trials. Spine 1998; 23: 717–725.

20 Alaranta H, Rytokoski U, Rissanen A, Talo S, Ronnemaa T, Puukka P, Karppi SL, Videman T, Kallio V, Slatis P. Intensive physical and psychosocial training program for patients with chronic low back pain: a controlled clinical trial. Spine 1994; 19: 1339–1349.

21 Mitchell RI, Carmen GM. The functional restoration approach to the treatment of chronic pain in patients with soft tissue and back injuries. Spine 1994; 19: 633–642.

22 van Tulder MW, Koes BW, Bouter LM. Conservative treatment of acute and chronic nonspecific low back pain. A systematic review of randomized controlled trials of the most common interventions. Spine 1997; 22: 2128–2156.

23 van Tulder MV, Goossens M, Waddell G, Nachemson A. Conservative treatment of chronic low back pain. In: Nachemson A, Jonsson E (eds) Neck and Back Pain: The Scientific Evidence of Causes, Diagnosis, and Treatment. Lippincott, Willams and Wilkins, Philadelphia, PA, 2000: 271–304.

24 Guzman J, Esmail R, Karjalainen K, Malmivaara A, Irvin E, Bombardier C. Multidisciplinary rehabilitation for chronic back pain: systematic review. Br Med J 2001; 322: 1511–1516.

25 Flor H, Fydich T, Turk DC. Efficacy of multidisciplinary pain treatment centers: a meta-analytic review. Pain 1992; 49: 221–230.

26 Basler H, Jakle C, Kroner-Herwig B. Incorporation of cognitive-behavioral treatment into the medical care of chronic low back patients: a controlled randomized study in German pain treatment centers. Patient Educ Couns 1997; 31: 113–124.

27 Nicholas MK, Wilson PH, Goyen J. Operant–behavioural and cognitive–behavioural treatment for chronic low back pain. Behav Res Ther 191; 29: 225–238.

28 Nicholas MK, Wilson PH, Goyen J. Comparison of cognitive–behavioral group treatment and an alternative non-psychological treatment for chronic low back pain. Pain 1992; 48: 339–347.

29 Waddel G. The Back Pain Revolution. Churchill Livingstone, Edinburgh, 1998, pp 351–367.

Medical Management of Acute and Chronic Low Back Pain. An Evidence-Based Approach
Pain Research and Clinical Management, Vol. 13
Nikolai Bogduk and Brian McGuirk
© 2002 Elsevier Science B.V. All rights reserved

CHAPTER 19

Precision diagnosis

1. Introduction

Pivotal to the reductionist approach to chronic low back pain is the ability to pinpoint an anatomical diagnosis. For this purpose, physical examination is neither reliable nor valid. Medical imaging provides little sound information. Even if MRI reveals a high-intensity zone (HIZ) or an endplate change (Chapter 15), the diagnosis is still not absolute.

2. Needle procedures

Although the discs and joints of the lumbar spine are not accessible to palpation, they are accessible to needles introduced onto or into these target structures under fluoroscopic control. Needles can be used to stimulate the target structure mechanically, with an injection of contrast medium; or to anaesthetise it, by injecting local anaesthetic into or onto the structure or onto the nerves that innervate it. By these means, needle procedures can be used to test if a particular structure is the source of a patient's pain.

Compared to palpation, needle procedures have the advantage that they can target a particular structure selectively and accurately. Radiography can be used to confirm that the target structure, and only the target structure, has been reached by the needle or by anything that is injected through it.

Compared to imaging studies, needle procedures can determine, physiologically, whether or not the target structure is painful. Imaging studies do not do this. In order to be diagnostic, imaging studies rely on a priori information, such as epidemiological data, that show that a particular feature is consistently associated with pain. Needle procedures provide this information directly, in each and every case in which they are used; and do not rely on a priori associations.

Most critically, needle procedures can be subjected to controls, in order to ensure the validity of the test in each and every patient. This virtue is not shared by physical examination tests, which lack valid controls that can be implemented every time that the test is used.

The singular disadvantage of needle procedures is that they require special facilities, such as fluoroscopy, and special skills, such as the ability to deliver a needle accurately and safely to the target structure. These requirements render needle procedures impracticable to most practitioners. However, that does not deter from their validity.

Three procedures are available for the investigation of chronic low back pain. They are provocation discography, zygapophysial joint blocks, and sacroiliac joint blocks. Each has been subjected to scientific scrutiny to determine their validity and diagnostic utility.

3. Provocation discography

Provocation discography is a procedure designed to identify a painful intervertebral disc. It involves introducing into the nucleus pulposus of the target disc a needle that is used to distend the disc from the inside with an injection of contrast medium in order to reproduce pain stemming from that disc (Fig. 1).

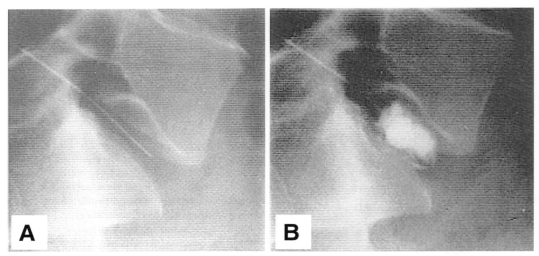

Fig. 1. Lateral views of an L5–S1 discogram. (A) Needle inserted before injection. (B) After injection of contrast medium, which outlines the internal morphology of the disc.

3.1. Principles

The premise upon which provocation discography is based is that if a particular disc is painful then stressing it should reproduce the patient's pain. If the disc is not the source of a patient's pain then stressing it either should not be painful or should produce pain that is not the patient's familiar or accustomed pain.

In this regard, provocation discography is analogous to palpation for tenderness. But as in the case of tenderness, provocation does not reveal pathology or the cause of pain; it only indicates the structure that when stressed reproduces the patient's pain. In order to reveal the responsible lesion, provocation discography must be supplemented by post-discography CT (Fig. 2), which has the ability to reveal the fissures characteristic of internal disc disruption (Chapter 14).

Because it is a provocation test, provocation discography is liable to false-positive results. In formal terms, provocation discography tests the hypothesis that if a disc is the source of a patient's pain, stressing that disc should reproduce their pain. The competing hypothesis is that, in patients with back pain, stimulation of any structure in the back will similarly reproduce their pain, and accordingly, stimulating any disc will reproduce their pain.

Simply reproducing pain by stimulating a single disc does not distinguish between the two hypotheses. Consequently, provocation discography at a single segmental level cannot provide a valid diagnosis of discogenic pain. For validity to be sustained in the first instance, provocation must be subjected to controls.

In order to refute the competing hypothesis, discs at adjacent segments to the target level must be stimulated on a single-blind basis. If all discs are painful, the test fails to refute the competing hypothesis that anything and everything in the patient's back hurts. Consequently, a diagnosis of discogenic pain cannot be rendered. In contrast, however, the validity of the diagnosis is enhanced if pain is reproduced when the target disc is stimulated, but no pain is produced if and when adjacent discs are likewise stimulated. Such a response is not compatible with the competing hypothesis that anything and everything in the patient's back hurts. Consequently, the hypothesis prevails that the target disc is the single and sole source of pain.

Accordingly, both the International Association for the Study of Pain (IASP)[1] and the International Spinal Injection Society (ISIS)[2,3] have recommended that in order to be valid, provocation discography must be subjected to anatomical con-

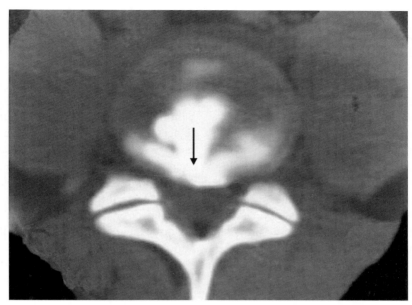

Fig. 2. A CT discogram of a lumbar disc showing a radial fissure (arrow) diagnostic of internal disc disruption.

trols. Specifically, the diagnostic criteria for disco-genic pain [1] are:

(1) that provocation of the target disc reproduces the patient's pain, but
(2) provided that provocation of adjacent discs does not reproduce pain.

Certain terms are used by discographers in reference to the response of the patient upon a disc being provoked. If the patient's accustomed pain is reproduced, the response is said to be concordant. If some other pain is produced, the response is said to be discordant. This distinction emphasises that the objective of provocation discography is not to find a painful disc, but to find the one that is responsible for the patient's pain.

The diagnostic criteria for internal disruption [1] are:

(1) that the patient has discogenic pain, and
(2) the affected disc exhibits a grade 3 or greater fissure, upon CT-discography.

Two further criteria have been developed by the International Spinal Injection Society in order to enhance the validity of provocation discography. One

requirement is that the patient's pain is reproduced to a significant extent. The ad hoc criterion is this regard is that the pain is of an intensity of at least 7 on a 10-point visual analogue scale. The second, additional criterion is that pain is reproduced at an injection pressure of less than 50 psi, and preferably less than 15 psi. This criterion guards against an asymptomatic disc being misdiagnosed as symptomatic simply because it was rendered painful by an extremely forceful injection.

3.2. Validity

Central hyperalgesia is a physiological phenomenon in which the perception of stimuli from a particular receptive field is facilitated by ongoing nociceptive activity arising from an adjacent, or nearby, but separate, receptive field. In clinical terms, a structure that is not actually intrinsically painful may appear to be painful when stimulated if there is a source of pain in some other structure innervated by the same spinal cord segment.

In this regard, a formal study has shown that in patients with no history and no symptoms of back pain, but with a painful donor site on the iliac crest, disc stimulation can produce back pain[4]. This observation warns discographers to beware of other possible sources of pain in patients undergoing disc stimulation. Without such attention, the response to disc stimulation may be false-positive. For these reasons, steps should be taken in obtaining a history, performing a physical examination, and assessing any available imaging studies, in order reasonably to exclude other possible sources of pain, before embarking upon disc stimulation. If doubts arise, other investigations may be more appropriate before undertaking disc stimulation.

Another study has warned of potential psychosocial sources of false-positive responses to provocation discography[5]. The study reported that the false-positive rate of provocation discography was 10% in asymptomatic individuals, 40% in patients with chronic pain, and 75% in patients with somatisation. Superficially, these figures are alarming and would seem to indicate that provocation discography lacks validity. However, closer inspection of the data reveals limitations and flaws[6].

Most significantly, the diagnostic criteria for discogenic pain, proposed by the IASP or by ISIS were not applied. The so-called false-positive rates pertained to the number of discs that were painful, irrespective of the pressure of injection and without regard to anatomical controls. If the requirement for controls is applied, together with the manometric criterion of 50 psi, the prevalence of false-positive response drops to 10% in asymptomatic individuals, 10% in patients with chronic pain, and 50% in patients with somatisation[6]. If the manometric criterion is increased to 15 psi, these figures become 0%, 0% and 25%, respectively.

These corrections do not eliminate false-positive response completely, but they reduce their risk to tolerable levels. In particular, they warn of a substantial risk of false-positive responses amongst patients with somatisation. In other patients, the false-positive rate is no worse than that of many other tests in medical practice that are not considered controversial.

3.3. Diagnostic utility

The diagnostic utility of provocation discography lies in its ability to establish the source of a patient's pain. Establishing a diagnosis has merits in its own right. The patient can be told that the source of their pain has been found; and no longer are they subject to accusations that there is nothing wrong with their back. Establishing a diagnosis also obviates and averts continued and futile pursuit of a diagnosis. Moreover, establishing a diagnosis of discogenic pain protects the patient from being subjected, by trial and error, to treatments that are inappropriate for discogenic pain, and which will not relieve their pain.

A formal study, following the diagnostic criteria of the IASP (see above), found that the prevalence of discogenic pain due to internal disc disruption was 39% amongst patients with chronic back pain[7]. Provocation discography is the only means by which to establish this diagnosis. Not using this procedure leaves this proportion of patients without a diagnosis.

3.4. Therapeutic utility

While protecting the patient from inappropriate treatments, establishing a diagnosis of discogenic pain allows the patient to be directed to appropriate treatments. What those treatments might be is, to some extent, a matter of choice. The options are considered in Chapter 21.

References

1   Merskey H, Bogduk N (eds). Classification of Chronic Pain. Descriptions of Chronic Pain Syndromes and Definition of Pain Terms, ed 2. IASP Press, Seattle, WA, 1994, pp 180–181.

2   Bogduk B. Proposed discography standards. ISIS Newsletter, Volume 2, Number 1. International Spinal Injection Society, Daly City, CA, 1994, pp 10–13.

3   Derby R. A second proposal for discography standards. ISIS Newsletter, Volume 2, Number 2. International Spinal Injection Society, Daly City, CA, 1994, pp 108–122.

4   Carragee EJ, Tanner CM, Yang B, Brito JL, Truong T. False-positive findings on lumbar discography: reliability of

subjective concordance assessment during provocative disc injection. Spine 1999; 24: 2542–2547.

5   Carragee EJ, Tanner CM, Khurana S, Hayward C, Welsh J, Date E, Truong T, Rossi M, Hagle C. The rates of false-positive lumbar discography in select patients without low back symptoms. Spine 2000; 25: 1373–1381.

6   Bogduk N. An analysis of the Carragee data on false-positive discography. ISIS Scientific Newsletter 2001; 4(2): 3–10. International Spinal Injection Society, Daly City, CA.

7   Schwarzer AC, Aprill CN, Derby R, Fortin J, Kine G, Bogduk N. The prevalence and clinical features of internal disc disruption in patients with chronic low back pain. Spine 1995; 20: 1878–1883.

4. Zygapophysial joint blocks

The lumbar zygapophysial joints are innervated by the medial branches of the lumbar dorsal rami [1,2]. Consequently, these joints can be anaesthetised by anaesthetising the medial branches that supply them. Complete relief of pain following such anaesthetic blocks constitutes evidence that the joints anaesthetised are the source of the patient's back pain.

Medial branch blocks are performed under fluoroscopic control. They involve introducing a needle onto each of the two nerves that innervate the target joint [3,4] (Fig. 3). Each nerve can be anaesthetised by injecting as little as 0.3 ml of local anaesthetic.

Medial branch blocks have been shown to have face validity. Local anaesthetic injected accurately onto the correct target points selectively infiltrates the target nerve, and does not anaesthetise any adjacent structures that might be an alternative source of pain to the zygapophysial joint [3]. Furthermore, medial branch blocks have been shown to protect normal volunteers from pain provoked experimentally from the anaesthetised joint [4].

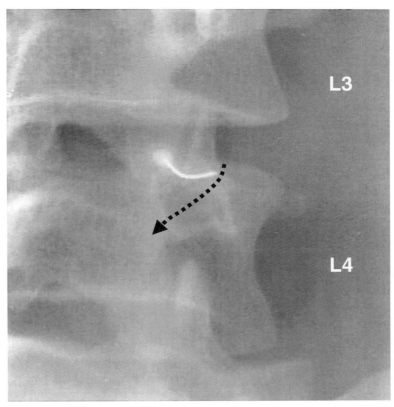

Fig. 3. A posterior oblique radiograph of a lumbar spine in which a needle has been placed onto the target point for the L3 medial branch. The dotted arrow shows the course of the nerve.

In order to have construct validity, medial branch blocks must be controlled. Single diagnostic blocks carry a false-positive rate of about 30% [5-7]. False-positive responses are reduced by performing controlled blocks in each and every patient [8]. The most convenient form of control is the use of comparative local anaesthetic blocks, in which the target nerves are anaesthetised, on separate occasions, with a different local anaesthetic agent. A positive response is one in which the patient obtains complete relief of pain on both occasions that the target joint (or joints) is blocked, but obtains long-lasting relief when a long-acting agent (e.g. bupivacaine) is used, and short-lasting relief when a short-acting agent (e.g. lignocaine) is used [8].

4.1. Diagnostic utility

Establishing a diagnosis of zygapophysial joint pain provides the patient with a valid diagnosis, and allays any concerns about the source of their pain. It also obviates the need for any further investigations in the pursuit of a diagnosis. It protects the patient from undergoing treatment that is not appropriate for zygapophysial joint pain.

Amongst older patients, the prevalence of zygapophysial joint pain is about 40% [5,6,9]. In younger, injured workers, it is only about 15% [10]. Not performing zygapophysial joint blocks prevents a diagnosis being made in this proportion of patients.

4.2. Therapeutic utility

Establishing a diagnosis of zygapophysial joint pain allows appropriate treatment to be instigated. To date, only one treatment for lumbar zygapophysial joint pain has been validated. It is discussed in Chapter 21.

References

1 Bogduk N, Wilson AS, Tynan W. The human lumbar dorsal rami. J Anat 1983; 134: 383–397.
2 Bogduk N. The innervation of the lumbar spine. Spine 1983; 8: 286–293.
3 Dreyfuss P, Schwarzer AC, Lau P, Bogduk N. Specificity of lumbar medial branch and L5 dorsal ramus blocks: a computed tomographic study. Spine 1997; 22: 895–902.
4 Kaplan M, Dreyfuss P, Halbrook B, Bogduk N. The ability of lumbar medial branch blocks to anesthetize the zygapophyseal joint. Spine 1998; 23: 1847–1852.
5 Schwarzer AC, Aprill CN, Derby R, Fortin J, Kine G, Bogduk N. The false-positive rate of uncontrolled diagnostic blocks of the lumbar zygapophyseal joints. Pain 1994; 58: 195–200.
6 Manchikanti L, Pampati V, Fellows B, Bakhit CE. Prevalence of lumbar facet joint pain in chronic low back pain. Pain Physician 1999; 2: 59–64.
7 Manchikanti L, Pampati V, Fellows B, Bakhit CE. The diagnostic validity and therapeutic value of lumbar facet joint nerve blocks with or without adjuvant agents. Curr Rev Pain 2000; 4: 337–344.
8 Bogduk N. International Spinal Injection Society guidelines for the performance of spinal injection procedures. Part 1: zygapophyseal joint blocks. Clin J Pain 1997; 13: 285–302.
9 Schwarzer AC, Aprill CN, Derby R, Fortin J, Kine G, Bogduk N. Clinical features of patients with pain stemming from the lumbar zygapophyseal joints. Is the lumbar facet syndrome a clinical entity? Spine 1994; 19: 1132–1137.
10 Schwarzer AC, Wang S, Bogduk N, McNaught PJ, Laurent R. Prevalence and clinical features of lumbar zygapophyseal joint pain: a study in an Australian population with chronic low back pain. Ann Rheum Dis 1995; 54: 100–106.

5. Sacroiliac joint blocks

The sacroiliac joint can be anaesthetised by injecting local anaesthetic into the cavity of the joint, under fluoroscopic control [1-4] (Fig. 4). Complete relief of pain following such anaesthetic blocks constitutes evidence that the joint is the source of the patient's back pain.

The face validity of sacroiliac joint blocks is established by injecting contrast medium into the joint in order to show that the needle has entered the joint cavity and that solutions that are injected do not escape from the cavity to reach other structures that might conceivably be an alternative source of pain. The construct validity of sacroiliac joint blocks is secured by performing comparative local anaesthetic blocks, as for zygapophysial joint blocks.

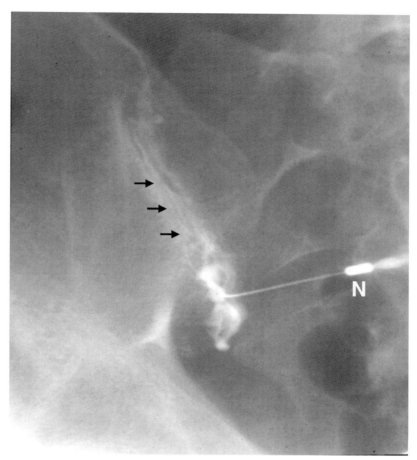

Fig. 4. An anteroposterior radiograph of a sacroiliac joint into which contrast medium has been injection in order to verify entry into the joint cavity. The arrows indicate the joint cavity. N, needle filled with contrast medium. Courteously provided by Dr. Paul Dreyfuss.

5.1. Diagnostic utility

When positive, sacroiliac joint blocks serve to establish a diagnosis of sacroiliac joint pain. Doing so curtails the futile pursuit of some other diagnosis, and protects the patient from undertaking treatment that will not relieve sacroiliac joint pain. Since the prevalence of sacroiliac joint pain is about 15% [3,4], not undertaking sacroiliac joint blocks prevents this diagnosis being determined in that proportion of patients.

5.2. Therapeutic utility

Unfortunately, at present, there is no proven treatment for sacroiliac joint pain. Consequently, sacroil-iac joint blocks do not have therapeutic utility. They do not lead to an effective treatment. However, because of their diagnostic utility, they do prevent the patient undergoing inappropriate treatment that is destined to fail because of an incorrect diagnosis.

References

1 Aprill CN. The role of anatomically specific injections into the sacroiliac joint. In: Vleeming A, Mooney V, Snijders C, Dorman T (eds) First Interdisciplinary World Congress on Low Back Pain and its Relation to the Sacroiliac Joint, San Diego, November 5–6, 1992. ECO, Rotterdam, 1992: 373–380.
2 Dreyfuss P, Michaelsen M, Pauza K, McLarty J, Bogduk N.

The value of history and physical examination in diagnosing sacroiliac joint pain. Spine 1996; 21: 2594–2602.

3   Schwarzer AC, Aprill CN, Bogduk N. The sacroiliac joint in chronic low back pain. Spine 1995; 20: 31–37.

4   Maigne JY, Aivaliklis A, Pfefer F. Results of sacroiliac joint double block and value of sacroiliac pain provocation tests in 54 patients with low-back pain. Spine 1996; 21: 1889–1892.

Medical Management of Acute and Chronic Low Back Pain. An Evidence-Based Approach
Pain Research and Clinical Management, Vol. 13
Nikolai Bogduk and Brian McGuirk

CHAPTER 20

An algorithm for precision diagnosis

1. Introduction

A risk associated with needle procedures is that they can be abused, if they are performed in an ad hoc, or arbitrary, manner. Indeed, it has been the undisciplined application of needle procedures, amongst other practices, that has concerned some critics of the reductionist approach [1]. Even if discography and diagnostic blocks are good procedures, they can be given a bad name if practitioners perform them in an undisciplined and unproductive manner.

One way of defining good practice is to establish an algorithm. An algorithm indicates to practitioners how investigations might best be applied in a responsible and efficient manner. By the same token, an algorithm serves to define, if not constrain, poor or inappropriate practice. If based on likelihoods, an algorithm promotes efficiency, by directing practitioners to the action that is more likely to be productive, and away from actions that are likely to be futile. Following an algorithm in this regard stands in stark contrast to practitioners performing procedures on the basis of whim or irresponsible habit.

2. Algorithm

The following algorithm for the investigation of chronic low back pain is based on the best available evidence on the epidemiology of various identifiable sources of chronic low back pain, and is designed to promote the efficient use of invasive investigations. It is not designed to achieve a diagnosis in each and every patient. Indeed, the algorithm contains several nodes that call either for a cessation of investigations, or for careful reconsideration of the propriety of proceeding. In this regard, the algorithm is based on the principles that:

- once an ambiguous or contradictory result has been encountered, it is wasteful of resources to venture to correct, overcome, or reverse that ambiguity by repeating procedures.
- the resources of a physician are better committed to investigating new patients who have a greater likelihood of obtaining a diagnosis than pursuing a diagnosis in patients in whom ambiguous or spurious results have been encountered.

In this regard, cardinal amongst the resources that can be so squandered are the skills and time of the physician who undertakes the investigations.

Otherwise, the algorithm is designed to provide a disciplined approach to the use of needle procedures for lumbar spinal pain, and to avoid haphazard use of the procedures. In this regard, the algorithm is predicated by the pre-test probabilities of various conditions, and invites investigation of the more common conditions first, rather than pursuing any condition arbitrarily.

2.1. Preliminary

The algorithm commences with and requires an MRI of the lumbar spine (Fig. 1). This serves two purposes. First, it provides a screening test for occult causes of back pain, such as tumours, infections, and metabolic disorders, that have not raised clinical

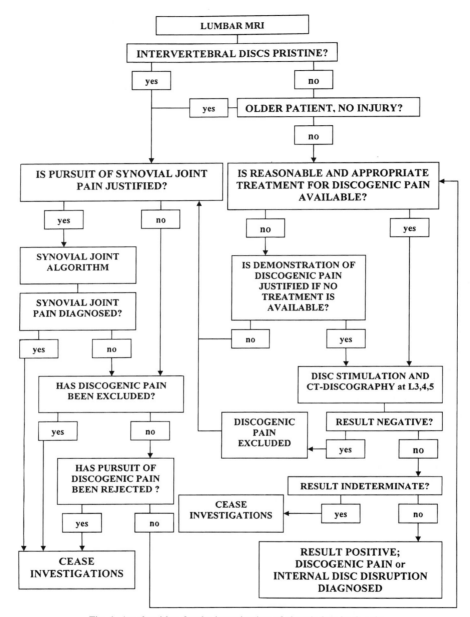

Fig. 1. An algorithm for the investigation of chronic low back pain.

red flag indicators. Because of the high sensitivity of MRI, not only will such a screening test detect these rare conditions, it will also exclude them. If the latter is the case, invasive investigations can be undertaken without fear of missing an undisclosed or unsuspected serious condition.

The second function served by an MRI is that it demonstrates whether or not the intervertebral discs are pristine, i.e. unaffected by disease or normal for age. This finding underlies, in part, a decision as to whether to direct investigations to or away from the intervertebral discs.

TABLE I

A contingency table correlating the results of MRI against the results of provocation discography as the criterion standard for a symptomatic lumbar disc

MRI	Provocation discography	
	Symptomatic	Asymptomatic
Abnormal	201	153
Normal	50	235

Based on the pooled data of Horton and Daftari [3], Osti and Fraser [4], and Simmons et al. [5]. Sensitivity = 0.80; specificity = 0.60; positive predictive value = 0.57; negative predictive value = 0.82.

Although discogenic pain can arise from discs that are normal on MRI this is uncommon [2]. If an MRI is normal, the odds are 3 : 1 against a disc being symptomatic (Table I). In the interests of efficiency, therefore, it is recommended that investigations of the disc not be undertaken in the first instance in patients with normal discs on MRI. Although this ostensibly disenfranchises those few patients who might have discogenic pain, but who have normal discs, the recommendation is critical. Without it, the absurd situation arises in which any and every patient becomes entitled to undergo provocation discography. Because of the low yield of discography in patients with normal discs, this constitutes a waste of resources. Physicians concerned about their patients with normal discs being disenfranchised, are nevertheless free to make a case for investigating the discs of these patients. For the most part, however, it is inefficient to do so.

If, on MRI, the intervertebral discs are normal, it is unlikely that the patient will have discogenic pain, but reciprocally it is more likely that they have some other source of pain. Therefore, the pre-test likelihood of pain from one or other of the synovial joints of the lumbar spine and sacrum becomes greater than base rates. Accordingly, the algorithm invites investigation of the synovial joints. If investigation of the synovial joints in due course shows that the pain does not arise from these joints, the algorithm allows a return to considering if it is worthwhile investigating the discs despite the normal MRI (Fig. 1).

A simultaneous consideration is the patient's age and history. In injured workers of younger age (35 ± 15 years), zygapophysial joint pain is uncommon, but internal disc disruption is far more common (Chapter 14). However, amongst older individuals, without a history of injury, zygapophysial joint pain is as common, or perhaps more common, than internal disc disruption. Therefore, in older patients, it may be equally efficient, or perhaps more efficient, to investigate for zygapophysial joint pain in the first instance, irrespective of the appearance of the MRI scan.

2.2. Discogenic pain

If, on MRI, one or more of the lumbar discs is abnormal, the decision to investigate should be predicated on whether or not reasonable and appropriate treatment is available, should the investigation of the discs prove positive (Fig. 1). The investigation of discogenic pain, using presently available techniques, is potentially harrowing for the patient, and carries a risk, albeit very low, of infection.

There may, however, be reasonable cause to test for a diagnosis of discogenic pain even though treatment is not available. Establishing a diagnosis of discogenic pain may prevent the futile pursuit of other diagnoses. The algorithm permits the use of discography for such purposes but calls for an active and conscious consideration of this indication (Fig. 1).

If reasonable and appropriate treatment is available, the discs should be investigated. This recommendation is based on the best available evidence which indicates that amongst patients with chronic low back pain, internal disc disruption is the single most common cause; it accounts for at least 40% of cases, and is far more prevalent than any other identifiable condition [6] amongst injured workers. In a patient with abnormal discs on MRI, internal disc disruption is the most likely diagnosis, and in the interests of efficiency should be the diagnosis first pursued. It constitutes a waste of effort and resources to undertake other investigations only to prove them negative in patients in whom those other investigations were never likely to be positive.

Disc stimulation and CT-discography is the only established means of pursuing discogenic pain. The techniques involved have been described in the literature[2], and criteria for a positive diagnosis have been established[6,7] (Chapter 19).

If the results of disc stimulation are negative, discogenic pain is excluded.

If discogenic pain is excluded, the question should be raised as to whether or not further pursuit of a diagnosis is justified. This decision relies on the judgement, inclination, or intuition of the physician involved. If further pursuit is not justified, investigations cease. Otherwise, the algorithm allows the patient to be investigated for sources of pain amongst the synovial joints of the lumbar spine and sacrum (Fig. 1).

If the results of disc stimulation are not negative, they may be indeterminate, i.e. not convincingly positive. This pertains to situations where many or all discs are positive to stimulation, or when no control disc is negative. Under these circumstances the algorithm recommends cessation of investigations (Fig. 1). The patient possibly does have discogenic pain; they may have discogenic pain at multiple levels. In that event, however, there is no valid treatment that might responsibly be prescribed. If the painful disc cannot be confidently identified, it cannot be targeted for treatment. If multiple discs are painful, there is, at present, no dependable treatment for multi-level discogenic pain. On the other hand, the patient's response may be false-positive. In that event, the indeterminate result constitutes a cue that any additional or further investigations may also be liable to false-positive results. Since there are no valid means of overcoming this possibility, the algorithm recommends cessation of investigations.

If the results of disc stimulation are neither negative nor indeterminate, by definition they will be positive. In that event a diagnosis of discogenic pain will have been made, and if the appropriate morphological features are evident on CT-discography, the diagnosis may be internal disc disruption.

2.3. Synovial joint algorithm

The algorithm for investigating the synovial joints of the lumbar spine and sacrum, commences with a set of clinical questions (Fig. 2). The first is whether or not the patient's pain is located in the very midline. The available evidence indicates that patients with this sort of back pain defy the investigations encompassed by this algorithm[8]. The yield from zygapophysial joint blocks or from disc stimulation is essentially nil. Therefore, the algorithm invites reconsideration of the propriety of pursuing investigations, and implicitly recommends that they cease.

Whether or not the pain is bilateral is an intermediate question (Fig. 2). Patients with bilateral back pain are unlikely to have bilateral sacroiliac joint pain. They are more likely to have bilateral zygapophysial joint pain. Therefore, the algorithm asks if there is good reason to believe or to credit that the patient might have bilateral sacroiliac joint pain. The expected, default answer is 'no', and the algorithm proceeds to assessment of the zygapophysial joints. Nevertheless, the algorithm does allow for consideration of bilateral sacroiliac joint pain.

The third question of the algorithm is whether or not the patient's pain is entirely caudal to the L5 level of the lumbar spine (Fig. 2). The basis for this question is that in patients proven to have sacroiliac joint pain, in all instances the pain is perceived caudal to the L5 level. Conversely, no patient with proven sacroiliac joint pain has been described who had pain extending above the L5 level[9]. Pain below L5 does not necessarily implicate the sacroiliac joint as the source[6]; but pain above L5 renders sacroiliac joint pain unlikely, and by implication, promotes the likelihood of zygapophysial joint pain. Consequently, this third question is pivotal to the efficiency of the algorithm. It is worth pursuing sacroiliac joint pain if the pain is entirely caudal to L5, but not if it extends above L5.

In the event that the patient's pain does not stem from the sacroiliac joint, that will be established at the expense of only one block. It is more efficient, therefore, to exclude the sacroiliac joint in

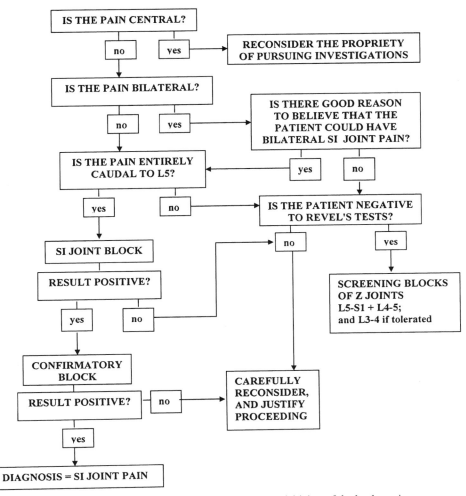

Fig. 2. An algorithm for the investigations of the synovial joints of the lumbar spine.

the first instance, than to exclude or pursue zygapophysial joint pain, for the latter may require multiple investigations.

If the patient's pain is entirely caudal to L5, a sacroiliac joint block should be undertaken.

If the block is negative, the patient is considered for zygapophysial joint blocks.

If the block is positive, a confirmatory block should be undertaken.

If the confirmatory block is positive, the diagnosis of sacroiliac joint pain is established.

If the confirmatory block is negative, a conundrum arises. Either the first block was false-positive, or the second block was false-negative. Since this conundrum cannot be resolved without multiple, repeated investigations, the algorithm recommends cessation of investigations, with the diagnosis remaining indeterminate.

Before allowing zygapophysial joint blocks the algorithm asks if the patient is negative to Revel's tests [10] (Chapter 15). These tests do not establish that the patient does, indeed, have zygapophysial joint pain, but they do increase the likelihood to a modest degree. The tests, however, are essentially negative in nature. They require the absence of certain features. If, however, any of the tests are positive, the likelihood of zygapophysial joint pain drops. Accordingly, the algorithm requires careful reconsideration of the propriety of summarily proceeding to zygapophysial joint blocks in a patient who is negative to Revel's tests. That negativity indicates that the likelihood of obtaining a positive result from blocks is low. To proceed with blocks should be justified on grounds greater than a guess or a whim.

If a patient is negative to Revel's tests, their zygapophysial joints can be investigated.

2.4. Zygapophysial joint blocks

The zygapophysial joints are entertained last in the algorithm because they are the least likely sources of chronic back pain in the working age population, with a prevalence of only about 15% [8].

A different guideline, however, applies to older patients without a history of injury. In these patients, because the pre-test likelihood of zygapophysial joint may be 40% or higher [11,12], zygapophysial joint blocks become a prime investigation, ahead of disc stimulation, and possibly ahead of sacroiliac joint blocks.

The low prevalence of lumbar zygapophysial joint pain predicates the design of the algorithm. Because zygapophysial joint pain may arise from any of a number of segmental levels, multiple investigations may be required to detect a symptomatic joint. However, the low prevalence of this condition means that the majority of such investigations will be negative and fruitless. It, therefore, becomes inefficient to pursue zygapophysial joint pain, one joint at a time, only to exclude all joints in the majority of cases. For this reason, the algorithm recommends a multi-level screening test (Fig. 3).

The virtue of a screening test is its negative predictive value. If the likelihood is that the majority of patients will not have zygapophysial joint pain, it

is efficient to establish this expeditiously. Not only are resources conserved, but the patient does not need to suffer repeated invasive tests in vain.

At a single sitting, both joints at L4–L5 and L5–S1, bilaterally if indicated, can be anaesthetised. If the patient can tolerate the additional steps required, the L3–L4 joints can be added.

If the result of this screening test is negative, zygapophysial joint pain will have been excluded, and investigations can cease.

If the result of the screening test is positive, zygapophysial joint pain is implied, but its exact source is not evident. That requires anaesthetising joints one at a time.

The algorithm recommends commencing arbitrarily at L5–S1 in order to pinpoint the exact joint that is the source of pain (Fig. 3). This segmental level is an appropriate starting point because it is one of the two levels most commonly found to be symptomatic [8,11]; and starting at L5–S1 predicates a systematic ascent of investigations, if required, from the lowest to higher levels in the lumbar spine.

If blocks of L5–S1 are negative, the L4–L5 joint should be considered and blocked, for this is the next, most commonly symptomatic joint.

If L4–L5 blocks are negative, the question is posed whether or not it is reasonable to suspect or to test L3–L4. The basis for this question is that L3–L4 is an uncommon source of pain [8]. The physician should, therefore, have good cause to suspect this joint, lest they perform investigations that in the majority of cases simply prove that it is not painful.

If at any time a block is positive, it should be followed by a confirmatory block.

If that confirmatory block is negative, investigations should cease. A negative response raises a conundrum. Either the first block was false-positive, or the second block was false-negative. Since this conundrum cannot be resolved without undertaking multiple further blocks, the algorithm recommends cessation of blocks, with the diagnosis remaining indeterminate.

If the confirmatory block is positive, a diagnosis of zygapophysial joint pain is established.

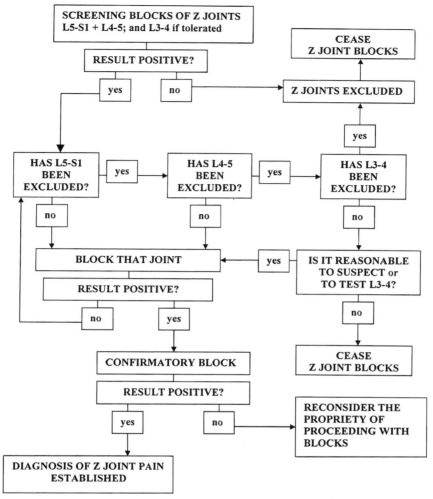

Fig. 3. An algorithm for the investigation of the lumbar zygapophysial joints.

If, at any time, a block of a single joint or of both joints at a single segment is partially positive, in that it provides complete relief of pain but only in part of the patient's region of pain, yet the patient responded to multi-level screening blocks, the response indicates zygapophysial joint pain at multiple levels. In that event, the next most likely joint should be blocked, in an effort to relieve that part of the patient's pain that was not relieved by the previous, single-level block.

If the response to the block of the second level is negative, the patient's responses to blocks should be carefully reconsidered, for their responses to screening blocks are not concordant with their responses to blocks at single levels. Their response to screening blocks may have been false-positive.

If the response to the block of the second level is positive, in that it relieves that part of the patient's pain that was not relieved by the first block, a diagnosis can be entertained prima facie that the patient has two-level zygapophysial joint pain. That diagnosis can then be confirmed with a control block in which both symptomatic levels are simultaneously anaesthetised, so as to reproduce and confirm the effect of the original screening block.

If the response to the control block is positive, the diagnosis of two-level pain is confirmed.

If the response to the control block is negative, the patient's responses to blocks should be carefully reconsidered, for their responses to blocks are inconsistent with two-level pain. Their responses to blocks may have been false-positive.

2.5. Efficiency

Under the operation of this algorithm, discogenic pain is excluded or confirmed within one step. Sacroiliac joint pain is excluded within one block, or confirmed within two blocks.

In patients in whom sacroiliac joint pain is not suspected, zygapophysial joint pain is excluded within one step — a screening block, or diagnosed within four steps: one screening block that is positive; one or two blocks at single levels to pinpoint the responsible joint; and one confirmatory block.

In patients in whom sacroiliac joint has been entertained but excluded, zygapophysial joint pain is excluded within two steps: the negative sacroiliac block, and the negative screening block for zygapophysial joint pain. Zygapophysial joint pain is established within a total of five steps: one to exclude sacroiliac joint pain, one screening block to implicate zygapophysial joint pain, one or two blocks to pinpoint the responsible joint; and one to confirm the response.

Given the pre-test probabilities that:

- internal disc disruption accounts for 40% of cases of chronic low back pain;
- sacroiliac joint pain accounts for 15% of cases; and
- zygapophysial joint pain accounts for 15%;

most patients under the algorithm would undergo investigations of their discs, with 40% proving positive and requiring no other investigations. Of the 60% remaining, not all will require sacroiliac joint blocks, but perhaps half will prove positive, and will not require zygapophysial joint blocks. Zygapophysial joint blocks will therefore be indicated in perhaps

only 30% of the original population. Perhaps half of these will prove negative on screening blocks. Only the remaining half should be subjected to multiple tests of the zygapophysial joints.

Accordingly,

- in about 30% of cases, sacroiliac joint pain will be diagnosed within one block plus a confirmatory block;
- in about 15% of cases, investigations will exclude sacroiliac joint pain and zygapophysial joint pain within two blocks;
- only 15% of cases may require up to four or five blocks to pinpoint a painful zygapophysial joint.

References

1 Loeser JD. Mitigating the dangers of pursuing care. In: Pain Treatment Centres at a Crossroads: A Practical ad Conceptual Reappraisal, Progress in Pain Management, Vol 7. IASP Press, Seattle, WA, 1996, pp 101–108.

2 Bogduk N, Aprill C, Derby R. Discography. In: White AH (ed) Spine Care, Volume One: Diagnosis and Conservative Treatment. Mosby, St Louis, 1995, pp 219–238.

3 Horton WC, Daftari TK. Which disc as visualized by magnetic resonance imaging is actually a source of pain? A correlation between magnetic resonance imaging and discography. Spine 1992; 17: S164–S171.

4 Osti OL, Fraser RD. MRI and discography of annular tears and intervertebral disc degeneration: a prospective clinical comparison. J Bone Joint Surg 1992; 74B: 431–435.

5 Simmons JW, Emery SF, McMillin JN, Landa D, Kimmich SJ. Awake discography: a comparison study with magnetic resonance imaging. Spine 1991; 16: S216–S221.

6 Schwarzer AC, Aprill CN, Derby R, Fortin J, Kine G, Bogduk N. The prevalence and clinical features of internal disc disruption in patients with chronic low back pain. Spine 1995; 20: 1878–1883.

7 Merskey H, Bogduk N (eds). Classification of Chronic Pain. Descriptions of Chronic Pain Syndromes and Definition of Pain Terms, 2nd edn. IASP Press, Seattle, WA, 1994.

8 Schwarzer AC, Aprill CN, Derby R, Fortin J, Kine G, Bogduk N. Clinical features of patients with pain stemming from the lumbar zygapophysial joints. Is the lumbar facet syndrome a clinical entity? Spine 1994; 19: 1132–1137.

9 Dreyfuss P, Michaelsen M, Pauza K, McLarty J, Bogduk N. The value of history and physical examination in diagnosing sacroiliac joint pain. Spine 1996; 21: 2594–2602.

10 Revel M, Poiraudeau S, Auleley GR, Payan C, Denke A, Nguyen M, Chevrot A, Fermanian J. Capacity of the

clinical picture to characterize low back pain relieved by facet joint anesthesia. Proposed criteria to identify patients with painful facet joints. Spine 1998; 23: 1972–1977.

11 Schwarzer AC, Wang S, Bogduk N, McNaught PJ, Laurent R. Prevalence and clinical features of lumbar zygapophysial joint pain: a study in an Australian population with chronic low back pain. Ann Rheum Dis 1995; 54: 100–106.

12 Manchikanti L, Pampati V, Fellows B, Bakhit CE. Prevalence of lumbar facet joint pain in chronic low back pain. Pain Physician 1999; 2: 59–64.

Medical Management of Acute and Chronic Low Back Pain. An Evidence-Based Approach
Pain Research and Clinical Management, Vol. 13
Nikolai Bogduk and Brian McGuirk
© *2002 Elsevier Science B.V. All rights reserved*

CHAPTER 21

Precision treatment

1. Introduction

If the algorithm for precision diagnosis is followed (Chapter 20), one of four endpoints will be reached.

(1) No diagnosis is established.
(2) A diagnosis is established of sacroiliac joint pain.
(3) Zygapophysial joint pain is diagnosed.
(4) Discogenic pain or internal disc disruption is diagnosed.

If no diagnosis is established, treatment will not be possible of a particular lesion or a particular source of pain. In that event, the only options for management are multidisciplinary therapy (Chapter 18) or one of the better monotherapies (Chapter 17).

If a diagnosis of sacroiliac joint pain is established, no treatment specific for this condition can be recommended, for none has been validated.

Some orthopaedic surgeons offer arthrodesis of the joint as a means of relieving the pain, but there are no data from controlled trials to show that arthrodesis is effective. Nor are there any compelling observational data to this effect.

Some pain specialists offer radiofrequency denervation of the joint; but likewise, no controlled studies have shown this to be effective. One observational study reported only a modest success rate: 32% of patients obtaining greater than 50% reduction of pain for 6 months[1]. Variations in the course of the nerves that innervate the joint prevent these nerves from being accurately and consistently targeted either for diagnostic blocks or percutaneous denervation procedures[2,3].

Some investigators have shown in controlled trials that various forms of manipulation, coupled with various forms of injection therapy, does relieve pain in patients diagnosed as having sacroiliac joint pain[4–9]. However, the diagnosis was made using clinical tests, not by controlled, precision diagnostic blocks. Evidence from other studies indicates that the clinical diagnosis of sacroiliac joint pain is not valid (Chapter 15). Therefore, although the results of these studies of manual therapy and injection can be taken as evidence of efficacy for the treatment of low back pain, they do not constitute evidence that manual therapy is effective explicitly for sacroiliac joint pain. No studies have yet assessed any form of conservative therapy for sacroiliac joint pain diagnosed by controlled blocks of the joint.

For the two other endpoints of the algorithm for precision diagnosis, specific options for treatment are available. Each is associated with some degree of evidence of efficacy.

References

1 Ferrante FM, King LF, Roche EA, Kim PS, Aranda M, De-Laney LR, Mardini IA, Mannes AJ. Radiofrequency sacroiliac joint denervation for sacroiliac syndrome. Reg Anesth Pain Med 2001; 26: 137–142.
2 Dreyfuss P, Akuthota V, Willard F, Carreiro J, Yin W, Bogduk N. Are lateral branch blocks of the S1–3 dorsal rami reasonably target specific? Proceedings of the 8th Annual Scientific Meeting of the International Spinal Injection Society, San Francisco, September 8–10, 2000. International Spinal Injection Society, San Francisco, 2000, p 25–29.
3 Dreyfuss P, Park K, Bogduk N. Do L5 dorsal ramus and S1–4 lateral branch blocks protect the sacroiliac joint from an

experimental pain stimulus? A randomized, double-blinded controlled trial. Proceedings of the 8th Annual Scientific Meeting of the International Spinal Injection Society, San Francisco, September 8–10, 2000, pp 31–36.

4   Blomberg S, Svardsudd K, Mildenberger F. A controlled, multicentre trial of manual therapy in low-back pain; initial status, sick-leave and pain score during follow-up. Scand J Prim Health Care 1992; 10: 170–178.

5   Blomberg S, Svardsudd K, Tibblin G. Manual therapy with steroid injections in low-back pain: improvement of quality of life in a controlled trial with four months' follow-up. Scand J Prim Health Care 1993; 11: 83–90.

6   Blomberg S, Tibbin G. A controlled, multicentre trial of manual therapy with steroid injections in low-back pain: functional variable, side-effects and complications during four months follow-up. Clin Rehabil 1993; 7: 49–62.

7   Blomberg S, Hallin G, Grann K, Berg E, Sennerby U. Manual therapy with steroid injections — a new approach to treatment of low back pain: a controlled multicenter trial with an evaluation by orthopedic surgeons. Spine 1994; 19: 569–577.

8   Blomberg S, Svardsudd K, Tibbin G. A randomised study of manual therapy with steroid injections in low-back pain: telephone interview follow-up of pain, disability, recovery and drug consumption. Eur Spine J 1994; 3: 246–254.

9   Ongley MJ, Klein RG, Dorman TA, Eek BC, Hubert LJ. A new approach to the treatment of chronic low back pain. Lancet 1987; 2: 143–146.

2. Zygapophysial joint pain

Three forms of treatment have been devised and promoted for pain stemming from the lumbar zygapophysial joints. Each has been subjected to controlled trials and other studies to assess its efficacy.

2.1. Intra-articular steroids

Intra-articular injection of corticosteroids is an attractive treatment for pain shown to be stemming from a lumbar zygapophysial joint. It is target-specific and easy to perform by trained individuals equipped with a fluoroscope. Several observational studies claimed success for this treatment[1–4], but controlled trials have questioned its efficacy.

One study[5] is often touted as evidence against intra-articular steroids for lumbar zygapophysial joint pain. However, this study[5] was not an appropriate test of the paradigm of zygapophysial joint pain. The patients enrolled in the study were, indeed, randomized to receive either intra-articular steroids or a control injection, but they were not previously diagnosed as having zygapophysial joint pain. Diagnostic blocks were not performed before treatment. The trial, therefore, shows only that indiscriminant injection of steroids without making a precision diagnosis does not work.

The best available study of intra-articular steroids for lumbar zygapophysial joint pain is that of Carette et al.[6]. In this study, patients were selected on the basis of diagnostic, intra-articular blocks of the lumbar zygapophysial joints, and only patients whose pain was relieved by such blocks were enrolled. The trial subsequently showed that the injection of steroids conferred no greater benefit than the injection of normal saline.

The one criticism of this study that protagonists of intra-articular steroids have raised is that the selection criteria used lacked specificity. Carette et al.[6] enrolled patients who had at least 50% relief of their back pain after a single diagnostic block of a lumbar zygapophysial joint. They did not use controlled blocks, and did not require complete relief of pain as the diagnostic criterion. Some, if not many, of their patients, therefore, may not actually have had zygapophysial joint pain. Protagonists of intra-articular steroids have not responded by repeating the study in a sample of patients with rigorously diagnosed lumbar zygapophysial joint pain. Unless and until such a study reveals efficacy, the study of Carette et al.[6] continues to cast a shadow of doubt over this intervention.

2.2. Medial branch blocks

Lumbar medial branch blocks were designed as a diagnostic procedure, and that remains their primary utility (Chapter 19). They were not designed as a therapeutic intervention. Local anaesthetic agents have a duration of effect that lasts no more than several hours. Consequently, any pain relief following medial branch blocks should cease as the effects of the local anaesthetic agent used wear off.

However, some investigators have adopted the technique of medial branch blocks for a therapeutic procedure. Instead of using local anaesthetic agents, they have added other agents designed to prolong the analgesic effect. One such agent is Sarapin (High Chemical, Levittown, PA), which is an extract of the pitcher plant (*Sarracenia purpurin*) in an alkaline solution. This agent is claimed to suppress C-fibre activity without causing motor weakness when injected onto a peripheral nerve[7].

An observational study[7] assessed the effectiveness of injections of Sarapin mixed with lignocaine in a series of 32 patients diagnosed as having lumbar zygapophysial joint pain on the basis of comparative local anaesthetic blocks. A parallel series of 41 patients, similarly diagnosed, was treated with injections of Sarapin mixed with local anaesthetic and methylprednisolone. Significant relief was defined as greater than 50% relief of pain. In both groups, significant relief lasted for a mean period of 6 weeks after one injection and up to 12 weeks each after a second or third injection. Some 80% of patients maintained significant relief for 4–6 months after a total of one to three injections. The authors argued that repeated injections could extend the duration of relief, and that doing so was cost-effective in comparison with other interventions for lumbar zygapophysial joint pain.

These data are not evidence that Sarapin is effective for lumbar zygapophysial joint pain, for it was not compared with either a placebo or a competitive treatment. However, they do raise the intriguing possibility that Sarapin could be a more expedient alternative to other means of treating lumbar zygapophysial joint pain. A randomised, controlled trial is needed to test this possibility.

2.3. Radiofrequency neurotomy

Radiofrequency (RF) lumbar medial branch neurotomy is a procedure in which the nerves that innervate a painful zygapophysial joint are coagulated in order to stop the perception of pain. The nerves are coagulated using electrodes inserted percutaneously, under fluoroscopic control, onto the target nerves. In essence, the procedure reproduces the relief obtained by blocking these nerves with local

anaesthetic agents during the conduct of diagnostic blocks, but the ensuing relief lasts longer because the nerves are coagulated, not just anaesthetised.

RF neurotomy has had a chequered history (see Bogduk et al.[8] for a comprehensive review). Early versions of the procedure, then known as 'facet denervation', used inaccurate target points, such that the medial branches of the dorsal rami could not have been coagulated[9,10]. Yet this did not prevent outstanding results being claimed for the procedure, in observational studies[8]. Furthermore, 13 years after the introduction of the procedure, it was found to be technically flawed. The original approach required electrodes to be introduced perpendicular to the target nerve, in the same manner as needles used to inject local anaesthetic onto the nerve. Laboratory studies[11] showed that this was inappropriate because the electrodes did not coagulate tissues distal to their tip; they coagulated circumferentially to the shaft of the electrode. Accordingly, in order to coagulate the nerves, the electrodes must be placed parallel to the target nerve (Fig. 1).

It took 26 years from when facet denervation was first introduced for the first controlled study of medial branch neurotomy to be conducted and published. That study[12] clearly showed that RF neurotomy was not a placebo. Patients who were treated with a sham lesion did not obtain pain-relief. Relief occurred only in patients who were treated with an active lesion. However, while this study did show that RF neurotomy was not a placebo, it did not demonstrate the true efficacy of medial branch neurotomy. The follow-up period was only short, and although patients benefited from the active procedure, the magnitude of relief was not great (barely a three-point improvement on a 10-point visual analogue scale). This limited effect could be attributed to suboptimal placement of the electrodes. Instead of being placed parallel to the target nerve, they were placed semi-orthogonally. This difference compromises how thoroughly the nerve can be coagulated.

A subsequent study[13] demonstrated the effectiveness of lumbar medial branch neurotomy. Fifteen patients were carefully screened, and diagnosed as having lumbar zygapophysial joint pain, using

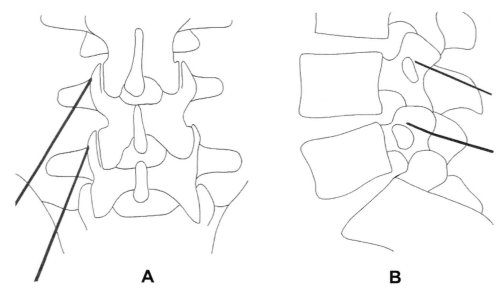

Fig. 1. Tracings of radiographs showing the placement of electrodes parallel to the medial branches of the L3 and L4 dorsal rami, for the conduct of RF neurotomy. (A) Posterior view. (B) Lateral view.

double local anaesthetic blocks. All obtained complete relief of their pain following these blocks. The painful joints were denervated by RF neurotomy, in which the electrodes were correctly placed parallel to the target nerves. Post-operative electromyography demonstrated that the nerves had indeed been fully coagulated. Patients were followed for 12 months after treatment. All showed major and sustained improvements in their pain (Table I), complemented by improvements in physical functioning [13].

This study does not constitute evidence of efficacy for lumbar medial branch neurotomy in general; nor does it vindicate how lumbar medial branch neurotomy is commonly practised. The study treated only patients who satisfied rigorous diagnostic criteria, which included complete relief of pain following each of two diagnostic medial branch blocks, and the absence of any co-morbidity. It used a meticulous surgical technique. Some practitioners do not abide by these standards. They allow less than complete relief of pain as the diagnostic criterion, and use variants of the procedure that have not been validated, such as not placing the electrodes parallel to the target nerves. There are no data to suggest that these variants are equally successful, and every reason to

TABLE I

The numbers, cumulative numbers, and proportion of patients, who, at 12 months after treatment with radiofrequency lumbar medial branch neurotomy, obtained the percentage improvements indicated in their visual analogue pain scores [13]

Change in VAS (%)	Number	Cumulative numbers	Cumulative proportion
100	5	5	0.30
90	2	7	0.47
80	2	9	0.60
70	2	11	0.73
60	1	12	0.80
50	1	13	0.87
40	0	13	0.87
30	0	13	0.87
20	1	14	0.93
10	0	14	0.93
0	1	15	1.00

believe that they are not. Nevertheless, the study of Dreyfuss et al. [13] sets a benchmark. In essence, at 12 months, some 60% of patients can expect to have at least 80% relief of their pain, and 80% of patients can expect more than 60% relief. This benchmark becomes critical when assessing other studies.

A recent, randomised, placebo-controlled study [14] has been heralded as evidence against the efficacy of RF neurotomy [15]. That study found no difference in outcome at 12 weeks after treatment between patients treated with active neurotomy and sham neurotomy. However, two factors confound this study.

The inclusion criteria were "significant relief of their low back pain. . . after intra-articular facet injections" [14]. Medial branch blocks were not used, and controlled blocks were not used. Consequently, readers cannot be certain that the patients enrolled actually had zygapophysial joint pain.

Perhaps more significantly, none of the patients who had active neurotomy obtained any clinically significant degree of relief, at either 4 or 12 weeks after treatment. At these times, the patients achieved only a 4% reduction and a 0.5% worsening of pain, respectively. This degree of improvement is not even remotely close to the benchmark established by Dreyfuss et al. [13], and effectively constitutes no

response. Indeed, at 12 weeks, the active group achieved less relief than the placebo group. This lack of effect indicates either that the patients did not have zygapophysial joint pain, or that the technique used by the investigators was inaccurate and ineffective. If the former obtains, then the study is not a proper test of treatment for zygapophysial joint pain. If the latter obtains, the study compared one sham therapy with another. In either case, the data are not evidence against the efficacy of RF neurotomy.

If performed meticulously in properly diagnosed patients, RF neurotomy can be a powerful therapeutic tool. Unlike monotherapies (Chapter 17) or multidisciplinary treatment (Chapter 18), RF neurotomy can provide complete or substantial relief of pain stemming from the lumbar zygapophysial joints. It is one of the few treatments for chronic low back pain that can produce sustained and major relief.

Key point

- For patients with lumbar zygapophysial joint pain, diagnosed by controlled medial branch blocks, lumbar radiofrequency medial branch neurotomy offers a good chance of obtaining worthwhile relief of pain, sustained for at least 12 months.

References

1   Lippit AB. The facet joint and its role in spine pain: management with facet joint injections. Spine 1984; 9: 746–750.

2   Lau LSW, Littlejohn GO, Miller MH. Clinical evaluation of intra-articular injections for lumbar facet joint pain. Med J Aust 1985; 143: 563–565.

3   Lynch MC, Taylor JF. Facet joint injection for low back pain. J Bone Joint Surg 1986; 68B: 138–141.

4   Murtagh FR. Computed tomography and fluoroscopy guided anaesthesia and steroid injection in facet syndrome. Spine 1988; 13: 686–689.

5   Lilius G, Laasonen EM, Myllynen P, Harilainen A, Gronlund G. Lumbar facet joint syndrome: a randomised clinical trial. J Bone Joint Surg 1989; 71B: 681–684.

6   Carette S, Marcoux S, Truchon R, Grondin, Gagnon J, Allard Y, Latulippe M. A controlled trial of corticosteroid injections into facet joints for chronic low back pain. New Engl J Med 1991; 325: 1002–1007.

7   Manchikanti L, Pampati V, Bakhit CE, Rivera JJ, Beyer CD, Damron KS, Barnhill RC. Effectiveness of lumbar facet joint nerve blocks in chronic low back pain: a randomized clinical trial. Pain Physician 2001; 4: 101–117.

8   Bogduk N, Aprill C, Derby R. Diagnostic blocks of synovial joints. In: White AH (ed) Spine Care, Vol 1: Diagnosis and Conservative Treatment. Mosby, St Louis, 1995: pp 298–321.

9   Bogduk N, Long DM. The anatomy of the so-called 'articular nerves' and their relationship to facet denervation in the treatment of low back pain. J Neurosurg 1979; 51: 172–177.

10   Bogduk N, Long DM. Percutaneous lumbar medial branch neurotomy. A modification of facet denervation. Spine 1980; 5: 193–200.

11   Bogduk N, Macintosh JE, Marsland A. A technical cause for clinical failure with percutaneous radiofrequency peripheral neurotomy. Neurosurgery 1987; 20: 529–535.

TABLE II

Criteria for successful outcome and success rates from observational studies of anterior interbody fusion for proven discogenic pain

Source	n	Duration of follow-up (months)	Criteria for successful outcome			Success rate (%)
			>75% Relief of pain	Return to work or normal ADLs	No opioid medication	
Lee et al.[4]	62	>18	+	+	+	87
Blumenthal et al.[5]	34	29[a]		+	+	74
Kozak and O'Brien[6]	69	>19	+	+	+	74
Gill and Blumenthal[7]	53	>24	+	+	+	66
Loguidice et al.[8]	85	>15		+		61
Knox and Chapman[9]	22	ns	+	+		35

n, number of patients studied; ns, not stated; ADLs, activities of daily living.
[a] Average, range not provided.

12   van Kleef M, Barendse GAM, Kessels A, Voets HM, Weber WEJ, de Lange S. Randomized trial of radiofrequency lumbar facet denervation for chronic low back pain. Spine 1999; 24: 1937–1942.

13   Dreyfuss P, Halbrook B, Pauza K, Joshi A, McLarty J, Bogduk N. Efficacy and validity of radiofrequency neurotomy for chronic lumbar zygapophysial joint pain. Spine 2000; 25: 1270–1277.

14   Leclaire R, Fortin L, Lambert R, Bergeron YM, Rossignol M. Radiofrequency facet joint denervation in the treatment of low back pain. A placebo-controlled clinical trial to assess efficacy. Spine 2001; 26: 1411–1416.

15   Deyo RA. Point of view. Spine 2001; 26: 1417.

3. Discogenic pain

The diagnostic criteria for lumbar discogenic pain are reproduction of the patient's pain by provocation discography, provided that stimulation of adjacent (control) discs does not produce pain (Chapter 19). There have been no studies of any conservative therapy explicitly for patients who have been shown to have this condition. The only treatment regarded as specific for discogenic pain is arthrodesis.

For various reasons, fusion has not been subjected to randomised, placebo-controlled trials. Not only is it difficult to blind patients as to whether they have surgery or not, the ethics of performing sham surgery as a placebo are questionable. The data on the efficacy of fusion for diagnosed discogenic pain, therefore, stems only from observational studies.

Only a few studies have described outcomes in patients shown to have discogenic pain. Some have assessed the efficacy of various forms of posterior or posterolateral fusion. Others have assessed anterior interbody fusion.

The results of posterolateral fusion for proven discogenic pain are not impressive. One study reported that only 39% of patients obtained a good or excellent result, at between two and four years after surgery[1]. Another reported only 46% of patients achieving a satisfactory outcome[2].

Better outcomes have been reported for discogenic pain treated with anterior interbody fusion (Table II). In the best-reported studies, the criteria for success included some combination of 'greater than 75% relief of pain', 'return to work' or 'resumption of normal activities of daily living', and cessation of the use of opioids for back pain. Other studies that have claimed that anterior interbody fusion is effective did not report data on each of these variables[3].

The majority of studies attest to at least 60% of patients achieving a successful outcome, at times greater than 15 months after treatment. Only one study[9] reported a success rate as low as 35%.

The literature on anterior fusion for discogenic pain should not be confused with the literature on fusion for back pain in general. The general literature describes the treatment of patients with a variety of diagnoses, such as degenerative disc disease, segmental instability, and spondylolisthesis, none of which is a valid diagnosis of low back pain (Chapter 14). Indeed, it would seem that such invalid diagnoses are still the most common indication for lumbar fusion [10].

The literature on anterior fusion for discogenic pain deals with the treatment of a specific condition, and has used more stringent outcome measures than the general literature. Even so, it reports better outcomes. This suggests that making a specific diagnosis makes a difference to outcome.

Purists, of course, would demand controlled trials to assess properly the efficacy of anterior fusion. However, such trials are unlikely to be forthcoming. Placebo-controlled studies of surgical treatment are just too difficult to mount. At best, one might expect a trial comparing fusion with some form of conservative therapy. Observational data, therefore, will remain the principal basis for judging the efficacy of anterior fusion for proven lumbar discogenic pain.

Key point

- If discogenic pain is properly diagnosed, the available literature would suggest that anterior fusion is a possible, therapeutic option. Patients could expect greater than a 60% chance of achieving 75% relief of their pain, associated with restoration of normal activities, and no further need for opioids.

References

1. Parker LM, Murrell SE, Boden SD, Horton WC. The outcome of posterolateral fusion in highly selected patients with discogenic low back pain. Spine 1996; 21: 1909–1917.
2. Wetzel FT, La Rocca SH, Lowery GL, Aprill CN. The treatment of lumbar spinal pain syndromes diagnosed by discography: lumbar arthrodesis. Spine 1994; 19: 792–800.
3. Penta M, Fraser RD. Anterior lumbar interbody fusion: a minimum 10-year follow-up. Spine 1997; 22: 2429–2434.
4. Lee CK, Vessa P, Lee JK. Chronic disabling low back pain syndrome cause by internal disc derangements. The results of disc excision and posterior lumbar interbody fusion. Spine 1995; 20: 356–361.
5. Blumenthal SL, Baker J, Dossett A, Selby D. The role of anterior lumbar fusion for internal disc disruption. Spine 1988; 13: 566–569.
6. Kozak JA, O'Brien JP. Simultaneous combined anterior and posterior fusion. An independent analysis of a treatment for the disabled low-back pain patient. Spine 1990; 15: 322–328.
7. Gill K, Blumenthal SL. Functional results after anterior lumbar fusion at L5–S1 in patients with normal and abnormal MRI scans. Spine 1992; 17: 940–942.
8. Loguidice VA, Johnson RG, Guyer RD, Stith WJ, Ohnmeiss DD, Hochschuller SH, Rashbaum RF. Anterior lumbar interbody fusion. Spine 1988; 13: 365–369.
9. Knox BD, Chapman TM. Anterior lumbar interbody fusion for discogram concordant pain. J Spinal Dis 1993; 6: 242–244.
10. DeBerard MS, Masters KS, Colledge AL, Schleusener RL, Schlegel JD. Outcomes of posterolateral lumbar fusion in Utah patients receiving worker' compensation: a retrospective cohort study. Spine 2001; 26: 738–747.

4. Internal disc disruption

Internal disc disruption is a more specific diagnosis than discogenic pain. In addition to the criteria for discogenic pain, internal disc disruption requires the demonstration of a radial fissure on CT-discography. Few studies have explicitly addressed the treatment of this condition. Although the studies of discogenic pain (outlined above) may well have included patients with internal disc disruption, those studies did not technically satisfy the criteria for internal disc disruption. They used discography, but did not include CT-discography.

The one study [1] of internal disc disruption that reported outcomes in detail, compared various forms of arthrodesis for this condition. It defined 'satisfactory result' as no pain or mild pain, with no use of medication or only occasional NSAIDs, and working with no restriction or only minimal restriction. It also reported the proportion of patients previously not working who returned to work. For the vari-

TABLE III

Outcomes after 2 years' follow-up of patients with internal disc disruption treated by various forms of fusion [1]

Type of fusion	n	Satisfactory result (%)	Return to work (%)
Posterolateral with facet screws	16	38	31
Posterolateral with pedicle screws	13	46	38
Anterior interbody	11	36	31
Anterior interbody with BAK cage and facet fusion	16	63	38

ous forms of arthrodesis, the outcomes were slightly different (Table III).

Although the outcomes appear to be better for anterior interbody fusion with BAK cage and facet fusion (Table III), the success rate of 63% is not significantly different statistically from the other success rates. Overall, these data indicate only a modest, if not marginal, success rate for fusion for the treatment of internal disc disruption.

Surgeons might respond that the literature specifically on discogenic pain overrides this one study of internal disc disruption. Furthermore, the small numbers of patients in the latter study, preclude drawing too strong a conclusion about what the representative success rate is of fusion for internal disc disruption. However, there are no other data on the success of fusion for patients explicitly diagnosed as having internal disc disruption.

Key point

- The limited data on surgical fusion for proven internal disc disruption do not paint a compelling picture of its efficacy.

References

1 Vamvanij V, Fredrickson BE, Thorpe JM, Stadnick ME, Yuan HA. Surgical treatment of internal disc disruption: an outcome study of four fusion techniques. J Spinal Dis 1998; 11: 375–382.

5. Intradiscal electrothermal anuloplasty

Arthrodesis is not a panacea for discogenic pain or for internal disc disruption. Although some reported success rates might seem attractive, a substantial proportion of patients do not benefit from this invasive and irreversible form of intervention. Meanwhile, no form of conservative therapy has been shown to be effective for proven discogenic pain or for internal disc disruption. This state of affairs has prompted investigators to develop and evaluate new, less invasive, and less destructive means of treating these conditions.

One such development has been intradiscal electrothermal anuloplasty (IDET). This procedure involves the insertion, under fluoroscopic control, of a flexible electrode into the painful disc. The electrode is maneuvered so as to pass circumferentially around the anulus fibrosus from one posterolateral sector, across the posterior sector, to the opposite posterolateral sector (Fig. 2). Once the electrode is properly placed, it is heated to 90°C. Heating the electrode putatively denatures the collagen of the anulus, seals the radial fissure and any circumferential fissure, and destroys the nerve endings in the anulus.

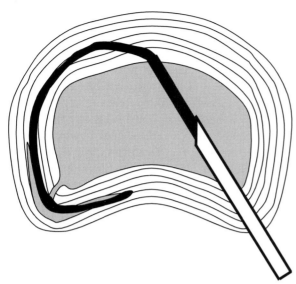

Fig. 2. A sketch of an axial view of an electrode inserted into a disc with internal disc disruption, for the conduct of intradiscal electrothermal anuloplasty.

5.1. Discogenic pain

Several observational studies have described the efficacy of IDET [1–3]. In all, the indication for treatment was discogenic pain, diagnosed by discography. CT-discography was not used to establish a diagnosis of internal disc disruption. In one study [1], the criteria for discogenic pain (Chapter 19) were not satisfied. The only criterion used was that the patient's pain was reproduced by provocation discography. Absence of pain from adjacent discs was not a stipulated criterion. In the other two studies [2,3], asymptomatic controls were required, and one of these studies [2] required the additional criterion of pain reproduction at less than 15 psi injection pressure (Chapter 19).

The smallest of these studies ($n = 23$), and the one with the shortest follow-up (6 months) [1], reported a decrease in the mean visual analogue scale (VAS) for pain from 6.2 to 3.9, on a 10-point scale. The other two studies followed patients for at least 12 months. The smaller studied 32 patients and reported a mean decrease in VAS of 1.84, and a mean improvement of 4 on the Roland–Morris Disability Questionnaire [2]. The larger studied 62 patients and

reported a decrease in VAS from 6.6 to 3.7; an improvement in physical functioning on the SF-36 from 39 to 59; and a return to work rate of 95% [3].

As presented, the data from these studies hint at a modest efficacy of IDET for discogenic pain. They attest to a reduction of mean pain scores, but they do not stipulate what proportion of patients was totally relieved of their pain. The standard deviations published suggest that some patients achieved major degrees of relief, not reflected by the mean change or mean scores, while others did not benefit.

5.2. Internal disc disruption

For the treatment of internal disc disruption, diagnosed by provocation discography and CT-discography (Chapter 19), there has been one controlled study [4]. This study used a convenience sample of 17 patients whose insurer denied treatment with IDET and who were treated by a standard rehabilitation program. Thirty-six other patients were treated with IDET.

At 3 months after treatment, only one of the control patients showed any clinical significant improvement in pain, and the median pain score of the group did not improve. In the IDET group, four patients obtained no relief, but the remainder achieved various degrees of relief. As a group, these patients improved their pain scores from a median of 8 to a median of 4 at 3 months.

The patients treated with IDET were followed for 12 months. At that time, 13 patients had not benefited from the procedure but the remainder achieved one of three grades of success. Of these patients, 14% achieved at least 50% reduction of their pain to a level of 3 or 4 on a 10-point VAS, and were working. Another 23% achieved at least 50% reduction of their pain to a level of 1 or 2 on the VAS, and were working. A further 23% achieved complete relief of their pain and were working. Table IV shows the cumulative proportions of patients who achieved particular degrees of pain relief. While 23% of patients obtained complete relief, 40% obtained at least 70% relief, and 60% obtained at least 50% relief.

These results do more than hint at a possible

TABLE IV

The numbers, cumulative numbers, and proportion of patients, who, at 12 months after treatment with intradiscal electrothermal anuloplasty, obtained the percentage improvements indicated in their visual analogue pain scores [4]

Change in VAS (%)	Number	Cumulative numbers	Cumulative proportion
100	8	8	0.23
90	1	9	0.26
80	3	12	0.34
70	2	14	0.40
60	5	19	0.54
50	2	21	0.60
40	1	22	0.63
30	1	23	0.66
20	1	24	0.69
10	5	29	0.83
0	5	34	0.97
+10	1	35	1.00

efficacy of IDET for internal disc disruption. The results are not as good as the better results reported for anterior interbody fusion for discogenic pain (Table II), but they are at least as good as the lesser results for fusion for discogenic pain or for internal disc disruption (Table III). Moreover, IDET is a far less invasive procedure than fusion, and leaves no impairment if it fails to work. For these reasons, IDET stands to be a valid alternative to proceeding summarily to arthrodesis for patients with internal disc disruption.

The cardinal limitation to the evidence concerning IDET is that it has not been submitted to a randomised controlled trial. As used in the one controlled trial of IDET, a convenience sample of patients denied treatment by their insurer could possibly suffer a nocebo effect, which would exaggerate the difference in outcome between IDET and control therapy. However, there is no evidence that patients with proven internal disc disruption undergo spon-

taneous remission with the passage of time [5], or that any conservative treatment achieves the same outcomes as IDET. Moreover, any nocebo effect in the control group does not affect the outcomes in the IDET group. Those are established by having thoroughly followed their outcomes.

At this point in time, IDET is an emerging technology. Studies into its efficacy have barely started. It is still an imperfect treatment. Not all patients benefit. However, this relatively simple intervention offers appreciable relief of pain in over 50% of patients, associated with return to work. Moreover, it offers one in five patients the prospect of complete relief of pain. Refinements of the technique, improved technology, and rigorous selection criteria stand to improve these success rates.

References

1 Singh V. Intradiscal electrothermal therapy: a preliminary report. Pain Physician 2000; 3: 367–373.
2 Derby R, Eek B, Chen Y, O'Neill C, Ryan D. Intradiscal electrothermal annuloplasty (IDET): a novel approach for treating chronic discogenic back pain. Neuromodulation 2000; 3: 82–88.
3 Saal JA, Saal JS. Intradiscal electrothermal treatment for chronic discogenic low back pain. A prospective outcome study with minimum 1-year follow-up. Spine 2000; 25: 2622–2627.
4 Karasek M, Bogduk N. Twelve-month follow-up of a controlled trial of intradiscal thermal anuloplasty for back pain due to internal disc disruption. Spine 2000; 25: 2601–2607.
5 Rhyne AL, Smith SW, Wood KE, Darden BU. Outcome of unoperated discogram-positive low back pain. Spine 1995; 20: 1997–2000.

6. Discussion

The cardinal problem with precision treatment of chronic low back pain is that its literature is limited

Key point

- For the treatment of internal disc disruption, intradiscal electrothermal anuloplasty is an emerging treatment with promising results that stand to rival those of arthrodesis for this condition.

in quantity and in quality. Although the interventions attract many adherents and proponents, they attract few investigators, probably because of their surgical nature. Consequently, there is far less evidence concerning precision treatment than there is for other interventions for chronic low back pain. However, that other evidence does not demonstrate that other interventions are patently superior, and therefore preferable to precision treatments.

A practitioner would be justified in feeling confused about what to do. In practical terms, they have a patient with chronic low back pain for whom something needs to be done. Yet in intellectual terms, they are faced with strong evidence that other measures are not particularly effective, and weak evidence that precision treatments might be effective. They might ask if it is at all worthwhile pursuing precision diagnosis if the ensuing treatments are not properly or not fully proven.

In the case of fusion for discogenic pain or for internal disc disruption, reservation would seem justified. Fusion constitutes a point of no return. Although fusion holds some prospect of achieving a good outcome, some 40% of patients, or more, will fail to benefit. In those patients, the effects of fusion cannot be undone.

Against that background, the prospect of patients benefiting from IDET becomes attractive. This rel-atively simple, and innocuous, procedure may afford significant relief to some 50% of patients, and thereby avert both the need for fusion and the need to decide about fusion. Otherwise, for patients with proven discogenic pain, the only option is to revert to conservative treatments, for which there is no evidence of efficacy for this particular condition.

Less of a problem pertains to the pursuit of lumbar zygapophysial joint pain. If this diagnosis is established, the treatment options are quite innocuous. When performed correctly, radiofrequency neurotomy is not associated with morbidity. At worst, it simply fails to provide relief. However, some 80% of properly diagnosed patients stand to benefit, and 60% of patients stand to benefit greatly.

Choosing to pursue precision diagnosis, and to pursue precision treatment, becomes a matter of offering patients options. If a diagnosis is established of internal disc disruption or of zygapophysial joint pain, specific treatments can be offered. None is perfect, but each offers a substantial chance of benefit, with little to no risk. If precision diagnosis is not pursued, patients are denied these chances. Their only option is to pursue, or to revert to, conservative treatments whose efficacy is palliative at best. This is the decision that practitioners and their patients have to take.

Medical Management of Acute and Chronic Low Back Pain. An Evidence-Based Approach
Pain Research and Clinical Management, Vol. 13
Nikolai Bogduk and Brian McGuirk

CHAPTER 22

An approach to chronic low back pain

1. Introduction

On the basis of what research studies have shown to be effective and ineffective interventions for chronic low back pain, one can elaborate an approach for its management. This approach, however, depends on the patient's previous history.

In the past, patients who developed chronic low back pain, as a rule, have not been managed well during their acute and subacute phases. Psychosocial factors have been ignored, and become entrenched by the time the patient presents with chronic pain. It is for this reason that psychologists and others have urged and have favoured a behavioural approach to the management of chronic low back pain.

However, if practitioners were to follow evidence-based principles for the management of acute and subacute low back pain, psychosocial factors would be addressed during the acute phase of illness, resulting in fewer patients becoming chronic as a result of, or because of, psychosocial issues. Under those conditions, those patients whose back pain persists will either have deep-seated psychosocial problems that need to be pursued, or a physical cause for their pain that needs to be found, and treated appropriately.

Accordingly, the algorithm that follows is contingent upon how well patients have already been managed. If they have not had the benefit of concerted management, including psychosocial assessment and behavioural intervention, there may be a prospect that implementing such an approach belatedly might still be effective. However, if patients have already been managed well, repeating the same approach would seem superfluous.

2. Algorithm

The algorithm (Fig. 1) commences with assessment (Chapter 15). Paramount is an assessment for red flags. If the history suggests a possibility of a serious disorder, this should be investigated using conventional means. If a serious condition is confirmed, the present algorithm no longer applies, and the patient should be managed for the condition detected. If a serious condition is excluded, the patient re-enters the algorithm.

If the patient has widespread pain, involving more than just low back pain (Chapter 15), the present algorithm does not apply. The approaches outlined subsequently are not appropriate for such patients. They require a different form of management. What that management should be, and whether it works or not, are matters beyond the province and ambition both of this algorithm and of this text. The algorithm is designed for patients with well-defined back pain.

That is not to say, however, that the algorithm does not apply to patients with multiple, concurrent musculoskeletal problems (Chapter 15). In such patients, if their back pain is perceived as a distinct and separate problem, there is no reason to presume that the back pain is not amenable to investigation and treatment. There is every prospect that if the source of their back pain can be found, it can be treated. Successful treatment of the back pain amounts to one less problem that the patient has to bear.

The algorithm calls for imaging. The investigation of choice is MRI. If MRI has already recently been performed, there is no need to repeat the study. The definition of 'recent' involves judgment. In a patient with a stable history extending over several

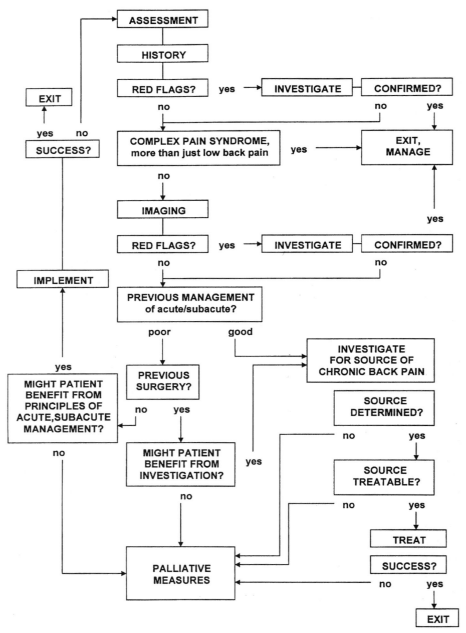

Fig. 1. An algorithm for the management of chronic low back pain.

years, an MRI obtained within the last 12 months may be sufficient. For patients with a shorter history, 3 months may be sufficient. If imaging has not been performed recently, or if the pain is escalating, an MRI should be requested.

The purpose of imaging at this stage is primarily to serve as a screening test: to exclude occult, sinister lesions that have not yet manifest features detectable on the red flag checklist (Chapter 15). If such lesions are detected, they should be managed appropriately;

and the patient leaves the algorithm. Excluding occult lesions allows the practitioner to proceed with the algorithm without fear of compromising the patient's welfare.

In addition, obtaining an MRI serves as the first step in investigating possible sources of chronic low back pain (Chapter 15). If a detectable entity such as a high-intensity zone (HIZ) or and endplate lesion is detected, there may be no need to confirm this as the source of pain. Conservative management might be applied, instead of invasive interventions, but on the basis of an organic source of pain having been determined.

Before embarking on treatment, the patient's previous management should be reviewed. If this management has been poor, either in the sense that it did not work, or that it did not follow evidence-based principles, consideration should be given to whether or not the patient might benefit from application of those principles. Although they are applied belatedly, there may be some prospect that explanation, reassurance, behavioural therapy, activation and exercises, could still serve to reduce the patient's distress, improve their disability, and reduce their pain, to acceptable levels, and thereby avoid pursuing the pain with invasive investigations. Even in patients with chronic low back pain, persisting fear may be the major and only problem. They may not want to pursue a diagnosis, once they understand that the cause of their pain is not threatening.

Intercalated in the assessment is whether or not the patient has had surgery. It seems unlikely that a patient who has failed surgery would respond to the simple measures appropriate for acute and subacute pain. But failed surgery is not a nihilistic endpoint. Publications soon to appear will indicate that a large proportion of patients who fail surgery have identifiable and potentially treatable lesions, that were not addressed by their original surgery. Not all 'failed backs' are unsalvageable. Nevertheless, hopefully, if more patients are treated according to evidence-based principles during their acute and subacute phases, the incidence of inappropriate surgery should fall.

For patients whose earlier management has been appropriate: whose fears, beliefs, and behaviours have been properly addressed, but whose pain and disability has persisted, the appropriate step would be to investigate the source of pain. These patients can be joined by those with failed back surgery for whom there is some prospect of finding a treatable lesion.

Investigations are undertaken according to the algorithm for precision diagnosis (Chapter 19). If a source is detected, and if it is treatable (Chapter 21), it should be treated. If the treatment is successful, the algorithm has worked, and the patient exits.

Various steps in the algorithm may have a null response. The patient may not be suitable for revisiting the principles of acute management; they may not be suitable for investigation; investigations may fail to disclose a treatable source of pain; treatment may fail. The algorithm draws these patients to a common endpoint that is called 'palliative measures'.

From a pragmatic perspective, the algorithm recognises that not all patients will have a detectable and treatable lesion; but some form of management is, nevertheless, required for these patients. Those measures are called palliative, for there is no evidence that these patients' pain can be eliminated. It may even not be possible to reduce the pain substantially, let alone to tolerable levels. The distress and disability of these patients, however, may nevertheless be improved. It is in this regard, that the evidence-base indicates that behavioural therapy may offer some gains (Chapter 17), notwithstanding what might be achieved in reducing the patient's pain with analgesics and even opioids (Chapter 17). However, none of these measures constitutes a cure, and for that reasons they have been labelled 'palliative' in the algorithm.

The optimal constituents of a palliative regimen have not been determined. Providers of such care, no doubt, will argue which interventions should be included and which should be shunned. For example, some providers might disavow combining opioids with behavioural therapy, while others might accept the combination.

From an ideological perspective, palliative measures should not be considered an endpoint of management. There is a need, but not for more of the same thing, or for proselytising that this is all that can be done. The prevalence of patients with intractable chronic back pain calls for new ideas to be developed and evaluated. In that regard, instead of constituting an endpoint, the node called 'palliative measures' should be construed as a starting point for the disciplined implementation of new interventions, so that additional arms can be added progressively to the algorithm and the population under palliative care reduced.

In graphic form, the measures and interventions that best apply throughout the acute, subacute, and chronic phases of back pain are summarised in Fig. 2. Simple measures are indicated, and are all that may be required for the acute phase (Chapter 11). They may be applicable for patients with chronic symptoms if they have not had appropriate treatment earlier. If patients respond, these measures can be reinforced, and the patient can continue to use them indefinitely.

Patients who do not respond to simple interventions may benefit from a more concerted approach. This may involve intensive exercises, undertaken in a cognitive–behavioural milieu (Chapter 12). If workplace problems persist, or have not been fully addressed previously, serious attention should be paid to them (Chapter 12). Yellow flag issues should be revisited, recognised, and addressed if they exist (Chapter 10). The evidence supports including certain forms of manipulative therapy at this stage (Chapter 12), but not the gratuitous application any form of manipulation, or the continued application of monotherapies (Chapter 12).

If appropriate measures are implemented during the acute and subacute phases, fewer patients, than has been the case to date, should progress to the chronic phase. Moreover, fewer patients should have had inappropriate treatments, fewer should have been subjected to prolonged passive treatments, and fewer, if not none, would have inappropriate surgery. Failed back surgery syndrome should become extinct.

Those patients whose pain persists can be investigated in order to determine their source of pain, but this should be undertaken in a disciplined, and not cavalier, manner. Patients successfully diagnosed using precision techniques, and successfully treated, will no longer add to the burden of illness.

For patients with persisting and intractable symptoms, palliative measures become the pragmatic next step, but all patients should be eligible for new interventions. Those interventions, however, should also be offered in a disciplined manner, so as to contribute to the evidence-base, instead of polluting the literature with still more untested claims, and instead of oppressing patients with unjustified and forlorn hope.

3. Discussion

This approach to chronic low back pain differs in some respects from those advocated and followed by others, but it is not fundamentally dissonant with them. It shares with other approaches the rejection of passive conservative therapies, and the futile persistence with monotherapies that do not work. It retains certain interventions advocated by others, but accords them a different emphasis and temporal location. These are complemented by interventions that others have rejected or ignored.

The present approach accords behavioural interventions, in the context of concurrent physical interventions, an important role in the management of acute and subacute low back pain (Chapter 11). Intensive exercises, in a cognitive milieu, are advocated for subacute pain (Chapter 12). The implication and expectation, however, is that these measures should have been implemented during the acute and subacute phase. The approach allows for implementation of these measures for patients with chronic low back pain, if they have not been treated well previously, but otherwise, it considers that repeating, or persisting with, this form of intervention will not make it any more successful.

Although others have portrayed behavioural and multidisciplinary treatment as the preferred and only treatment for chronic back pain, the evidence indicates that their efficacy is limited (Chapters 17 and 18). They do not stop pain, but they may reduce it. They do not restore function fully, but may im-

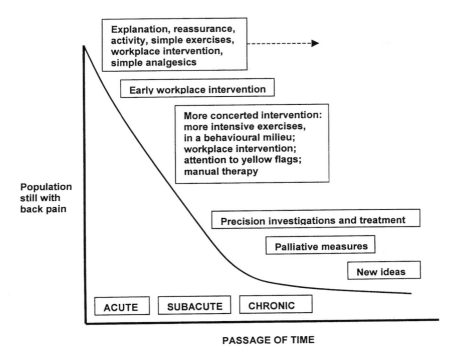

Fig. 2. The implementation of interventions for the various stages of low back pain.

prove it. They do not eliminate psychological and behavioural problems, but they may reduce them. For these reasons, behavioural and multidisciplinary interventions have been interpreted as legitimate, palliative measures, in the present approach. These interventions are not shunned or disparaged, but they are accorded a different status.

Where the present approach departs markedly from those advocated by others is in its allowance for the pursuit of precision diagnosis of chronic low back pain. The approach does not mandate that every patient should be investigated. Nor does it expect that every patient will be investigated. Yet, it allows the pursuit of a diagnosis with the prospect of offering a treatment that can stop the back pain, or reduce it far more greatly than other measures. Doing so may, of itself, restore the patients' function to satisfying levels (Chapter 21), or may render the patient more amenable to functional restoration programs.

In this regard, two important caveats apply. Foremost, the approach insists that precision diagnosis be undertaken in a responsible and disciplined manner.

For that purpose, a detailed algorithm is provided (Chapter 20). That algorithm strives to avoid the indiscriminate use of invasive investigations. It strives to base decisions on the best available epidemiological data, instead of whim or arbitrary physician-preference. If, and as, newer data become available the algorithm can be amended or fine-tuned. But in the meantime, the algorithm for precision diagnosis is designed to allow practitioners to find treatable sources of chronic low back pain, in a responsible manner, instead of assuming either that such a source cannot be found or that it cannot be treated.

The second caveat is that the precision treatment of chronic low back pain is still in its infancy. Pundits might argue that the evidence is too weak to advocate precision treatment. In certain respects, this is true. However, the main purpose of advocating precision diagnosis and precision treatment is to redress the imbalance that has emerged amongst approaches to chronic low back pain.

At present, the prevailing favoured approaches are essentially nihilistic. They claim that nothing can be found and nothing can be done, biophysically. This is not true. The advent of precision diagnostic techniques has shown that sources of chronic low back pain can be found, under controlled conditions, in substantial proportions of patients. Furthermore, options for treatment have followed.

Even if the data on precision treatment are regarded as weak or preliminary, they are nonetheless encouraging in principle. Chronic low back pain is not a terminal sentence. In some patients, it can be stopped. Even if the present options for precision treatment prove to be suboptimal or weak, the prospect remains for better interventions to be developed.

In promoting the present approach, this text stands as an advocate for optimism in the face of contemporary nihilism and a sense of defeat. Instead of simply relegating patients summarily to behavioural intervention and intensive exercises as the only option, it invites the disciplined pursuit of a diagnosis, and availing patients of treatments that possibly can eliminate their pain, or reduce it to degrees far greater than possible with conventional measures. But, moreover, the optimism does not stop there. The approach does not consider chronic low back pain to be an endpoint. It not only allows, but also calls for, patients to be the beneficiaries of new ideas, provided that they are implemented in a responsible manner. There is no reason to assume that what we have at present is the best there is, or all there is. The future holds promise, and will necessitate revisions of this and like texts.

Medical Management of Acute and Chronic Low Back Pain. An Evidence-Based Approach
Pain Research and Clinical Management, Vol. 13
Nikolai Bogduk and Brian McGuirk

Appendix 1: Elementary biostatistics

1. Introduction

Statistics can be used to determine and to describe how well a device works. In clinical practice, that device may be a diagnostic test or a treatment. Different statistics apply to diagnostic tests and to treatments, but they each have in common the objective of expressing, in a single number, just how well the test or treatment works. This appendix provides a short explanation of terms used in this text in the evaluation of various diagnostic tests and treatments used for low back pain.

2. Diagnostic tests

There are two, separate determinants of how well a diagnostic test works. One is *reliability*. The other is *validity*. For a diagnostic test to be held to 'work', it must be both reliable and valid. Conversely, the test cannot work if it lacks either reliability or validity.

2.1. Reliability

Reliability is the extent to which two observers obtain the same results when using the same diagnostic test on the same sample of patients. It is determined by having two observers independently apply the test on the same patients, and recording the results in a contingency table (Table I).

In such a table, the total number (N) of patients in the sample is $a + b + c + d$; 'a' constitutes the number of patients in whom both observers found that the test was positive; 'd' is the number of pa-

tients in whom both observers found that the test was negative; 'b' is the number of patients in whom observer one found the test to be positive, but observer two found it to be negative; and 'c' is the number of patients in whom observer one found the test to be negative, but observer two found it to be positive. Such a table shows that the observers agreed that the test was positive in 'a' cases, and agreed that the test was negative in 'd' cases. Their apparent rate of agreement is $[(a + d)/N] \times 100\%$.

The apparent rate of agreement, however, is not an accurate measure of how good the test is, for it incorporates agreement that might have occurred by chance alone. The true agreement is provided by discounting the apparent agreement for agreement by chance. This is illustrated in Fig. 1.

This figure illustrates that if there is not complete agreement in all cases, the observed agreement (P_o) is less than complete agreement by the extent to which there is disagreement. The figure also illustrates that complete agreement consists of two, hypothetical parts: the agreement expected by chance alone (P_e) and the range available for possible agreement beyond chance alone ($1 - P_e$).

TABLE I

A contingency table from which the reliability of a diagnostic test can be derived

Observer one	Observer two	
	Positive	Negative
Positive	a	b
Negative	c	d

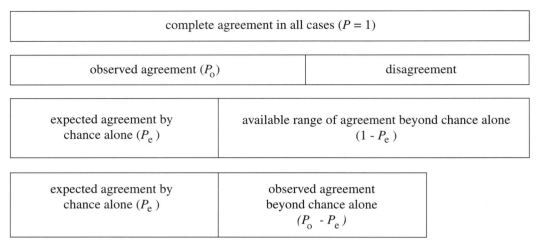

Fig. 1. The distinction between observed agreement and agreement beyond chance.

The observed agreement consists of one portion due to agreement by chance alone, and another portion that is the agreement beyond chance alone $(P_o - P_e)$. In determining the reliability of the test, credit is not given to the observers for that agreement which they achieved by chance alone. Their true skill, and the strength of the test, is determined by how well they agreed beyond chance alone.

That is established by measuring how far their observed agreement extends into the range of agreement available beyond chance alone, and is expressed by a statistic called 'kappa', where

$$\text{kappa} = (P_o - P_e)/(1 - P_e).$$

In words, kappa is the extent to which the observed agreement (discounted for chance) fills the range of possible agreement available (also discounted for chance).

An example to help understand this concept is a multiple choice examination. If there are 100 questions each with four choices, a candidate could, on the average, answer one in four questions correctly simply by guessing. By chance alone, they could score 25%. A candidate who scores 65% has not demonstrated a proficiency of 65%, for 25 of those 65 marks could have been gained by chance alone. Their true skill is demonstrated by how well they performed beyond chance alone. Accordingly their raw score (65) is discounted by the number of ques-

tions that they could have answered correctly by chance alone (25), which yields 40. Similarly, the total number of questions (100) is discounted by the number of questions that might have been answered correctly by chance alone (25) to yield the available number of questions that might have been answered correctly beyond chance alone (75). The true skill of the candidate then is the proportion of the available number of questions (75) that the candidate correctly answered (40), i.e. 40/75 = 53%. The true skill of the candidate, discounted for chance, is 53%, not the raw score of 65%.

Not obvious in the determination of reliability is how the expected agreement by chance alone should be estimated. This is based on what the two observers find, on average, which is shown by the sums of the columns and rows of the contingency table (Table II).

This table shows that, overall, observer one

TABLE II

A contingency table from which agreement can be derived

Observer one	Observer two		Totals
	Positive	Negative	
Positive	a	b	$a+b$
Negative	c	d	$c+d$
Totals	$a+c$	$b+d$	$N = a+b+c+d$

recorded positive findings in $(a+b)$ cases. The proportion of cases that this observer found to be positive is $(a+b)/N$. On average, therefore, this observer would record positive findings in $(a+b)/N$ of all cases presented to him. Meanwhile, observer two found $(a+c)$ cases presented to him to be positive. If these cases were presented to observer one, the number that would be expected to be recorded as positive, by chance alone, would be $(a+c) \times (a+b)/N$.

Similarly the proportion of cases that observer one recorded as negative is $(c+d)/N$. The number of cases that observer two found to be negative is $(b+d)$. If these cases were presented to observer one, the number that would be expected to recorded as negative, by chance alone, would be $(b+d) \times (c+d)/N$.

These derived numbers provide an estimate of the agreement expected by chance alone (P_e), i.e.

$$P_e = [(a+c)(a+b)/N + (b+d)(c+d)/N]/N$$

which is different from the observed agreement (P_o), viz.

$$P_o = (a+d)/N.$$

From these equations, P_o, P_e, $(P_o - P_e)$, and $(1 - P_e)$ can be calculated, and hence, kappa can be calculated. Readers interested in further reading about kappa can consult the original literature [1] or various other educational resources [2,3].

For practical purposes, however, readers should understand that once calculated, kappa can range in value from 0 to 1, or from 0 to −1. Negative values of kappa indicate abject disagreement, which occurs only for very unreliable tests. For most tests, the values are positive. A value of 0 indicates no agreement beyond chance alone. A value of 1 indicates complete, i.e. perfect, agreement.

Values between 0 and 1 can be accorded a range of verbal descriptors (Table III). The kappa values indicate quantitatively, and the descriptors indicate qualitatively, just how reliable the diagnostic test is.

If practitioners use diagnostic tests with high kappa scores, they can be confident that the reliability of the test is good. However, if the kappa score is low, practitioners should realize that the diagnostic

TABLE III

Verbal translations of kappa scores

Kappa value	Descriptor
0.8–1.0	very good
0.6–0.8	good
0.4–0.6	moderate
0.2–0.4	slight
0.0–0.2	poor

test does not work well; that someone else using the same test on the same patient is not likely to obtain the same result. Consequently, they have grounds to question or to doubt the result that they have obtained.

The kappa score does not, and cannot, determine which of two observers is correct. It measures only how consistent any two observers are, or might expect to be. But if consistency is lacking, the test, or how it is used, is defective. In essence, diagnostic tests with low kappa scores just do not work well enough to be reliable. Their results are little better than guessing, and do not reflect professional proficiency.

2.2. Validity

Validity is the measure of how well a diagnostic test actually establishes both the presence and the absence of a condition that it is intended to detect. It is determined by comparing the results of the diagnostic test with those of another test — called the criterion standard — which provides more direct evidence of the presence and absence of the condition. For diagnostic tests based on physical examination, the criterion standard could be the results of X-ray examination, surgical findings, or post-mortem findings.

The numerical properties of a diagnostic test can be derived by constructing a contingency table, in which the results of a diagnostic test are compared to the results of the criterion standard when both are applied to the same sample of patients (Table IV). Two fundamental statistics can be derived from the columns of such a table.

TABLE IV

A contingency table from which the validity of a diagnostic test can be derived

Diagnostic test	Criterion standard	
	Positive	Negative
Positive	a	b
Negative	c	d

The *sensitivity* of the test measures how well the test correctly detects positive cases. It is also known as the *true-positive rate*. It is calculated as $a/(a+c)$, where $(a+c)$ is the number of cases that truly have the condition, and 'a' is the number of these cases that the test correctly detects. By inference, 'c' is the number of cases with the condition that the test failed to detect.

The *specificity* of the test measures how well the test correctly detects the absence of the condition. It is also known as the *true-negative rate*. It is calculated as $d/(b+d)$, where $(b+d)$ is the number of cases that truly do not have the condition, and 'd' is the number of these cases that the test correctly detects. By inference, 'b' is the number of cases without the condition that the test failed to detect correctly, and which the test incorrectly found to be positive instead of negative. Accordingly, the ratio $b/(b+d)$ is the *false-positive rate* of the test. By simple arithmetic it can be shown that

$$\text{false-positive rate} = [1 - \text{specificity}],$$

viz.

false-positive rate	=	$b/(b+d)$
specificity	=	$d/(b+d)$
$(b+d)/(b+d)$	=	1
$b/(b+d)+d/(b+d)$	=	1
$b/(b+d)$	=	$1-d/(b+d)$
false-positive rate	=	$1-\text{specificity}.$

Upon finding the result of a test to be positive, practitioners should not assume that the result is truly positive. The result might be false-positive. Just how good a test is depends on the balance between the true-positive rate and the false-positive rate. This is reflected by a third statistic known as the *positive likelihood ratio*.

Conceptually, the positive likelihood ratio (+LR) is defined as the true-positive rate discounted by the false-positive rate, i.e.

$$+\text{LR} = \text{true-positive rate}/\text{false-positive rate}.$$

Numerically it becomes:

$$+\text{LR} = \text{sensitivity}/[1 - \text{specificity}].$$

The utility and power of the likelihood ratio emerges from the following considerations.

If *diagnostic confidence* is defined as the chances of a diagnosis being correct, then it transpires that diagnostic confidence is a function of two factors: the *prevalence* of the condition being diagnosed, and the *power* of the diagnostic test being used to detect it, i.e.

$$\text{diagnostic confidence} =$$
$$\text{function(prevalence; diagnostic test)}.$$

Because of certain mathematical idiosyncrasies, this relationship becomes complicated if diagnostic confidence and prevalence are expressed as percentages. However, it becomes very simple if diagnostic confidence and prevalence are both expressed as odds. In that event, it can be shown [2,4] that:

$$\text{diagnostic confidence} =$$
$$\text{(prevalence)} \times \text{(positive likelihood ratio)}.$$

In verbal terms, this equation states that: the odds that the diagnosis is correct is the product of the odds that the condition is present and the positive likelihood ratio of the test used to detect it.

This equation underscores an important realization: that *diagnostic confidence is not dependent solely on the result of the test; it is also determined by how common the condition is.* Thus, for example, if the prevalence of a condition is 80%, the odds in favour of it being present are 80 : 20; and without applying any diagnostic test a practitioner can be 80% certain that the condition will be present. If the prevalence is only 10%, the odds in favour of the condition being present are only 10 : 90, and without applying any diagnostic test a practitioners can be only 10% confident that condition will be present.

For a diagnostic test to be worthwhile, it must have the ability to increase substantially the diagnostic confidence based on prevalence alone. In this regard, the equation reveals what value the likelihood ratio of the test must have in order for the test to be worthwhile.

If the likelihood ratio is only 1.0, the diagnostic test has no value. The diagnostic confidence is no greater than that which was available on the basis of prevalence alone. Just how large the likelihood ratio should be depends on the prevalence of the condition in question and how confident the practitioner wants to be.

Thus, if the prevalence of a condition is 40%, and the practitioner wants to be 80% certain in their diagnosis, the required likelihood ratio can be calculated as follows.

Prevalence = 40%
Prevalence odds = 40 : 60
Desired confidence = 80%
Desired confidence odds = 80 : 20

diagnostic confidence =

(prevalence) × (positive likelihood ratio)

$$80 : 20 = 40 : 60 \times LR$$
$$LR = 80/20 \times 60/40$$
$$= 6$$

If the prevalence is 10%, and the practitioner wants to be 80% certain in their diagnosis, the likelihood ratio is calculated as:

Prevalence = 10%
Prevalence odds = 10 : 90
Desired confidence = 80%
Desired confidence odds = 80 : 20

diagnostic confidence =

(prevalence) × (positive likelihood ratio)

$$80 : 20 = 10 : 90 \times LR$$
$$LR = 80/20 \times 90/10$$
$$= 36$$

If, in the preceding example, the desired diagnostic confidence is 90%, the required likelihood ratio becomes 81.

These examples illustrate that the desired likelihood ratio is not a singular figure; it depends on the

context. The less common the condition, the larger must be the likelihood ratio; and the greater the desired confidence, the larger must be the likelihood ratio.

Conversely, consider how little diagnostic value tests provide if their likelihood ratio is small. If the prevalence of a condition is 40%, and the likelihood ratio is 1.2, the diagnostic confidence is:

$$\text{diagnostic confidence} = 40 : 60 \times 1.2$$
$$= 48 : 60$$

If expressed as a percentage,

$$48 : 60 = 48/(48+60)$$
$$= 48/108$$
$$= 44\%$$

Such a likelihood ratio increases the diagnostic confidence by a meagre 4%. Even if the likelihood ratio is increased to 1.5, the diagnostic confidence rises only to 50%.

These examples indicate that diagnostic tests with small likelihood ratios (i.e. close to 1.0) confer little change to diagnostic confidence. In other words, diagnostic tests with small likelihood ratios do not work well enough to improve diagnostic confidence to a worthwhile extent.

A corollary of these properties is that if the positive likelihood ratio is less than 1.0, the test actually decreases diagnostic confidence to less than what it was on the basis of prevalence alone.

2.3. Odds ratio

The odds ratio is a statistic that is sometimes used by investigators to describe data in a contingency table that relates two variables (Table V). In such a table, if there is a relationship between the two variables,

TABLE V

A contingency table from which the odds ratio can be calculated

Variable one	Variable two	
	Present	Absent
Present	a	b
Absent	c	d

the values in the '*a*' and '*d*' cells should be greater than the values in the '*b*' and '*c*' cells. The odds ratio seeks to reveal this difference.

Explicitly,

$$\text{odds ratio} = ad/bc = (a/b)/(c/d) = (a/c)/(d/b).$$

In one sense, the odds ratio describes the 'balance' between the two rows. It describes the extent to which the ratio of '*a*' as to '*b*' is greater than the ratio of '*c*' as to '*d*'. Similarly, it describes the 'balance' between the columns. It describes the extent to which the ratio of '*a*' as to '*c*' is greater than the ratio of '*d*' as to '*b*'. In another sense, it describes the balance between the two diagonals. It describes how much the product of '*a*' and '*d*' is greater than the product of '*b*' and '*c*'. Each of these interpretations reflects by how much the '*a*' and '*d*' values are greater than the '*b*' and '*c*' values. The greater the 'imbalance' between these values, the stronger is the putative relationship between the two variables.

Historically, odds ratios have been used in epidemiological studies to determine the strength of association between exposure to a risk factor for a disease and the subsequent development of that disease. However, it is quite legitimate to use the odds ratio to compare other variables, such as two clinical signs, or the outcomes of two different treatments.

An odds ratio greater than 1.0 indicates that there is some relationship between the two variables; and the greater the odds ratio, the stronger the relationship. Alone, however, the odds ratio does not indicate how clinically significant that relationship might be. In general, relationships start to become clinically significant when the odds ratio exceeds 3.0. Values greater than 1.0, but less than 3.0, reflect a definite, but only slight, relationship.

Mathematically, it can be shown that the odds ratio (OR) is related to the likelihood ratio (LR). Thus,

$$\begin{aligned} \text{OR} &= ad/bc \\ \text{LR} &= [a/(a+c)]/[b/(b+d)] \\ &= (a/b)[(b+d)/(a+c)] \end{aligned}$$

If we let '*d*' be some multiple of '*b*', and '*a*' be some multiple of '*c*', i.e.

$$\text{if} \quad b = md \quad \text{and} \quad a = kc,$$

then

$$\begin{aligned} \text{LR} &= (a/b)[(md+d)/(kc+c)] \\ &= (a/b)[d(m+1)/c(k+1)] \\ &= (a/b)(d/c)[(m+1)/(k+1)] \\ &= ad/bc(m+1)/(k+1) \\ &= \text{OR}(m+1)/(k+1) \end{aligned}$$

Thus, whenever, '*a*' is greater than '*c*', and '*d*' is greater than '*b*', the odds ratio will be greater than the likelihood ratio.

The advantage of the likelihood ratio, however, is that it is directly related to prevalence and diagnostic confidence and so, can be used to compute diagnostic confidence directly (as described above). The odds ratio could be used to the same effect, but would need to be reduced by the coefficient $(m+1)/(k+1)$ in order to obtain the correct arithmetic result.

3. Treatment

When someone declares that a treatment "works", it begs several subsidiary questions. Paramount amongst these are: "how much?", "for how long?", and "in what respects?". Other questions can be: "for what types of patients?", "in whose hands?", and "according to whom?".

These latter questions pertain to important details about a treatment and the study that claims to have shown that "it works". A treatment might work for certain types of patients with a given presenting complaint, but not for others. For example, it might work for patients with mild back pain, but not severe back pain; or for motivated patients, but not for unmotivated patients. A treatment might work if it is administered by experienced and expert practitioners, but not in the hands of less experienced practitioners. Furthermore, although a practitioner might believe and claim that a treatment is successful, this may not be the case if the results are assessed by an independent observer.

These considerations, however, are of secondary

significance to the leading questions: "how much?", "how long?", and "in what respects?". These questions address how well the treatment works, in the first instance, before considering the context in which the treatment might be applied.

The literature on back pain often fails to address these critical questions. Studies may report "how much?" but not "for how long?". They may report an effect on pain but not on other variables such as restoration of function or return to work. In the absence of complete information it is difficult for a demanding consumer to credit that a treatment really "works". It might "work" to some degree, or for some period of time, or in some respects; but it may not constitute a worthwhile treatment if its effects are meagre, short-lived, or make little difference to the patient's function.

3.1. How much?

The tradition, or habit, of research in the past has been to report mean figures for outcome variables, usually improvements in pain. Thus, at baseline, a sample of patients may have a mean pain score of 6 out of 10, and after treatment they have a mean pain score of 4 out of 10. If the scores are significantly different statistically, a t-test produces a P-value of less than 0.05. Such P-values have been used to constitute proof that the treatment works.

A P-value of 0.05 simply indicates that there has been a statistically significant change in the variable. Whether or not that change is clinically significant, or worthwhile to the patients, is another matter. That depends on the raw figures. A change from a mean score of 6 to a mean score of 4 may be significant statistically but it is not necessarily significant clinically. After all, the sample has remained in pain. There has been an improvement but not necessarily a resolution of the problem. Thus, the treatment 'works' but only to a limited extent.

Furthermore, such group data provide little insight, for the practitioner or the patient, into what the chances are of a given patient obtaining a worthwhile response to the treatment. That information is better provided by categorical data that report what number

TABLE VI

The results of a treatment for low back pain

Relief (%)	n	P	Sum P
100	5	0.33	0.33
90	2	0.13	0.47
80	2	0.13	0.60
70	2	0.13	0.73
60	1	0.07	0.80
50	1	0.07	0.87
40	0	0.00	0.87
30	0	0.00	0.87
20	1	0.07	0.93
10	0	0.00	0.93
0	1	0.07	1.00
Worse	0	0.00	1.00
Total	15		

N, number of patients. *P*, proportion of patients. Sum *P*, cumulative proportions.

and what proportion of patients achieved different grades of response.

An example of such information is shown in Table VI. It reports the number of patients who obtained various degrees of relief following a treatment. For example, 5/15 patients obtained 100% relief, 2/15 patients obtained 70% relief, and 1/15 patients obtained 20% relief. The table also provides the proportion of patients that achieved particular degrees of relief, and the cumulative proportions. Thus, 33% of patients obtained 100% relief; a further 13% of patients obtained 90% relief; and another 13% of patients obtained 80% relief. Adding these proportions yields 60% of patients obtained at least 80% relief. Similarly, 87% of patients obtained at least 50% relief.

From such data, a reader can determine exactly how well a treatment works. The data show how many patients were completely relieved, how many were partially relieved, and to what extent. The outcomes are transparent, and not obscured under a single group mean. Given such data, a practitioner can determine what the chances are of a given patient obtaining a specified level of outcome.

Unfortunately, few studies of treatments for low back pain have ever reported such categorical data.

Consequently, they do not reveal the complete picture of how well a treatment works.

Categorical data also allow a revealing statistic to be calculated. If the categorical results of a treatment and a control treatment are provided, the *number needed to treat* (NNT) can be calculated. This statistic measures how effective a treatment is beyond non-specific effects of treatment[5,6].

If $P_{control}$ is the proportion of patients who respond to the control treatment, and P_{treat} is the proportion of patients who respond to the index treatment, the difference between these proportions ($P_{treat} - P_{control}$) is the attributable effect of the treatment, i.e. the proportion of patients who responded because of effects greater or other than the non-specific effects of simply having had treatment. The NNT is the reciprocal of this proportion, i.e.

$$NNT = 1/(P_{treat} - P_{control}).$$

Conceptually, NNT is the number of patients who must be treated before one patient, on the average, can be claimed to have responded because of the specific effects of that treatment. When the NNT is large, it means that, on the average, the responses to treatment are largely due to non-specific effects, and not due to the specific effects of the treatment. Good treatments that work because of specific effects have NNTs of less than 3.

Table VII provides an example of NNT. It records the results of an index treatment and a control treatment, together with NNT for different grades of outcome. This table shows that 8% of patients achieved complete relief of pain following the index treatment, but no patient having the control treatment obtained this degree of relief. For achieving 100% relief of pain, the attributable effect is 0.08, and the NNT is 13. (Arithmetically the NNT is 12.5, but since one cannot treat 0.5 of a patient, the NNT is rounded to the next highest integer.)

Of the patients undergoing the index treatment, 28% achieved at least 80% relief of their pain. Only 6% of patients achieved this response following control treatment. The attributable effect of the index treatment, for achieving at least 80% relief is 0.22, and the NNT is 5. This means that five patients

TABLE VII

The results of a treatment for back pain compared to those of a control treatment

Relief of pain (%)	Cumulative proportion		AE	NNT
	Control	Index		
100	0.00	0.08	0.08	13
90	0.00	0.08	0.08	13
80	0.06	0.28	0.22	5
70	0.06	0.42	0.36	3
60	0.06	0.50	0.44	3
50	0.06	0.64	0.58	2
40	0.06	0.67	0.61	2
30	0.06	0.81	0.75	2
20	0.24	0.86	0.62	2
10	0.24	0.94	0.70	2
0	0.53	1.00		
Worse	1.00			

The cumulative proportion pertains to the proportion of patients achieving the degree of relief indicated or better. AE, attributable effect; NNT, number needed to treat.

would need to be treated before one could be claimed to have responded explicitly because of the effects of the index treatment.

However, for achieving at least 50% relief of pain, the index treatment has an attributable effect of 0.58 and an NNT of 2. This means that, on the average, only two patients would have to be treated before one could be claimed to have responded, when 'response' is defined as at least 50% relief.

In this manner, if and when comprehensive categorical data are provided, a reader can determine for themselves what the attributable effect and NNT are for whatever level of outcome they consider to constitute a success. For some readers, that level might be 50% relief of pain; for others it might be complete relief. This facility is not provided by results that simply offer mean scores and a *P*-value.

3.2. How long?

Lack of follow-up plagues many studies of pain treatment. Some studies report outcomes immediately after treatment, but not thereafter. This leaves unanswered the question of how long the effects of treatment last. Short-term follow-up — 4 weeks or even 3 months after treatment — is little better. Regardless of how effective a treatment is in the short term, it is of little value if the patient's symptoms and disabilities promptly return.

How long the effects of a treatment should last depends on the nature of the treatment. Pharmaceuticals have a very short effect, but they can be re-administered on a regular basis, at relatively low cost. In contrast, it is unpalatable to recommend surgery on a recurrent basis, if the operation relieves symptoms, but for only 3 months at a time. A grey area pertains to conservative and manual therapies, with respect to how often, and at what cost, should they be repeated if their effectiveness is short-lived.

There is no magic number for the required period of follow-up. In some instances, 3 or 6 months might be enough. In other cases, 12 months or more might be required. A guideline, however, can be applied. Patients should be followed for as long as it takes for any decay in the outcome to plateau. This means that the follow-up should not be so short as to show no decay in the outcome. Conversely, once decay has been demonstrated, and the outcomes have stabilized, further follow-up would seem superfluous, for the behaviour of the outcomes has been clearly quantified.

3.3. In what respects?

Patients with back pain not only suffer pain, they are also disabled. Ostensibly because of their pain, there are things that they cannot do. Furthermore, simply relieving pain does not necessarily result in an improvement of disability.

A treatment, therefore, cannot be held to "work" simply because it improves pain scores. For a treatment to "work" it should also improve other measures of the patient's status. These may include psychological status, physical ability, and perhaps most critically — return to work.

In this regard, too few studies of back pain have reported comprehensively on the success of treatments. While some studies report pain scores, they do not report disability or return to work. Others base 'success' on improvements in psychological status, but not in pain, disability, or return to work.

4. Evidence-based medicine

The precepts of evidence-based medicine adopted in this text are that:

> evidence-based medicine is medical practice that uses techniques of proven reliability, validity, and efficacy; and which shuns techniques that lack reliability, validity, or efficacy.

Accordingly, the various chapters on diagnostic techniques refer to the available research data on reliability and validity. Those procedures that are reliable and valid are highlighted and recommended. Those that have been shown to lack reliability or validity are identified and shunned, regardless of how entrenched they may be in conventional practice, and despite the beliefs of their adherents that these techniques do work. The data show otherwise. It is for uncommitted readers that the data are provided, in order to show why these techniques should not be used.

For treatment techniques, those that are recommended are those for which there is strong evidence of efficacy: data that do answer "how much", "for how long", and "in what respects". Treatments are not recommended if the evidence is weak or lacking, despite what the original authors may have concluded and, at times, despite what authors of systematic reviews have concluded. In that respect, a P-value of less than 0.05 is not accepted as sufficient evidence that a treatment "works" if the data do not indicate just how well the treatment works, and for how long, or if it works in some respects, but not others.

For some treatments, there is no evidence. Proponents of such treatments have introduced them into the market on the basis of assertion or insistence that they work.

They defy academic accountability on the specious grounds that no-one has disproved them;

or by arguing that no evidence of efficacy does not constitute evidence of no efficacy. But assertion does not constitute evidence. Unless and until the treatment is tested, the assertion could just as well be wrong as it could be right. In the case of untested treatments, consumers can decide for themselves if they choose to believe assertions or not. In the present text, some treatments based on assertion are mentioned, but none are recommended. They await formal evaluation.

References

1   Cohen J. A coefficient of agreement for nominal scales. Educ Psychol Meas 1960; 20: 37–46.

2   Sackett DL, Haynes RB, Guyatt GH, Tugwell P. Clinical Epidemiology. A Basic Science for Clinical Medicine, 2nd edn. Little, Brown and Co., Boston, MA, 1991, pp 119–139.

3   Bogduk N. Truth in musculoskeletal medicine. II. Truth in diagnosis: Reliability. Australas Musculoskel Med 1998; 3: 21–23.

4   Bogduk N. Truth in musculoskeletal medicine. Truth in diagnosis — validity. Australas Musculoskel Medicine 1999; 4: 32–39.

5   Cook RJ, Sackett DL. The number needed to treat: a clinically useful measure of treatment effect. Br Med J 1995; 310: 452–454.

6   Laupacis A, Sackett DL, Roberts RS. An assessment of clinically useful measures of the consequences of treatment. New Engl J Med 1988; 318: 1728–1733.

Medical Management of Acute and Chronic Low Back Pain. An Evidence-Based Approach
Pain Research and Clinical Management, Vol. 13
Nikolai Bogduk and Brian McGuirk

Appendix 2: How to label acute back pain

1. Introduction

Acute low back pain attracts a variety of diagnostic labels in clinical practice. Some, such as 'lumbago' or 'lumbalgia' are simply translations of 'back pain' into another language. Others, such as 'segmental dysfunction' and 'lumbar insufficiency' are little more than metaphors, for they have no reliable or valid biological correlate other than the patient has back pain. Some terms, such as 'zygapophysial joint pain' or 'discogenic pain', express a diagnosis in anatomical terms, but these entities cannot be diagnosed clinically (Chapter 14); they require invasive investigations, such as controlled diagnostic blocks or discography (Chapter 19), neither of which are appropriate for the investigation of acute low back pain. Other terms, such as 'spondylosis', 'disc degeneration', or 'osteoarthrosis' attribute the pain to pathologic findings seen on radiographs, but this is neither valid nor legitimate. Spondylosis, disc degeneration, and osteoarthrosis are simply age-changes. They are common in asymptomatic individuals and correlate poorly, if at all, with the presence of pain (Chapter 8). Regardless of how popular their use has been in the past, they do not constitute valid diagnoses.

When composing the second edition of the taxonomy of the International Association for the Study of Pain [1], the subcommittee on taxonomy wrestled with the classification of spinal pain. It recognised certain entities drawn from the osteopathic, physical medicine, and mainstream literature, but set stringent criteria for their diagnosis. The objective in doing so was to ensure that if these conditions were to be accorded legitimacy, their diagnosis should be consistent, disciplined, and accountable. Moreover, many of the criteria were cast premeditatedly in such a way that they could not possibly be satisfied using history and examination alone, or even using conventional investigations. The purpose of setting such stringent criteria was to prevent presumptive diagnosis, and to indicate where research was necessary to establish the reliability and validity of traditional, diagnostic practices.

In essence, the exercise established that a patho-anatomic diagnosis or any other traditional diagnosis of back pain could not be made in the majority of cases. Accordingly, the subcommittee advocated the use of the term – 'lumbar spinal pain of unknown or uncertain origin' [1]. This term constituted an intellectually and clinically honest diagnosis. It serves well enough for the purposes of classification and coding. However, it is a long term and is, therefore, cumbersome and unattractive for everyday use. Moreover, it conveys the sense that the doctor does not really know what is going on. In that respect, it is perhaps excessively nihilistic in its honesty.

Diagnostic labels are important for a variety of reason. First, patients expect a diagnosis. It indicates to them that the doctor knows what is wrong with them. Simultaneously a diagnosis reinforces the doctor's self-image by implying that he or she has, indeed, determined what is wrong. However, a diagnosis should not be illegitimate or fallacious, lest it lead to therapeutic misadventure. On the one hand, an illegitimate diagnosis may provide a false sense of security and result in delays in establishing the correct or better diagnosis and treatment. On the other hand, an illegitimate diagnosis may result in the patient being subjected to inappropriate treatment and the attendant risks of morbidity, which include the morbidity of failed treatment. In this regard, some diagnostic labels may be outrightly deleterious as well as being fundamentally illegitimate. 'Degenerative disc disease' may imply to the patient that they are disintegrating, which they are not. 'Instability' may imply that they will fall apart, which they will not. 'Disc bulge' is not a cause of back pain, but may attract unnecessary and subsequently failed surgery.

One development has been the introduction of the term 'red flag' condition, to apply to serious causes of low back pain, such as tumours and infections (Chapter 6). Mercifully, such conditions are rare in primary care. In the vast majority of cases of acute low back pain, the cause is not serious. But there is no satisfying, official term for these instances that properly conveys the notion of non-serious back pain.

Another introduction has been the concept of 'yellow flags' (Chapter 10). This term pertains to what the patient believes about their back pain and what they do about it or because of it. The patho-anatomic cause is nevertheless non-serious.

2. The requirements

What is needed is a term that is satisfying to practitioners and is easy to use, yet at the same time conveys to the patient a reassurance that there is nothing seriously wrong with their back, and that they can resume normal activities of daily living without fear of deterioration or of doing further injury. This term cannot be dismissive. To tell a patient that they simply have back pain is telling them nothing new, and implies that either the doctor has no expertise or does not care. Both erode the confidence that the patient should have in their doctor. To tell a patient that they have 'lumbar spinal pain of unknown origin' may be correct officially, but sounds ostentatious or obfuscating. The label may be disheartening to the patient for, despite its honesty, it communicates that the doctor does not know what is wrong. Worse, it

may reinforce or amplify the patient's fears, on the grounds that if the doctor does not know, there may still be something seriously wrong.

Perhaps an expert committee could scour the English language in an attempt to find the correct term. Perhaps the committee could search for neologisms derived from Greek or Latin to mean back pain whose cause is not serious and not deserving of worry. Existing words and new words are elusive. 'Uncomplicated back pain' might convey the correct patho-anatomic sense, but fails to satisfy the requirement of positive encouragement. 'Non-serious back pain' conveys how the patient and the doctor might both feel about the pain, but still falls short of encouragement. 'Mechanical low back pain' is commonly used in this situation, but is far from satisfactory. Fundamentally, it means no more than pain that is aggravated by movement. Implicitly it used to pertain to non-serious causes of back pain, but the term does not expressly convey the sense of a non-serious and surmountable cause. Moreover, it carries the risk of implying that ergonomic factors, particularly work and overuse, are the cause of pain, for it is by overuse that other mechanical devices typically break down.

3. A solution

The acceptance of 'red flags' and 'yellow flags' predicates and invites a classification of back pain that is simple and which potentially satisfies all the requirements of a good diagnosis. It is:

Red back pain:
   back pain that requires serious medical attention and perhaps investigation.

Yellow back pain:
   back pain that requires concerted interaction between the patient and their doctor in order to resolve fears and misconceptions about their pain.

Green back pain:
   back pain about which the patient should have no grounds for fear, and from which they can expect recovery with straightforward, even minimal, management.

The advantages of such a taxonomy are several. For physicians, the three terms satisfactorily rank back pain into categories of seriousness that are already recognised. They allow for shades of colour, such as green back pain that is becoming a little bit yellow; or red back pain that has become green after the results of investigations return as negative. For patients, the analogy with traffic lights should be a meaningful metaphor. Red means stop; there may be danger. Yellow means proceed with caution. Green means it is quite safe to proceed; there is no danger.

In practice, the terms can be readily and innocuously introduced, and used to convey to the patient the implications of each condition. The following illustrate possible introductions to patients.

Red back pain

"I have examined your back, and I have carefully considered your history. While I can find nothing obviously wrong in your back, there is one thing [or, there are a few things] in your history that we call 'red flags'. These are things that suggest that we need to stop and think. In your case the red flags are [stipulate red flag as appropriate]. These mean that [explain implication]. The chances that anything serious is wrong with your back are still very low; the odds are that it is fine. But the red flag means that we have to take certain actions. Just to be certain we might [will need to] run some tests. In the meantime, there are some things that we can do to ease your pain, and some measures to get you as mobile as possible, while we get the tests done. Once the results are back we can review the situation, and make new plans."

Yellow back pain

"I have examined your back, and I have carefully and thoroughly considered your history. I can find nothing wrong, and I am confident that there is no serious cause for your pain. However, I notice that you have some concerns, [or that you are worried] about this pain. We call this 'yellow back pain'. It means that we don't have to be alarmed, and

that we can proceed carefully at this stage. What is most important, however, is that you and I need to talk about [what you think is causing your pain; why you are worrying; getting back to work (as appropriate)]. Foremost, we don't need to do any special tests. In the meantime, we can do something to ease your pain, and look at ways of getting you moving and back to a normal life."

Green back pain

"I have examined your back, and I have carefully and thoroughly considered your history. I can find nothing wrong, and I am confident that there is no serious cause for your pain. You have, what we now call, 'green back pain'. It means that we don't have to worry about what is causing the pain; that we have a green light to get on with life. We have every prospect that you can, and you will, recover from this episode of pain. There is no need to use fancy tests to find out exactly what is wrong. In the meantime, there are some simple things that we can do to ease the pain while it gets better of its own accord, and things that we can do to get you moving and back to work. And the sooner the better."

Such introductions endow the new terms with legitimacy. They come from the doctor, with confidence and authority, and their meaning and implications are explained. Individual practitioners could embellish or elaborate the introductions and explanations according to their own style and preferences.

4. Discussion

From a clinical perspective the term 'green back pain' is resistant to criticism. Technically, it provides a competent and legitimate diagnostic label, which is easy to use. If the term is confidently explained, it should be satisfying to the patient, for it does explain what is, or rather what is not, wrong. Moreover, using a familiar metaphor, the term conveys the required notion of safety to proceed; and thereby should be reassuring.

The one disadvantage of the term is its seeming, childish, absurdity. However, the absurdity does not lie intrinsically with the term. It lies in how it is portrayed or perceived. Individuals may be reluctant to use a term on the grounds that it sounds childish and that they will be ridiculed by their peers. But if that ridicule is not forthcoming, there are no grounds for embarrassment, and no grounds for not using the term. However, if conversely, the term is approved by one's peers, it is summarily dignified; and even an ostensibly childish term can rapidly become an official one. The physicists had no difficulty adopting the terms — up, down, charm, strange, truth and beauty, to describe the 'colour' of quarks. Consensus, therefore, and the absence of sarcasm, are the means of overcoming the sense of embarrassment that might apply to using a seemingly trivial term.

Subsequently, if used in a dignified manner by doctors, the term will be perceived as dignified by their patients.

Critics should address carefully whether their resistance to this suggestion is based on the term itself being inadequate, or on an emotional reluctance to sound silly. Until a better, new word is found that more elegantly, but no less efficiently, conveys the same comprehensive meaning, non-serious back pain should become known as green back pain. Please consider.

References

1   Merskey H, Bogduk N (eds). Classification of Chronic Pain. Descriptions of Chronic Pain Syndromes and Definitions of Pain Terms, 2nd edn. IASP Press, Seattle, WA, 1994.

Medical Management of Acute and Chronic Low Back Pain. An Evidence-Based Approach
Pain Research and Clinical Management, Vol. 13
Nikolai Bogduk and Brian McGuirk
© 2002 Elsevier Science B.V. All rights reserved

Subject Index

Lumbar
– insufficiency, 215
– spinal pain, 5, 215

Magnetic resonance imaging, *see* MRI
Magnets, 152
Malingering, 131
Manipulation, *see also* Manual therapy
– chiropractic, 95
Manipulative therapy, 145–147, 150
Manual therapy, 96–99
Massage, 152
McKenzie
– assessment, 43, 44, 129
– therapy, 95, 104
Medial branch blocks, 188–189
Minnesota Multiphasic Personality Inventory, *see* MMPI
MMPI, 24
Mobilisation, *see* Manual therapy
Morning stiffness, 30
Motion
– intervertebral, passive, 43
– range, *see* Range of motion
MRI
– acute low back pain, 37–38, 58–60
– application, 115, 177–179, 199–201
– arachnoiditis, 119
– cancer, 38
– chronic low back pain, 135
– endplate changes, 136
– high-intensity zone, 135–136
– internal disc disruption, 136
– reliability, 59
– screening test, as a, 37, 135
– utility, 58–60
– validity, 59, 60
Multidisciplinary treatment, 78, 140, 163–166
Muscle relaxants, 90–91, 144
Myeloma, 32, 38

Narcotics, *see* Opioids
Natural history, *see* Acute low back pain
Nerves, clunial, superior, 42

Neuroma, 119
Night sweats, 31
Non-steroidal anti-inflammatory agents, *see* NSAIDs
NSAIDs, 89–90, 143–144
Number needed to treat, 212

Odds ratio, 53, 209–210
Operant conditioning, 105
Operant treatment, 156
Opioids, 90, 144
– intraspinal, 154–155
Osteoarthritis, 50, 215
Osteomyelitis, 13, 31, 38, 54
Osteoporosis, 32, 34, 50, 54
Outcomes, 210–213

Paget's disease, 32, 38, 50
Pain
– discogenic, 9, 170–172, 179–180, 192–193, 195, 215
– gluteal, 6, 9, 10
– loin, 6, 28
– low back, 6, 28
– lumbar spinal, 5
– lumbosacral, 6, 28
– – acute, *see* Acute low back pain
– – chronic, *see* Chronic low back pain
– – recurrent, 7
– – subacute, *see* Subacute low back pain
– neurogenic, 8
– quality, 30
– radicular, 6, 10, 28–30, 44, 45, 129
– referred, 8
– severity, 30
– somatic referred, 8, 9, 28–30, 44
– spinal,
– – lumbar, 5, 215
– – sacral, 5
– – thoracic, 6
– sacral spinal, 5
– sacroiliac, 9
– thoracic spinal, 6
– visceral referred, 8